HEALING POLITICS

HEALING POLITICS

A Doctor's Journey into the
Heart of Our Political Epidemic

ABDUL EL-SAYED

FOREWORD BY ADY BARKAN

ABRAMS PRESS, NEW YORK

Library of Congress Control Number: 2019939904

ISBN: 978-1-4197-4302-3
eISBN: 978-1-68335-813-8

Printed and bound in the United States
10 9 8 7 6 5 4 3 2

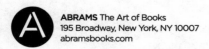

ABRAMS The Art of Books
195 Broadway, New York, NY 10007
abramsbooks.com

In the name of God, Most Merciful, Most Gracious,

To Emmalee and her sisters and brothers
in humanity, our hope.

Indeed, I was sent to perfect the good in human character.
—The Prophet Mohamed, peace and blessings be upon him
(author's translation)

Medicine is a social science, and politics is
nothing else but medicine on a large scale.
—Dr. Rudolf Virchow

Contents

Foreword by Ady Barkan   xi

Prologue   I

PART I: PRACTICUM

CHAPTER 1:   Home Away from Home   II

CHAPTER 2:   An Imperfect Science   18

CHAPTER 3:   Matched-Pair   25

CHAPTER 4:   Privilege   39

CHAPTER 5:   Complex Causes   48

CHAPTER 6:   Ideals and Institutions   56

CHAPTER 7:   Not That Kind of Doctor   69

CHAPTER 8:   Contagion and Miasma   78

CHAPTER 9:   Home Again   83

CHAPTER 10:   Doctoring Detroit   97

CHAPTER 11:   Running for Our Lives   II2

PART II: AMERICA'S INSECURITY EPIDEMIC

CHAPTER 12:   The Syndrome   129

CHAPTER 13:   Insecure Health   141

CHAPTER 14:   Insecure Households   150

CHAPTER 15:   Insecure Communities   166

CHAPTER 16:   Insecure Places   175

CHAPTER 17:   Insecure Economy   188

CHAPTER 18:   Insecure Politics   196

CHAPTER 19:   The Spread of Insecurity   216

PART III: HEALING POLITICS

CHAPTER 20: Toward a Politics of Empathy   229

CHAPTER 21: Them and Us   234

CHAPTER 22: Empathy Policy   248

CHAPTER 23: Thirteen Ideas to Heal Our Insecurity   256

EPILOGUE: Empathy for Our Future   290

NOTES   293

ACKNOWLEDGMENTS   327

INDEX   331

FOREWORD

by Ady Barkan

Over the past few months, my vision has become increasingly blurry. The problem has varied throughout the day, and some days have felt better than others. But the trendline seems clear. It's been particularly frightening for me because I am already suffering from a deadly, debilitating neurological disease called ALS, which has paralyzed my whole body and left me dependent on a ventilator to breathe, a wheelchair to move, and 24/7 home care to survive. For some unknown reason, ALS does not affect the eye muscles, and so they are now the only part of my body that I can control. I use them, and excellent eye-tracking technology, to write and speak. Without my eyes, life would be impossible. So the deterioration of my vision has been particularly frightening. Was it a result of ALS? Or of some fluke, particularly tragic other problem?

It took me two trips to the ophthalmologist and about twelve weeks to discover the real culprit: I had developed a mild case of farsightedness, which could be solved by a simple pair of +1.25 reading glasses, which now are perched stylishly on the bridge of my nose.

What is so notable about this minor saga is that it took me so long to resolve the issue, despite the tremendously high stakes, my access to good medical care, and the simplicity of the solution. Inertia, uncertainty, and fear had kept even me from going to the local drugstore and trying on a pair of twenty-dollar glasses.

Although the particulars of my story are tragic, my failure to get reading glasses is, I learned from Dr. Abdul El-Sayed in the pages that follow, completely routine and commonplace. Every morning, children sit in classrooms and cannot see what is on the blackboard. Their education, their career prospects, our collective investment in them as members of civil society—all undermined by a simple problem (with a simple medical solution) that we are failing to address because complicated, multifaceted social and political obstacles stand in our way.

That is what this book is about. It is about our public health, and the ways in which our lives are constrained and cut short because of the collective choices we make, and fail to make. As the commissioner of health for the City of Detroit, Abdul worked to change those choices, change those outcomes, put glasses on the bridges of many more young noses. With limited resources and political constraints, what is a public health official to do? Abdul has lived that challenge, and he recounts it with insight and humility.

But this book is also about so much more. It is about the broader illnesses facing our society and our body politic, and the options we have for curing them. Abdul brings to this exercise the rigor and skepticism of an elite epidemiologist, eschewing the easy answers in favor of those that recognize the interconnectedness of our systems and lives and politics.

This book is also about the man who has written it. Abdul's parents immigrated from Egypt to the United States, like millions before and after them, in search of stability and security and a better life for their children. And so Abdul grew up buoyed by privilege and burdened by prejudice. In the aftermath of 9/11, he was a star student whose name screamed out "Muslim." He learned to navigate the dual identities, the high and offensively low expectations of him, and emerged as a shining example of the best America has to offer.

Abdul trained as a scientist and a doctor. But I met him when he had become a different kind of public servant. On the campaign trail in the summer of 2018, with our democracy under grave threat, I witnessed his charisma and brilliance and power. His compassion. His vision. And his optimism. I witnessed how Michiganders responded to it. And I also witnessed how the political establishment responded; how the forces who felt threatened by Abdul defended their status quo.

And so, ultimately, this book is about the future. Or at least one future. A future where evidence informs our analysis. Where empathy guides our politics. Where people like Abdul are our leaders. Can we reach that future? The answer depends on us.

Ady Barkan
Santa Barbara, California
December 2019

PROLOGUE

About two weeks after I launched my campaign for governor of Michigan, Sarah, my best friend and wife of eleven years, suggested we grab some dinner. Rather than a casual meal at home, she opted for something more special, and chose one of my favorite spots: Supino Pizzeria, in the heart of Detroit's Eastern Market, just steps from where I had launched the campaign.

Sarah had news to share. After we finished off the last slice, she grabbed both of my hands and looked me in the eyes: "You're going to be a father."

I had figured that this was the news. After years of waiting to finish our educations—Sarah's also a doctor, and we were in college when we got married—we had started trying to get pregnant a few months back. But nothing prepares you for the emotion that comes with those words. Some odd combination of elation and fear swept over me as we hugged. We were going to be responsible for a tiny human life—some part each of us, but altogether new. But there was also a third emotion I had not expected: inspiration.

I had always been circumspect about the idea of having children. After all, there are so many parents struggling to care for their own kids. I wanted to dedicate my life to supporting them. Would having a child of my own detract from that mission? And then there are so many children who don't have parents at all. Why bring a child into this world when there are so many who need parents already?

Then my cohort of friends started to have kids. I noticed that when they talked about the downsides, they used language I could relate to: you don't get any sleep; they're expensive; you're no longer the person your partner is most interested in. But when they described the benefits, their words were emotional, hazy: "It's just this . . . feeling, this love," one said.

As a scientist, I tried to deduce what I could from this observation. If my friends could all describe the negatives in very clear, relatable language but could only describe the positives in far less specific terms, then having a child must be a unique human experience, unlike any other.

My work has always been about supporting and protecting children and their parents, whether it is understanding the circumstances of their births—and deaths—as a researcher focused on prematurity and infant mortality, or in preventing those things from happening as a public health official. And yet, hearing my friends, I came to appreciate that while I could understand that people love their children—and will do anything for them—I had never known the love of my own child, an experience for which it seems I could simply find no analogue.

Of course, Sarah had gotten there far faster. She'd always wanted children—which is why I probably would have ended up having them anyway—but, as usual, her emotional intelligence far surpassed my own. We were having a baby. And on the Sunday after Thanksgiving in 2017, when Emmalee was born, with her first tiny whimper, she took my breath away. I performed the Muslim traditions of birth, reading the call to prayer in her ears and chewing a small piece of date to feed her—the tears flowing down my face salting the sweet taste of the date in my mouth. Sarah, tired after eleven heroic hours of labor, held her to her skin.

I was carrying a lot of guilt that day. In recent months I hadn't been the kind of supportive husband and future father I'd aspired to be. In fact, I was hardly ever there at all. I had been crisscrossing the state of Michigan, spending evenings and weekends at town halls and county fairs. Every night I'd call Sarah, checking in to see how she was doing. We had long since moved in with her parents, and her mother—half angel, half maternal ninja—was a far better supporter than I could ever be. But I like to imagine there is something about a partner's presence and love that's uniquely comforting, and I was rarely there to provide it during her pregnancy.

In truth, there was some small risk I wouldn't be there for her at all. Our campaign had received a surprising number of death threats: people from all parts of the country had taken to Facebook to tell me that I was taking my life in my hands. As the first Muslim-American to make a serious run for governor in any state, I knew what I was getting into. But only after our campaign started to pick up national attention did the hatred rise to a level that warranted serious concern. There's still a Facebook chain post floating around that reads "Don't say you weren't warned—'He IS on his way' . . . PRESIDENT ABDUL EL-SAYED? Etch this man's name in your mind. His name is Abdul

El-Sayed . . . He is handsome, articulate, charismatic and smart . . ." Perversely flattering, maybe, but our campaign decided to invest in a full-time bodyguard. And just in case the future didn't work in my favor, I wrote a long letter to my unborn child to be opened on her eighteenth birthday. In the letter, I ventured to introduce myself and explain the world as I see it. At best, it would be a personal time capsule we could read together in eighteen years. At worst, it would serve as an introduction to a father she'd never get to know.

Months later, well after the campaign had ended, I thought about the letter again when I got a concerned call from my father-in-law. A Detroit police officer had come by the house and said that he needed to speak with me. I was in no trouble but I should call him as soon as possible. I called my lawyer and asked if she might reach out on my behalf. When she called me back, I could hear the fear in her voice. "Are you sitting down?" she asked.

"Yeah. What's up?" I responded, concerned.

"You know that guy who mailed all those bombs to CNN and Democratic politicians?" She was talking about Cesar Sayoc, a Florida man inspired by Donald Trump, who pleaded guilty to having mailed sixteen explosive devices to various Democratic politicians, Democratic supporters, a former director of national intelligence, a former CIA director, and CNN in October 2018. "Well, you were in his list of Google searches. And they wanted to make sure you know." I'm grateful that it was a police officer—and not an explosive—that came to our door. My daughter lived behind that door.

* * *

That day at Supino's, I asked Sarah if she wanted me to drop out of the race. I had quit my job as health director of the city of Detroit to campaign full-time, meaning I had no income. We were relying on Sarah's psychiatry residency salary. That would have been fine for just the two of us, but caring for a child was another matter entirely.

Sarah said no. Our daughter's name, Emmalee, means "my hope" in Arabic. She is ethnically half Egyptian and half Indian—and 100 percent American. She's growing up in a Muslim household. I know many of the ways she will be told that she's not enough: I experienced some of them firsthand.

"The best thing you can do for this kid is go out and win that race," she said. Once again, Sarah had gotten there far faster than I did.

* * *

On the campaign trail one day, a woman who looked like a seventy-year-old Shirley Temple grabbed my face, squeezing my cheeks. Her light brown eyes radiated a warmth and honesty. "Son," she asked, "are you listening to me?" She had waited in a reception line after a town hall at a church in suburban Detroit. Her blue "HELLO, my name is" sticker gave her name, "Sally," in big, bold, curling cursive.

"Ma'am, with all due respect, you've got your hands on my face. Yes, I'm listening to you," I said through my smooshed lips. *I'm already feeling kinda young,* I thought to myself, *and this lady's making me feel like I'm twelve.* To be sure, campaign stop eight that day had just become the most notable.

"Son, you've got a great smile," Sally said. "And I hope you keep smiling. A lot of people are going to say terrible things about you—I've already heard it—but you gotta keep smiling. Because it's really hard to hate someone who's smiling at you."

On the one hand, it would have been easy to react to this Pollyannaish advice with sarcasm. *You think a smile is going to solve racist death threats?* But on the other, I had been coming to the same conclusion.

Sally was reminding me that people *are* good—even if sometimes the things they say and do are not. Everything that Trump has unleashed in our politics is motivated by fear. And there is something about the empathy in an honest smile that uniquely melts through fear and cuts through hate.

And in a small way, this is what I was trying to do. Even though I was a thirty-two-year-old Muslim-American named Abdul and a doctor who had never been elected to office, I declared my candidacy for governor of Michigan in February 2017. I had served the city of Detroit as health director—my only government experience—having rebuilt the Health Department after it was privatized in 2012, when Detroit was facing municipal bankruptcy. Prior to that, I had been an epidemiology professor. But in the aftermath of the Flint water crisis and Donald Trump's election, I felt that perhaps my skills as a physician and epidemiologist could help heal my state—and my campaign as the son of an Egyptian immigrant and the stepson of a Daughter of the American Revolution could remind us who we are as a country.

Over eighteen months, I visited more than one hundred fifty cities and nearly all of the eighty-three counties in the state of Michigan. I had thought that I was leaving the epidemiologist in me behind when I chose to become a candidate for office. Rather, I found myself subconsciously applying my scientific training across the thousands of people I met.

As an epidemiologist, I was trained to coax stories from inanimate lines of data to find the elemental truths buried within them. As a candidate, I was hearing those stories in living color. I would listen to a single mother, or a retired Iraq War veteran, or a little eight-year-old girl sharing story after story of pain or hardship, of pride and triumph. I could watch their eyes, appreciate the emotional weight that hunched a back, and feel the emphasis in the extra squeeze of my hand.

I found myself during the long car rides back from distant parts of the state trying to identify the patterns in what I'd learned, to test my hypotheses. In Marquette, an older gentleman, Jake, told me how he deeply believed in gun rights, having gone hunting every year since he was a child. But his little girl had been murdered by her ex-husband, using a gun that a man with a history of domestic violence should never have had.

Rebecca from Grand Rapids told me her son Jason had already beaten cancer twice; he was eight. She fears it'll come back when he's older and worries that even if he beats cancer a third time, he could be bankrupted by the cost of medical care.

Shaun came out as transgender in high school and began his transition in the face of hatred and bullying. And yet he graduated at the top of his high school class. His mom worries about how they'll afford his college tuition.

Keisha was one of the top graduates from her high school in Flint, but she had to drop out because the job at McDonald's that pays her bills won't give her regular hours. Unable to afford auto insurance, she has to take the bus, tacking an extra hour to and from work onto her already precarious work schedule. She's taking online classes but doesn't know if she'll ever get her degree.

My heart ached for these folks, for the struggles they have endured, for their futures hanging precariously in the balance. My mind raced to make sense of them.

On those long car rides, those endless days of campaigning, I came to appreciate that the justice each of us wants is simple. We want to know that we can work an honest job, make a fair wage, afford the roofs over our heads, and put meals on our tables—and have a little something left over to enjoy. But more than that, we want the peace of mind to look at our children and believe that their lives will be just a little bit better than ours. And we want to know that we can enjoy these things together, as communities. This is the American dream as I understand it.

It's not a tall order, yet so few in our society have it. The median household income in Michigan—the amount the Michigander right in the middle makes—is $49,847 per year.[1] After taxes, that's about $3,311 per month.[2] The median mortgage sits at $1,217, leaving about $2,100 per month. If you have student debt, that'll be an average of $304 off the top every month.[3] Silver plan health insurance takes another $305. The average car payment for a used car is $381—not to mention auto insurance and gas.[4] Then there's groceries and utilities and any necessary childcare or senior care. The costs add up fast.

And that's the *middle* household. Poverty—defined as earning less than $24,600 for a family of four—afflicts nearly one in six Michiganders. For children under five years old, it's one in four.[5] Poverty is not borne equally. In Michigan, nearly 30 percent of Black-Americans live in poverty. Contrast that with the fact that Michigan's twelve billionaires—all white—have a combined net worth of nearly $41 billion.[6]

As a candidate, I reflected on these realities, the women and men whose hands I was shaking, and the girls and boys they worry about. As an epidemiologist, I was coming to a clear pattern of what ailed them—what ails us all. We are suffering a collective epidemic that threatens our social, economic, and political futures. It's an epidemic that is fundamentally reshaping our politics. It affects nearly all of us, eroding our chances of achieving the American dream, and it has the potential to erode our highest national ideals. It is an epidemic of insecurity.

Yet, as a doctor, it's not enough to diagnose a disease; one has to treat it. This epidemic of insecurity leaves us in need of a new politics, one that recognizes the structure, culture, and consequences of insecurity—a new politics that equips us with the moral and tactical tools to address our most serious problems.

That's what I hope this book can offer. In Part I, I intersperse chapters introducing myself and my science—and how epidemiology helped me make sense of my own life. In Part II, I diagnose the insecurity epidemic and its causes, working outward from the individual to society and tracing its mechanisms of spread. And in Part III, I reflect on how we'll need to reframe our politics around empathy if we aim to take on insecurity and dismantle the systems that have perpetuated it.

I am writing to share my vantage point on America as a first-generation son of Egyptian immigrants, raised in a mixed household, from which I came to understand who I was—and who we are. Calling on my training as a scientist, a doctor, and my work in public health and politics, I want to share the evidence I've collected about how our epidemic of insecurity is squandering the potential we have—and what we'll have to do to cure it. And underlying all this, I want you to see that both appreciating the challenges we face and then doing the work to address them will take a reframing of our politics around something we've been starved of for a long time: empathy. I hope to show you why America is ailing, and why *all of us* must do all we can to heal her.

PART I

PRACTICUM

CHAPTER 1
Home away from home.

In June 1998, I waited in Detroit Metropolitan Airport to board a flight to Egypt for just the second time in my life. I was thirteen. This would be my first visit in ten years—since I had spent a few months there after my parents' divorce. This time I was traveling without any immediate family. I was nervous. My parents thought it was about time for me to reconnect with the family I had not seen in so many years and to brush up on Arabic—my first language. As a hyphenated-American kid, I had all but jettisoned this native tongue. *What was Arabic good for, anyway?* I reasoned. No accent meant less teasing. Never mind the worlds and the people it could connect me to.

I boarded the plane to the harmonizing tune of Puff Daddy's Notorious B.I.G. elegy, "I'll Be Missing You," a track on the "Abdul's Summer Mix" CD my friend had burned for me. If I was going to be leaving America, I was at least going to take a piece of it with me.

I am Egyptian-American. In some ways I am both, in some ways neither.

That summer, some small part of me worried that the balance across the hyphen would shift indelibly—that I would forget how to be American. I was afraid that I'd have to start all over when I got back home—from "home"—in the fall.

Although hyphens are short, they take up a lot of space in the minds of hyphenated kids. W. E. B. DuBois, writing about the psychic load Black-Americans had to bear, called this a "double-consciousness." Not only must you move in your spaces aware of the world, but you must also be aware of the way the world is aware of you. It's a lot of work, especially for a kid.

For me, nothing quite reflects that double-consciousness like my name. Most everyone knows me as Abdul. But that's not my full name, which is Abdul-rahman. It means "Devotee of the Most Merciful." In the Muslim tradition, it is one of God's most beloved names, which is why my parents chose it (before they realized I would be growing up in America). I love my name, reflecting a connection to a character of the divine that is so lacking in humanity: mercy.

I didn't become "Abdul" until about a week before I started preschool. My stepmom, Jackie, realized that with its full complement of eleven letters "Abdulrahman" might be a challenge. She gingerly broached the topic with my father, Mohamed.

The traditional Arabic nickname for "Abdulrahman," "Boody," pronounced like the body part, was a non-starter for obvious reasons. That was the summer of 1989. Billboard's number-one hit song was . . . "Straight Up," by Paula Abdul. And Kareem Abdul-Jabbar had just wrapped up his stellar basketball career. Unlike "Abdulrahman," with its deep meaning, "Abdul" is nonsensical in Arabic, roughly translating to "Devotee of the," but given its references in pop culture, it took on meaning in America. So on my first day of preschool in 1989, I introduced myself as "Abdul," and I've been Abdul to most of the world ever since. I still prefer Abdulrahman, if people can say it. One person, two names. Two consciousnesses.

Hyphens connect things—people, places, ideas—but they also bisect, separating out the pieces of those things. I prefer to think of my hyphen as a connector. But that, too, takes work—the constant upkeep of belonging. I imagine that, for most folks, home is an effortless place to be. The rules are automatic. For the hyphenated, home is not *one* place but many places, and with each home there's a different set of rules. Make a mistake, break a rule, and you'll show yourself to be an outsider, even in your own home.

As I boarded that plane, I imagined the home I would find at the other end of my journey. My father had left Egypt behind in his mid-twenties to pursue a PhD in mechanical engineering at Wayne State University in Detroit. Like many children of immigrants, I grew up hearing the legend of my parents— first in their class at this and that. My father was the archetype. After finishing at the top of his class at his public high school in Alexandria, he finished near the top of his class in engineering at Alexandria University, all while working full-time to support his family. He was chosen to join the teaching faculty, where he excelled in front of the classroom. But his political agitation against Egypt's increasingly brutal military dictatorship, coupled with his proximity to young minds, made him a threat to the regime.

He had to leave. There were a few options. But Detroit, Michigan, was the most compelling. Detroit was, after all, in the United States of America, where his name, the color of his skin, and how he prayed shouldn't matter. He could be just as American as anyone else. America was also the home of democracy, that thing he had so wanted for Egypt. And Detroit was synonymous with the car, a mecca for this budding automotive engineer. Besides, if it didn't work out, he didn't intend to stay forever anyway. He figured that after he'd gotten his fancy American degree, he'd be free to return to Egypt and have his pick of good jobs.

Detroit's near-arctic winters felt like a personal insult to my father, whose childhood was saturated with the warmth of the Mediterranean sun, but he found Wayne State welcoming. Still, he was lonely. His heart had been broken a number of times before his transatlantic migration, so he decided to apply the exactitude of his engineering training to the work of finding love. He wanted to find a partner who shared his faith-driven values and his intellectual ambitions and who might join him in Detroit while he finished his PhD. My grandmother started to work the horn on his behalf, in a process that sounds more like the pre-auction marketing of a prized bull than romantic courtship.

She kept hearing about Fatten, a medical student and leader on campus. She was the eldest daughter of a biologist and had spent most of her childhood abroad after her mother passed when Fatten was thirteen. Fatten was a mother figure to her siblings and a loving, devoted daughter to her father. She, too, was a top student. Smart, warm, and charismatic, she seemed the right match, at least on paper. They met in person only once when my father had come back to Egypt over the summer. Under the watchful eyes of their parents, they chatted for twenty minutes. Everything looked to be in order. My father was smitten—perhaps less with the complex reality of the person he met than with the *idea* of her. She was equally taken with the idea of him.

But the future started to flicker. Both of their fathers were strong-willed, uncompromising men who wanted only the best for their eldest children. My paternal grandfather had already scuttled two relationships over petty slights at twenty-minute meetings that devolved into all-out feuds. My father was determined not to lose a third. Mohamed and Fatten married by phone a few months later.

My parents both take after their fathers. Both are strong-willed, charismatic, charming—and both are uncompromising, not only in their beliefs, but also in their approaches to life and their way of doing things. Their traits may make for excellent leaders and empowering parents, but they did not make them excellent life partners for each other. They divorced within a few years. My parents' relationship had one lasting outcome: me. I comfort myself by thinking that if my parents were a band, they would have been a "one-hit wonder."

My father decided to stay in America, and after finishing his degree he went to work for General Motors. He would never admit it, but he is a hopeless romantic. He was always destined to marry for love, not convenience. And he met—and soon married—a colleague at GM, one who could not have come from a more different a world. Jackie Johnson was the eldest daughter of Judith Ann and Jan Johnson. Her family has had roots in America since before the Revolution—she being a distant descendant of Abigail Adams. Jackie's connection to the lands of mid-Michigan was generational. She had been born in Flint, while my Grandma Judy was in nursing school and my Grandpa Jan was studying at General Motors Institute (now Kettering University). Although they moved often, they raised their children in the Midwest. For people like my grandparents, home is etched into who they are. Jackie is smart, hardworking, and warm, a tenacious counter to my father's hard-driving character.

Mohamed and Jackie met over a conversation about an obscure engineering concept: Mohr's circle, a graphical representation of how an object changes under varying external stresses. My siblings, Osama and Samia, and I became a sociocultural application of that concept. We grew up in the home they made together, children raised by an immigrant from Egypt and a Daughter of the American Revolution.

My mother remarried as well, to a translator with whom she would live all over the world. Tragically, he passed young, the victim of a heart attack. I have two sisters on that side, Eman and Arwa, as well as a stepbrother, Adam. Collectively, I have five half- or stepsiblings; our love is whole, even if the bloodlines are not.

* * *

On the other side of my two-leg, fifteen-hour journey, I came home to the working-class neighborhood in Alexandria where my father grew up. For a kid raised largely in the bland suburbia of 1990s America, this other "home"—one I had only imagined—offered a glorious assault on the senses, from the street vendors hawking *mish*, a caramel-brown fermented cheese dip that looked and smelled like a bad moment on the toilet; to the soot of the air polluted by the tailpipes of 1970s-era Soviet Ladas; to the majesty of watching the sun set from the Corniche over the rocks jutting out of Alexandria's Mediterranean waterfront; to the mystic cacophony of every muezzin's *adhan* simultaneously calling the pious to prayer. The place didn't even really wake up until after the sun went down; people filled the cafés and restaurants until well past 2:00 a.m. The manicured lawns and strip malls of Detroit's sleepy suburbs were no match for the energy and authenticity of this place.

Yet poverty and its consequences abounded. The ubiquitous beggars and garbage pickers who spent their days sorting through the refuse of the lives of others were the visible tip of an iceberg of poverty. Egyptian society is seg- regated, though differently than ours is. To be sure, there are posh neigh- borhoods, exclusive to the ultra-rich, yet many wealthy Egyptians live on the upper floors of apartment buildings shared by a cross-section of all of Egyptian society. At the very bottom were the *bawab*s, an army of doormen who serve as the social mortar that holds together the bricks of Egyptian life.

The face of Ali, our *bawab*, bore the crags of his many days under an unmerciful sun spent fetching this or haggling over that. Ali wore the tra- ditional Egyptian galabia, a gray, loose-fitting, collarless version of the robes made famous by the Saudis. Ali's family had been in the *bawab* business for a generation, and he became my Sherpa, helping me decode the sights and sounds of Egyptian life. Because his role was to be the monitor, arbiter, and catalyst of all that went on in building, he knew the secrets held just beyond each apartment door. He knew about the crooked businessman on the eighth floor—and his mistress younger than his daughter—and the young woman on the fourth whose parents wouldn't let her go to medical school. When I had questions that I was too embarrassed to ask my family, I would ask Ali.

"Why can't the farmers who bring their goods to market on a donkey afford a truck?"

"Why is there a group of young women who come to that coffee shop a few blocks away every night, and why do they leave with different men?"

"Why does that man beat his son?"

His answers were almost always the same: "*Miskeen.*" Because, Ali said, they were poor.

I began to realize just how narrow was the tightrope my predecessors had walked, how circumstances had threatened to knock them off at every turn—and just how fortunate I was that they never fell off. My people, too, had been poor.

Teta, my grandmother, was illiterate. She is the wisest, most intelligent person I have ever met, but she never spent a day in a classroom. She was denied that right. The fifth of nine children born to a streetlamp repairman and his illiterate wife, my grandmother grew up between her parents' home and that of an eccentric couple without children who lived a few floors up. The husband was an inventor who had made his money designing quick-action cameras that could be used to snap photos of tourists on the Corniche.

Though separated only by a few floors, the two homes might as well have been different worlds. A far cry from the overcrowded rooms downstairs, the upstairs flat was a local salon for intellectuals and activists of the moment. Teta, an apprentice of sorts to the matron, would help with odd jobs around the house. With guests from all over Egypt, North Africa, Europe, and the Levant, she learned to cook in their various styles. Her proximity to the conversations shared over her meals gave her an ease with ideas and viewpoints to which few young women in her social circumstances would have been exposed. They were ever impressed with her wit, her memory, and her grace. And yet it never occurred to any of them that this intelligent, precocious, and charming young woman should be given access to formal education. I often wonder what my grandmother might have achieved had she been born in a different place in a different time.

Teta married my grandfather, then eighteen, when she was just fifteen. Giddo, my grandfather, had an eighth-grade education and sold tomatoes at a local fish market. He had spent much of his childhood as the eldest son of a wealthy landowner in Alexandria. But his father died when Giddo was thirteen, and when his uncles moved in for his inheritance, he was powerless, forced onto the street to fend for his mother and siblings. Although he was a rough man, ground down by life's misfortunes, my grandfather loved my grandmother, for whom he reserved all the softness left in him. Teta had an extraordinary temperament. She was never angry, only disappointed—and not with you but with the version of you that you were choosing to be at the moment. She had the rare gift of seeing the best in you even when you could not see it in yourself, charming it out with a friendly parable or a caress of the hand. She was a natural leader, a towering figure of all of five feet one inch and much shorter in her usual pose, squatting over a little burner stove from which she would coax feasts of Egyptian cuisine. She'd hold court in that kitchen, helping a cousin with marital issues or settling a dispute between friends—always with a smile on her face, a story on her lips, and her heart firmly on the side of the powerless.

My father had a special reverence for his mother, and among the many gifts she gave me—the one for which I am most thankful—is the capacity for tenderness she showed me in him. My father was the eldest of her eight children, two of whom died before their first birthdays. My grandmother wanted him, her eldest son, to be a doctor. But watching two infant siblings die in hospitals left him with a lifelong aversion to the medical institutions that had failed them. He would oblige her somehow, though, ultimately earning a different kind of doctorate on a path he paved with books. He would start his day in the local market, helping set up my grandfather's tomato stall before heading off to school, where he was expected to be the best student in his class.

My grandfather wanted better for his kids but knew only one way of wringing it from them: brute force. As you can imagine, my dad would dutifully make his way back to the market after school to help break the stall down. By the time he'd finish his chores in the market, the sun would have gone down. With only one bedroom for a family of eight, he was left to study on the rooftop, by the light of a streetlamp. Night after night, alone on that rooftop, my father studied my future into existence. That summer I often sat in his place, imagining the other versions of my life that might have been had he not sat there so many nights, so many years ago.

CHAPTER 2

An imperfect science.

Most of the time, when I tell people that I am an epidemiologist, they think I'm a skin doctor. It's a fair mistake, owing to the similarity between the words "epidemiologist" and "epidermis." We're not skin doctors, and we don't make nearly as much money.

Epi is Greek for "what is upon," and *demos* means "the people." Epidemiologists want to understand "what is upon the people," what is plaguing them. Epidemiology is the basic science of public health, the study of the distribution and determinants of disease in populations. We count things having to do with why people get sick so we can understand how often—and why—they happen so that we can stop them from happening.

To get a sense of why this matters, consider this: if I asked you what the biggest health risk was among women, you'd probably think it was breast cancer. After all, everything turns pink every October for breast cancer awareness. But the most common killer in women is actually heart disease. That matters, because it should dictate how and where we apply our resources, concentrating our efforts on the health risks that affect the most people most profoundly. Of course, that is not to say that less common problems are not important, but we want to spend limited resources efficiently.

Our ability to count things systematically and make sense of them is relatively new, because it's actually quite hard to do. First, we have to collect complete and reliable data about people over time. That requires the infrastructure to keep track of people and make sure we're measuring what we want, when we want it. That only became possible with the advent of organized, efficient bureaucracies across larger, settled societies. Second, you need the mathematical and technological tools to make sense of all that data. That requires modern statistics.

As far as we know, those two things didn't converge until 1662, when John Graunt, an English haberdasher, published an analysis of all of the deaths in London and its surroundings to understand the causes of plague.[1] That

means we've been systematically counting disease for only 350 of the estimated 300,000 years that humans have existed—about 0.1 percent of our
time here on earth.

But there's another side of this coin. Methodically counting disease isn't
just a matter of the ability to do so; it's also a matter of the *need* to do so. Only
since humans have concentrated in cities has counting disease even been
necessary. Before then, massive outbreaks were generally uncommon, because
mass contagion requires the kind of population numbers and density that only
cities provide. Worse, a serious contagion in a small band of roving nomads
would have left no one to ask what happened.

The first known epidemiologic study arose out of the need to understand
how and when bubonic plague outbreaks might occur.[2] After the first major
outbreak in 1347, regular outbreaks of plague became a major hazard, killing
thousands of people at a time and forcing those with the means to do so to
head for the hills. With authorities fleeing to the countryside, rioting and loot-
ing rocked cities and social upheaval destroyed towns and villages. The worst
suffering was sustained in low-income enclaves where poverty exacerbated
outbreaks and left people the most vulnerable. Not knowing how or when
disease might strike left people feeling insecure. Epidemiology was created to
reduce this insecurity.

Step one meant trying to predict when an outbreak might be on the horizon. To do so, though, you would need to be able to identify disease in real
time. Beginning in 1603, England's Queen Mary ordered the Church of England to initiate the first "disease surveillance system" wherein elderly women
in local communities would investigate houses where deaths had occurred,
sometimes with a surgeon in tow. They would report to the clerk of the local
parish, and every parish's findings would be collected and collated by the clerk
of the City of London, then published weekly as the "Bills of Mortality": data
about every death in London, by parish, every week. These bills were predecessors to the county-level mortality data we still collect and analyze today.

But beyond simply collecting data, one has to analyze it, revealing the
patterns buried in the numbers. That's what Graunt did in 1662. He collected
fifty years' worth of data—nearly 2,500 volumes—and then pulled up Micro-
soft Excel, and . . . ha, nope! Graunt had to painstakingly make his calculations
by hand, a time-intensive, tedious, error-prone process essential to rendering

the discoveries that the fifty years of data might afford. He observed the jagged pattern of mortality that you would expect from an infectious, outbreak-driven illness like the plague. But, perhaps more interestingly, he found that deaths by other causes—"chronical diseases"—were relatively stable.[3]

We still call them chronical—okay, "chronic"—diseases today. And by contrasting these to the plague, with its much more variable mortality pattern, Graunt was able to demystify the disease that had devastated European cities for three centuries. Immediately his observations all but destroyed (extremely problematic) theories about Jews, Muslims, or lepers poisoning the wells, or the planets aligning, focusing attention, rather, on the circumstances in local communities where outbreaks emerged. At its core, Graunt's first epidemiologic analysis used systematic, comprehensive, and relatively reliable data to count how often and under what circumstances a disease occurred—and therefore to offer clues to what the causes of that disease might be.

Others built on this approach, counting and analyzing the probability of disease to understand what might cause it. Dr. John Snow, whom I'll talk about later, is often credited as being the "Father of Epidemiology" for his use of a similar line of reasoning to trace the cause of a cholera epidemic that struck Soho in London in 1854 to a water pump on Broad Street.[4]

You can imagine that epidemiology has changed dramatically since the days of Graunt. Revolutions in modern computing have fundamentally changed how we collect, store, and analyze data. Today we can, almost in real time, collect terabytes of data about people in the places they live, learn, work, and play, and we can fit complicated statistical models to this data that allow us to identify complex correlations between factors.

But the central question in epidemiology remains the same: What *causes* disease in populations? And although our tools are more powerful than Graunt could have ever imagined, definitive answers to that question remain elusive.

* * *

To give you a better sense of how hard it can be to tease causation from mere correlation, let's consider an example we've all heard before. We know that smoking is generally really bad for your health, and we can identify how a previous history of cigarette smoking during pregnancy may predict the probability of a premature birth. Our technological tools have allowed us to ascertain this correlation quite easily. But to go from saying there is a correlation between cigarette smoking and premature births to saying that cigarette smoking *causes* premature births is not a technological problem; it's a logical one.

But shouldn't it be obvious that smoking causes premature births? There is a strong and consistent statistical correlation between smoking and prematurity. We observe it in almost every study that has ever considered the predictors of prematurity or the consequences of smoking. That's really strong evidence, to be sure, and it's why we spent so much time trying to empower Detroit moms to quit when I was health director at the Detroit Health Department. To prove causation, however, we would have to run an experiment. It might look something like this: An epidemiologist would identify a woman who is pregnant who has never previously been exposed to cigarette smoke and then expose her to a controlled number of cigarettes over a prescribed period of time. Then the scientist would record the gestational period of the child.

Here's where it gets wild. To ascertain whether or not smoking causes prematurity, the scientist would have to *go back in time*, find the same woman under the same circumstances, *not* expose her to the cigarettes, and then record the length of gestation of the child.

To understand why our epidemiologist would have to go back in time, suppose the scientist just waited until the next time the same woman got pregnant to record and compare her babies' gestational periods. A lot of things would have changed: she would be older and would have had the previous baby, and perhaps she would have changed jobs, moved, or undergone other major life changes, like the stress of caring for a child, all of which could influence her probability of delivering prematurely—not to mention the fact that she was *already* exposed to cigarette smoke during her first pregnancy, which could have had lasting effects. And those are just the changes *she* sustained. The world around her might have also changed in the meantime. Perhaps the second pregnancy did not occur in the same season as the first, or perhaps the first pregnancy was during a period of stability and prosperity, while the second was during a recession or a war.

If we can't quite master time travel, what about just running the experiment with two women who are the same exact age at the same exact time? I imagine you're already starting to see the flaw: these two women would have different genetics and different life experiences—and that's before we even consider the matter of smoking. All of these differences are called confounders, and they make elucidating causation—and the science of epidemiology—really hard.

But then there's also the fact that it's hard to measure *how much* smoking matters. To see why, consider this possibility: What if in the impossible time travel experiment I proposed, despite the different smoking habits of the mother, there was no change in gestational length? Could we say that smoking did not cause prematurity? Well, no. We could only say that *that amount* of smoking did not cause it.

I also have yet to mention the fact that even if the time travel experiment were possible, it would be completely unethical: once you postulate that a given factor might hurt someone, it's morally unethical to direct a subject to do it. You can see how that might pose a serious challenge for a science attempting to understand what's bad for you. It gets even harder when you're talking about factors that are impossible to expose someone to, like racism.

Taken together, you can see the central challenge of epidemiology: that it's nearly impossible to generate real experiments that allow us to disentangle causation from correlation. Yet because we still want answers to help us stop epidemics, prolong life, and ease suffering, we make do with imperfect study designs that allow us to *infer* causation, and most of them stem from two basic types: randomized controlled trials (RCTs) and natural experiments.

Most people have heard of RCTs, but fewer know why they're so powerful. They have two key characteristics: comparison of the effects of a treatment on those who received it with a "control" group that didn't, and random allocation of participants into those two groups. That second part—randomization—is as close to magic as epidemiologists get. I'll explain. But first, let's set up our RCT.

Because we can't ethically ask someone to do something that we think is bad for them, like smoking, we'll test the inverse. So let's say we want to know the effects of a nicotine patch on total weeks of gestation among women between ages eighteen and forty who have smoked at least a pack a day for at least three years prior to pregnancy. Remember, the ideal experiment would have considered the same exact person under the same exact scenario with only one difference: the treatment. That's not possible because we can't go back in time. So instead we test our treatment on several different women. But as we discussed, we can't know if differences in the outcome are because of the differences in their treatment or because of the initial differences between the women.

We can't do anything about the differences between individuals, but randomization—epidemiologist magic—fixes that by doing something about differences between *groups* of women. How? Consider this: Find a quarter and flip it twice. You might expect that you would get one head and one tail. Statistically, though, you're just as likely to get all heads or all tails. Flip the quarter one hundred times, however, and you'll probably get something very close to fifty heads and fifty tails. Unlike when you flipped it twice, your likelihood of getting all heads or all tails is so infinitesimally small (1 in 1.2 nonillion) as to be zero. What explains the difference between two flips and a hundred flips? It's called the central limit theorem. It stipulates that the larger the number of flips, the closer you will get to a statistical approximation of the natural probability of an outcome—in this case fifty-fifty heads or tails.

If we randomize enough people to treatment versus control, we will distribute all the possible characteristics of people that could differ and confound our study results—like age, race, income, education, wealth—across the treatment and control groups of the study and evenly between each group. The more people we recruit, the closer we get to perfectly even, as with the quarter flips. So, even if the individuals in the study may differ, the treatment and control groups do not. See, magic (or statistics)!

After recruiting enough people into our study, we then give the treatment group their treatment and the control group a placebo. Often the study is blind (meaning that the subjects don't know whether or not they're getting the treatment or control) or double-blind (meaning that the study administrators don't know, either), because the human mind is a powerful thing, and the placebo effect is real. If people think they're taking something that will help them, it usually helps them.

Finally, we wait . . . and tally the results. We compare the average gestational period between groups and interpret our findings. Simple enough, right?

But there are some catches to an RCT. First, because you still can't ethically give someone something if you think it will hurt them, instead of exposing nonsmokers to smoking, we exposed smokers to something that would reduce their smoking. Were we really answering the question we set out to ask?

Second, we still can't use an RCT to study things that are impossible to randomize and assign, like race, or the neighborhood someone grew up in, or if a grandparent was exposed to trauma. That's where the second study design comes in: the natural experiment.

Natural experiments help us observe what happens when nature assigns a particular exposure to someone, even when we cannot. For example, imagine you want to understand the influence of the neighborhood in which a child is raised on their probability of having diabetes at the age of thirty. It's unethical, of course, to assign a child to a low-income neighborhood at birth so that some epidemiologist can study how that will shape her life. But imagine you identify identical twins, separated at birth, who happened to grow up in different homes. They are alike in many ways, right down to their DNA. But at the time of separation their circumstances began to differ. This kind of study, called a "matched-pair analysis," allows us a unique lens into how environment shapes health over the long term.

Natural experiments, of course, have their flaws. You have to find one. And finding two good subjects for comparison is like looking for a needle in a haystack. Worse, there are still confounders. For example, in the matched-pair analysis I described above, there are many things about the twins' experiences that differed beyond their neighborhoods, like the parents who raised them or the incomes of their households. Nevertheless, these studies provide us with profound insights into how circumstances can shape our health.

There are no perfect experiments in epidemiology. Instead, rendering scientific truths from imperfect studies forces epidemiologists to be more imaginative than our fellow scientists: we have to imagine the world as it might have been, compare it with the world as it is, then ask how we can design studies or identify unique natural experiments with the ultimate goal of understanding what makes people sick—to make them healthier.

CHAPTER 3
Matched-pair.

I like to think that I was destined to become an epidemiologist. From an early age I learned how to imagine different worlds, how to use each piece of knowledge to fill in the gaps; it was a matter of social survival for a hyphenated kid. But there was something more. In epidemiology we ask questions about why people get sick, how they die, and what we can do about it. None of our questions matter, though, unless we are committed to making use of the answers.

Many with privilege can recognize, in the abstract at least, that poverty and the suffering it creates are a scourge and that we should work to end them. But without ever having lived in poverty, they may not appreciate its wiles, how it penetrates every aspect of a life. Many more do live in poverty, but because the nature of poverty is to disempower and distract, the burdens of their daily lives limit their capacity to act. Few have both an intimate understanding of the day-to-day reality of poverty—the suffering it causes—and the privilege to address it. The profound responsibility of those in this last category abides.

I live in that last category. That's because I was born into a matched-pair epidemiological study of sorts. Until that summer in Egypt, I had been blinded as a subject in this study. Unblinded, I learned just how lucky I was to be receiving the treatment: the security of privilege, the chance to grow up in a high-income society with guaranteed social and political rights, being raised with two parents, never wanting for access to clean water or medical care, my health and safety protected by laws and regulations, and with incredible educational opportunities. My treatment was a level of security that relatively few in the world can imagine.

My cousins were on the opposite side of the matched-pair natural experiment in which we were all unknowing subjects. My *ammu*, just a year younger than my father, was by all accounts more charming, better-looking, and just as smart as his brother. But he lacked his grit or patience. Rather than pursue a college degree after his mandatory year of army service, Ammu chose to pursue a get-rich-quick scheme. He's been pursuing it ever since—while driving a cab my father bought.

He had six kids, four near my age and two others much younger. That summer I spent several weeks with Ammu's family in their apartment in Kardasah, a low-income neighborhood somewhere off the tourist trail between Cairo and Giza. Although their apartment featured a balcony with a breathtaking view of the pyramids on the horizon, it didn't have a working toilet. My uncle petitioned me to lobby my dad for the extra money to buy one.

* * *

I would learn what it meant to *have rights* that summer. Teta had warned me several times that the free speech I took for granted at home simply didn't exist in Egypt. I tested her admonitions anyway. Amid the bustle of the afternoon market one day, I shouted the choicest Arabic words my cousins had taught me about the then dictator, Hosni Mubarak. That evening, plainclothes cops came to our apartment looking for me. It was the first time I saw fear on my grandfather's face.

"Go get me your passport," he told me calmly, his eyes adding the emphasis. Holding my American passport in his hands like a talisman against evil, he went to the door: "This boy is an American. You can't talk to him."

Even beyond the borders of my own country, my American passport protected the freedom of my speech. Had my cousins pulled the same stunt, they would have been detained and possibly disappeared.

In the twenty years after that visit, I would go on to graduate from a phenomenal public high school in a well-to-do Detroit suburb and then from the University of Michigan, one of the world's great public universities. I would earn two doctoral degrees, from Oxford and Columbia, paid for by a Rhodes scholarship and the U.S. government's Medical Scientist Training Program fellowship. I would teach at an Ivy League university, lead the rebuilding of Detroit's health department, and then run for governor of Michigan.

My cousins in Egypt were just as smart and just as capable as I was. They were kindhearted and ambitious. They deserved every shot that I had. They did not get them. My cousin Ahmed was twenty-five when he died in an auto accident in the chaotic traffic of modern Cairo in 2017. Mohamed, a few years older than me, supports his kids for a month on what might buy a nice pair of sneakers in the United States.

When I was born, the local health department had me registered. I was vaccinated for a series of infectious diseases that still plague many in Egypt. Whooping cough, for which I was vaccinated, killed one of the two children my grandmother lost: Badriyyah, who would have been my aunt.

The water from my tap in the United States ran clean, so my gut never had to adjust to the kinds of microorganisms that live in the drinking water in Egypt. (When I made the mistake of drinking the tap water in Egypt, I was sick for days.) The streets I traveled as a child—still travel—have speed limits, stop signs, traffic lights, and other safety features that quite possibly saved my life at some point. Their absence killed my cousin.

The U.S. government subsidized my education through graduate school, affording me a world-class education. My cousins would have had to pay much more to attend the same schools. The stipends I received spared me from having to choose between going to graduate school or supporting myself: I got to do both.

When I got frustrated with the leadership my state government offered me, I declared myself a candidate for governor and ran a vigorous political campaign—a right my cousins could never dream of.

* * *

But my improbable life at home has another side. It meant being a person of color in an America grappling with its diversity.

An elementary school teacher was the first to teach me a lesson in hate. I was seven, an eager kid who wanted my teacher to like me; I think all kids do. But she never did. No matter how many questions I got right or what I did to earn her affection, I couldn't earn the warmth she seemed to give the other kids so readily.

On our way back from lunch one day, a boy began teasing me about my name. I told him to stop. He wouldn't. He pushed me. I pushed him back. He hit me. I hit him back. He cried. I didn't.

Our teacher swooped in to pull the other boy behind her, as if to protect him from me, and shot me a look I will never forget: cold, dead eyes. I was sent to the principal's office alone, and my parents were told that I had hit a defenseless kid. When they asked me for my side of the story, I was ashamed. "It's not fair" just couldn't carry the weight of what I wanted to tell them. "It's not *just*" would have been more appropriate—but those are words they don't teach you in second grade.

It wouldn't be my last lesson in how the world viewed me because of my skin color, my name, or my faith. Another one came when I went out with my friends to play basketball one night. I was sixteen.

To be sure, I *was* wrong that night, but only because I had lied to my parents. My teenager's angsty self-obsession had frayed our relationship, and I had told my dad I was going to spend all night praying at our masjid when I was actually off to spend the night at my friend's house after a night of partying. I did neither in the end.

Nothing went right that night. We ended up back at his house early. At about 12:30 a.m. we concocted one of those ideas only sixteen-year-old boys could think was good: we decided to head to the local middle school, which had an outdoor court. The other boys were a diverse bunch, their parents hailing from Puerto Rico, Bangladesh, the Philippines, and India. We also had one white friend with us.

None of us had brought any athletic gear, so we had to improvise. Earlier in the week I happened to have lent my friend a pair swim trunks, which he had washed, so I put those on in lieu of gym shorts. On my feet were the Doc Martens boots I had gone out in that evening. I was also wearing a ribbed A-shirt—a "wifebeater" in the offensive early-2000s vernacular—under my sweater.

We were walking down the street on our way to the court, well past a curfew we didn't even know existed, when a cop car rolled by. My friends, suitably anxious, suggested we should run if the car came by again. Thinking, *Running from the cops is the universal sign of guilt*, I argued we should stay put and just tell the cops what we were up to.

We hadn't achieved any consensus when the car rolled by again. My friends booked it. Before I realized what had happened, the Crown Vic had come to a screeching halt about twenty-five feet away. Adrenaline flooding my brain, I booked it, too. Two dogs bolted out of the car. I was deathly afraid of angry dogs, having been chased by one when I was younger. So I put my hands up and turned around, not wanting to know what would happen if those dogs caught me out of view of their masters.

The next thing I knew, I was being thrown to the ground by two cops, both white. I was a wrestler in high school, and the instinct for any wrestler who gets taken down is to get right back up. I did—and that's when I caught one of the cop's eyes, cold and dead. Then one of the officers struck me over the head with a pepper spray bottle, knocking me right back down on the lawn of some poor family whom I'm sure we had awakened at that point.

"What are you doing in this part of town?" yelled the cop who had hit me, now cuffing me as I lay facedown in that front yard.

"I live in this part of town," I said.

"*What are you doing in this part of town?*" he screamed again, clearly implying that I was lying.

"I was playing basketball with my friends—"

"I'm going to ask you *one more time*: What are you doing outside of Mexicantown?"

"Sir, I'm Egyptian. I live a mile away, and I was going to play basketball with my friends." Although I was trying to maintain whatever shreds of dignity I had left, tears started flowing down my face. At sixteen, I wasn't a boy anymore—not to these cops, at least. But I wasn't a man, either; they had made sure I understood that.

They took me home. I was still in cuffs, flanked by both cops, when my dad opened the door. He was wearing his galabia. His eyes widened when they caught the flashing lights silhouetting me.

"Sir, is this boy your son?"

"Yes, sir. I'm sorry for whatever he did. Thank you for bringing him home."

At that point the cop who had rapped me with the pepper spray can began to uncuff me. I couldn't look up at first. I didn't want to look my dad in the eye, but I wanted to be loved—even if it was the love of disappointment—so I raised my head to face him. His eyes were brown and warm and sad. After the door closed, I tried to explain, but Baba was already halfway up the stairs.

The only thing my father ever said was that he was disappointed. Sometimes I wonder with whom and what for. In me for lying, certainly, but perhaps also for subjecting myself to that kind of humiliation. We both knew that my punishment had been too severe and had come at the wrong hands. There was nothing left to do but be disappointed.

I saw that cop once again at my high school's graduation awards ceremony. He was on assignment, in uniform. When he noticed me, the officer approached my family and me, and with the same dead stare he said, "I'm glad we straightened you out." *He* had straightened me out?

* * *

Three weeks after my run-in with those cops, I watched terrorists with names like mine attack my country in the name of my faith. Three thousand of my fellow Americans were killed in the craven terrorist attacks in New York, Washington, D.C., and Pennsylvania. The attack devastated me.

For me, as a Muslim-American, the trauma of that day was compounded by having my names and faith targeted. When the Twin Towers fell, so did any pretense I had of ethnic anonymity; I wasn't just another Brown kid anymore. That morning I had strutted into school with the confidence it takes sixteen years to develop and only a moment to take away. Within a few hours of the attack, Mom called me on my blue Nokia brick to tell me that she was going to be picking up my brother from school. His name is Osama. I could come home if I wanted to.

"No, Mom. I'm going to stay, just in case."

"In case what?"

"I don't know . . . in case anyone gets picked on." I had already started to hear epithets buzzing around. "Those damn Muslims did this. Fucking ragheads . . ."

At my school of approximately a thousand students there were about fifty Muslims—many more than in most public high schools, but too few to feel as if we had a presence. To be sure, there was little I *could* do if someone got picked on, but being there might help. It was the first time I felt responsible to people who shared my identity—because it was the first time our identity had been singled out on such a broad stage.

I heard the new brand of hate that would follow me after 9/11 for the first time a week later, on the football field. A hardworking if not gifted athlete, I made up for my deficits in size and speed—and generally everything else—with a decent mind for the game and the will to work harder than my peers. On defense, I often got double-teamed to make sure I couldn't make plays or to prevent me from seeing the field. That day I was double-teamed the entire game—and when and the refs weren't looking, the players on the other side would punch and kick me, calling me names like "sandnigger" and "towelhead." On more than one occasion, though, I saw a ref look right at us—and do nothing.

I was getting frustrated. After one play in the middle of the third quarter, one of the opposing players grabbed my face underneath my face mask, screaming, *"Go home, Osama!"*

For the first time the entire game, I hit back, socking the kid with an uppercut underneath his helmet. I'm not sure why I did it. It might have been the anxiety I knew my brother's name was causing my family. It might just have been sheer frustration. We were winning the game, for God's sake. I regretted it the minute I made contact.

The ref had turned around just fast enough to see me land the punch. His yellow flag went flying. I got yanked from the game.

Our defensive coordinator—who looked like Popeye's forearms grew a human—grabbed my face mask and pulled it so close I could smell his Old Spice aftershave.

"What the hell was that?" he asked, his blue eyes piercing through mine.

"Coach, he was—"

"Son, I don't care what the hell he was doing, what the *hell was that*?"

"I lost my temper, Coach."

"Damn obvious you did, son!"

"They were hitting me off play the *entire* game, and they were calling me names and making fun of my religion, and—"

His eyes warmed, his tone that of someone who didn't want to have to tell you something that circumstances were forcing out of him: "Son, let me tell you something: you're going to be Abdul El-Sayed for the rest of your life. You can either use it as an excuse or you can use it as motivation."

I often reflect on that lesson, however unfair and frankly accommodating of bias it might seem in hindsight. Motivation toward what, exactly?

To me it has become the motivation to make this place more loving and kinder to the next kid with a funny name—my own child, perhaps. It's too easy to become the mirror image of those who hate you: equal in hatred, opposite in direction. I have met too many who are so consumed by the hatred of those who hate them that they *become* them. Both sides of hate use the same words—"us versus them"—to frame their hatred in all-or-nothing terms. But hatred cannot be defeated with more hatred: hatred begets hatred. One can only be bigger than it.

I would learn this over time. In college, when we played lacrosse against a small liberal arts college in California, a group of about twenty or so of their fans heckled me mercilessly throughout the game, using the same collection of racial and religious epithets that followed me onto nearly every playing field. I wouldn't hit back this time. Instead of my coach pulling me, the opposing coach would board our bus to personally apologize for the abuse.

This heckling wasn't limited to the lacrosse field. In the spring of 2007, Young Americans for Freedom, a reactionary student group at the University of Michigan, hosted an event with "the Three Ex-Terrorists": three Arab men who claimed to have had ties to terrorist organizations but were now telling their stories of "enlightenment and escape" and giving away the secrets of a plot to overthrow America that all of us olive-complexioned Moorish folk were ostensibly party to.

They were part of a post-9/11 traveling circus of "native informants": dark-skinned, thick-accented people with foreign names who prostituted their identities to help make the case for the U.S.-led war in Iraq. To counter the images of bombed-out apartment complexes, emaciated babies, and prisoners with their genitals clipped to electrical wiring, these native informants were there to reassure everyone that the natives actually *liked it*—that Western military invasions were the means to freedom and democracy.

We had come to interrupt. As Arab- and Muslim-American student leaders, we weren't about to let this orientalist warmongering go unopposed. Because of the buzz surrounding our opposition to the speakers, local right-wing groups blasted notice of the event to their email lists to attract attendees from outside the University of Michigan.

As a security measure, the university planned to close the doors fifteen minutes into the event. So we came forty-five minutes early, all wearing yellow ("maize" being the brighter of our two school colors, so we knew every student would have something to wear). We occupied the front third of the auditorium, and once the doors had been closed to newcomers, we got up and walked out en masse.

Growing up, I had attended protests with my parents, but this was my first time helping to organize one. As we filed out of the auditorium, I was helping to usher our protestors out, reassuring them in the face of the hecklers.

"*Go home!*" one woman screamed at me, her eyes iced like my grade school teacher's all those years ago.

"Ma'am, I *am* home," I said calmly. "I'm a student here—"

"Well, I don't pay taxes so that people like you can come here and take my kid's spot in college! *Go back to your own country!*"

"Ma'am, this *is* my country. I was born here. My parents pay taxes, and—"

More yelling. More vitriol. She wasn't there to understand.

"Just stay calm," I reminded my fellow students. "Justice is on our side. Don't dignify their hatred with a response."

Many of the students had never had to look that kind of hatred in the eyes before. It's an odd experience, confronting such raw animosity. You hear the words and your mind recognizes them for what they are. But you do a double take. Your heart doesn't believe—doesn't *want* to believe—they are being directed at you.

I believe that people are generally good. Hatred like this doesn't occur naturally; it has to be manufactured, a hard and bitter alloy forged of fear and ignorance and anger. To hate, people have to convince themselves that the object of their hate is the "other," maybe even *not human*. This dehumanization sits at the core of humanity's worst crimes against itself—war and slavery and genocide. To justify the transatlantic slave trade, for example, American slaveholders had to erect an entire social and ideological infrastructure to delude themselves that the people who worked their fields, cooked their food, and raised their children weren't actually people at all. That cognitive dissonance is what Frederick Douglass targeted every time he spoke his simple refrain: "I am a man." He was. They knew it. And yet admitting it would have forced them to come to terms with the crimes they had perpetrated on him and people like him.

The woman who yelled at me couldn't have imagined that I was raised by a woman whose American "heritage" was probably deeper than her own by generations—or that some of the protestors who had walked out with us in solidarity and who were now being told to go back to "their country" were Native-American Michiganders whose original claims to the very land we were on predated my stepmother's by millennia. After all, that woman had come to reassure herself that people like me weren't, in fact, equally human. And despite having to confront our humanity on display, by God, that was what she was going to do.

But the most damaging forms of hatred don't yell; they're coldly institutional. As the country struggled to respond to its wounds, I learned to look out for the dreaded "SSSS" on my boarding pass when I flew. It stood for "Selected for Secondary Security Screening," a signal to the TSA that I should be screened before boarding flights from abroad to the United States. Imagine riding in an airplane for eight hours with a man who fits every profile of a terrorist you've been taught to fear, whose body and belongings you just watched get searched for contraband authorities thought might be used to bring that airplane down. Imagine *being* that man.

* * *

The notion that somehow what I said or did might count for more than myself that I felt for the first time after 9/11 has stayed with me. That struggle with the perceived responsibility of being an "ambassador" for people who look like me or pray like me is one I struggle with, as do so many people of color.

But nobody alive today speaks for *all* Muslims. Nobody could speak for a global community of 1.8 billion people, nearly a quarter of the world's population. They include 1.8 billion different combinations of race, ethnicity, nationality, sect, interpretation, and perspective.

The millions of American Muslims mirror that global diversity. Estimates suggest that there are about 3.5 million Muslims in the United States. But this is probably an underestimate, as many Muslims aren't willing to "out" themselves.

I can only speak to what my faith means to me as a Muslim-American. I've had a complex and ever-evolving relationship with my faith. I was raised in a conservative Muslim household. We moved quite a bit, and so I grew up between many different Muslim communities—almost always ethnically diverse but almost never racially or socioeconomically so. The plurality of

Muslim-Americans is Black, but immigrant communities who came here after the 1965 immigration reforms have almost never sought to include them in their suburban community centers, opting shamefully to mimic the segregation they found when they got here. My generation—their children—hasn't done much better.

I grew up between these immigrant Muslim communities, where at any given prayer you might see a Moroccan immigrant in his Fez next to a Pakistani in *shalwar kameez* being led by a Kuwaiti in a blinding white *thawb*. My friends' parents were immigrants from all over the Middle East and South Asia—Morocco, Libya, Egypt, Syria, Lebanon, Iraq, Pakistan, Afghanistan, India, and Bangladesh—with a smattering of West Africans from Senegal or the Ivory Coast, and white converts like my stepmom. As communities grew, they would often subdivide even further—first by ethnicity, Arabs with the other Arabs, South Asians with the other South Asians, and then further still by nationality.

Although I grew up attending the mosque and the requisite Sunday school that went along with it, I often felt alienated by the wrote, Draconian pedagogy. There was no space for debate or dialogue—just dogma. I was naturally curious. But curiosity usually led to punishment, and I got punished. A lot.

It wasn't that I didn't appreciate the teaching of Islam's core tenets, but as I would only come to grasp later, this educational method missed the central point of faith: that, rather than some sterile set of ideas, faith ought to inspire how we maneuver the dramas of our daily lives. This dogmatic teaching style left you memorizing facts rather than understanding ideals.

Through middle and high school, I always strongly identified as Muslim, but it didn't induce me to follow any sort of daily practice. I didn't eat pork or drink and I fasted during Ramadan, the Muslim Holy month, but that was about it. I didn't pray the five daily prayers, and I stayed well outside of the strict bounds of good behavior I was taught that a good Muslim boy should follow.

But by college, with the stifling gaze of my local community replaced by the glare of post-9/11 public attention on my identity, I started to explore my faith for myself. Beyond the dogma and the idealized images of bygone times in Arabia that I had been taught at Sunday school, I started to ask questions about what Islam meant for me *today*.

I found a faith that was radiant, relevant, and real. I studied the life of the Prophet Muhammad, peace and blessings be upon him, and about how he summarized his message simply: insistence upon the good of human character. I learned how this message had been a hallmark of the teachings of the prophets before him—Abraham and Jacob and Moses and Jesus, peace be upon them all—and was always intended to apply to real problems in real places.

It was a simple but profound message: Believe in one God, who created and sustains you. And recognize that if God is greater, then everyone in the eyes of God is equal. Such a belief cannot sit and stagnate. It should uplift the needy and the poor, feed the orphan, stand up to the oppressor, and fight for the equal dignity of all classes of people, just as the Prophet fought to guarantee the dignity of all—which, more than 1,400 years ago in Arabia, was a revolutionary act.

I learned about the man—how he would visit the homes of people who bitterly opposed him when they were ill, and how he was always in service of his family when at home. I learned about how he would greet great leaders and orphan children with the same humility and respect, kneeling to look a child in the eye—even getting on all fours so that they could play on his back. And I learned to find comfort and solace on a prayer mat at the end of a long day, feeling the weight of my worries fall away in prostration.

I read the history that has shaped how so many view our faith today, Muslims or not. I learned about how the House of Saud, from which the Saudi monarchy descends, has invested billions in exporting an extreme, literalist interpretation of the faith meant to sterilize it. And I learned how that interpretation has been warped into the Wahhabi ideology, which is behind some of the greatest atrocities committed in the name of Islam.

I believe in an Islam that emphasizes God and my responsibilities to his creation. I believe in the words of Imam Ali, the Prophet's nephew and one of the most important figures in Muslim history, who said: "All people are either your siblings in faith, or your equals in humanity." And the Islam I practice doesn't judge people; it seeks to empathize with and empower them. Along with making my daily prayers, fasting, and giving to charity, my faith also means treating all people with the same dignity. It means humility among those without power—and strength among those with it. And it means reflecting on the fact of my own mortality—the recognition that I will meet a Creator who will ask what I chose to do with what I was given while I was here. I believe in the faith of my Teta.

Sarah and I think a lot about how we live our faith in public and how to raise our daughter on these tenets. But faith is in the practice, the constant effort to understand and grow. We're grateful to have family of many faith backgrounds, including my grandparents, who are deacons at their Presbyterian church. I admire the practices that connect people of all faiths and the genuine human goodwill that binds us all. And I'm deeply grateful for the Muslim community and the role it has played in our lives, even as we work to make it better, more inclusive, more empowering, and more empathetic.

But one thing is certain: being a member of the Muslim-American community today is harder than it's ever been. The incidence of hate crimes against Muslims has risen consistently, with a spike after Donald Trump's political rise and election to the presidency. Each of these instances has an outsized influence on the psyche of American Muslims, reinforcing the idea that America is a dangerous place for us. And every time we hear about a terrorist attack, a mass shooting, or a pickup truck ramming into a crowd, Muslim-Americans know the blur of dissonant emotions that ensues: grief for the victims, to be sure, then the immediate search for the perpetrators' names, hoping to God they aren't Ahmed or Ibrahim or Mohamed or Abdul. The privilege of individualism—being held accountable for your actions and your actions alone—is among the most elusive for people of color.

Although the vast majority of terror incidents in America are committed by white men, they aren't usually labeled "terrorists": their terrorism is excused and written off as the result of mental illness or a "troubled youth." They get to be individuals. But if the perpetrator's name is Ahmed or Ibrahim or Mohamed or Abdul, we brace for the inevitable bloviating by talking heads about why "they" hate "us." That's particularly hard when, to us, "they" and "us" are the same people.

Experiencing hatred and fear unstitches Muslim-Americans from the fabric of our society, decreasing interaction with the vast majority of Americans, who prefer inclusion to hatred. That, in turn, drives the cycle: the lack of meaningful interactions between Muslims and non-Muslims leaves everyone that much more susceptible to hate propaganda.

Given my family, I grew up with the "everyday Americans" whom the racists and bigots claim to speak for. And I know from firsthand experience that the vast majority of Americans are open-minded, curious, and thoughtful—more interested in what Muslims pray for than *how* we pray. They recognize that when we embrace our shared humanity, our differences enhance our relationships rather than impede them.

CHAPTER 4
Privilege.

My relative privilege was clear. Although I was learning what it meant to be a Brown Muslim-American named Abdul in a post-9/11 America, I was the son of PhD-educated parents, growing up in a safe suburban upper-middle-class neighborhood. I hadn't been killed or permanently injured by those cops that night, only embarrassed. I always got to board my flights after those extra searches.

Most Americans of color don't have my privilege. I learned that on so many Saturday trips with my father to the Eastern Market, one of America's biggest and oldest (and best) outdoor markets. Detroit has had an ongoing farmer's market since 1841. The original site downtown was a center for whole-sale trade for hay and wood. Over the next several decades it sprouted offshoots like the one about a mile northeast of downtown—hence "Eastern." The pace and feel of the market, with the sounds of barter and the sights and smells of fresh produce trucked in from the countryside, must have taken my newly arrived father back to his father's tomato stall. I think that's why he's always had such an affinity for the place—that, and the fact that in those days he still didn't quite trust the produce sold at the American-style supermarkets, where produce was optimized for shape and color rather than smell and taste. Instead, he could walk to the Eastern Market, only a few miles from Wayne State's campus, and get produce whose provenance he could see in the faces of the farmers who had grown it.

Whenever he could, my father would take us to the Eastern Market on Saturday mornings when I was growing up. The thirty-five minutes it took us to travel twenty-six miles down the Lodge Freeway from the suburbs to Detroit was like crossing between worlds. The difference in life expectancy that I would travel in those thirty-five minutes was nearly a decade—the same difference in life years between my home and Egypt. We would walk the market, sample the fresh produce, and procure our provisions for the week. At home, my father would transform them into the same dishes his mother would cook, albeit conforming to whatever the current diet fad was at the time. (His keto-friendly pita is particularly interesting.)

But first he would make sure that we shared our provisions with folks in need. He would buy a little bit more meat than we required and have it packed separately, then drive us around to distribute it among his old friends.

Baba has always had a profound appreciation for the restorative work of charity—mostly for the giver. As children, when we would pass people begging in the street, he would hand one of us some money to give them. He would instruct us to give it with our hand below the hand receiving it—never above. God, he would remind us, was above us both. In the Muslim tradition, the act of giving, itself, was a privilege. One should give with gratitude and humility.

I remember meeting Ammu Othman for the first time. *Othman* was a name he had adopted while in prison after he became Muslim. *Ammu* is Arabic for paternal uncle—an honorific bestowed upon a man of my father's generation. Ammu Othman knew how to use nunchucks, which was absolutely the coolest thing to a kid obsessed with the Teenage Mutant Ninja Turtles. Ammu once gave me a training pair after a quick demonstration. He probably cost the house at least one lamp and lost some of my mom's affection, but he forever earned mine.

Ammu was a Black man in a country whose unkindness to Black men I would only come to understand over time. With several children to feed, he had struggled to make ends meet for them since his release from prison. Although he was constantly searching for work, the modern version of a scarlet letter he bore for having spent time in a broken criminal justice system kept him from ever finding it. He met my father at Friday prayer services at one of the mosques where my dad, a part-time volunteer imam, would preach. It would be years before I would fully appreciate that so many Black and Brown people in America, like Ammu Othman and his family, don't benefit from the privileges that my life had provided me.

I got to know Ammu Othman's kids, who would invite me to play with them when we would stop by. His eldest daughter, Aisha, was my age. She couldn't always play with the rest of us. When we started running around as kids do, or she'd get too excited, she'd wheeze, the preamble to a coughing fit. She'd have to use the inhaler her mother always had on hand.

"Now, Aisha, what'd I tell you about that? You don't want to have to go to the hospital again, do you?" Aisha's mother would ask, the sound of the inhaler spritzing new life into Aisha's wheezing lungs. In the 1990s, Detroit kids faced a probability of being hospitalized for asthma that was nearly seven times that of kids from the suburbs.

Ammu Othman's kids didn't have many toys, but the few they had were marked with years of love as they were passed down from one child to another. And they always shared. My cousins were the same way. I have always found that those who have the least share the most—a consistent irony of poverty.

* * *

I could empathize with the constant struggles of people like my cousins and Ammu Othman's kids—people whom I could have been. But privilege shielded my family from having just less than we needed to survive, from always having to balance immediate needs, like heating an apartment or paying its rent, feeding a child or paying for her glasses, paying the bus fare or losing the hour of work that might pay that fare for the next week.

And although Alexandria and Detroit were separated by thousands of miles, I began to notice that the patterns in each of those communities were strikingly similar, as if created by the same processes. I began to read incessantly about the history of race and racism, poverty and structural inequality in America; Alex Haley and Malcolm X, Howard Zinn and Noam Chomsky, filled the blanks left in the sanitized history I encountered in school. I began to connect the struggle for equality and justice at home with my own experiences as a person of color—and connect America's long history of international folly with the events unfolding in the aftermath of 9/11.

All the while, I did well in my science classes—as any good child of immigrants raised by two engineers should. To my father, there was math and science, and there was the fluff. He didn't have much respect for the idea of well-roundedness. You'd only end up doing one thing for a living, anyway, he reasoned. But we were still expected to excel in the fluff, because, well, an A was the only acceptable grade—on anything. We didn't go to art museums or see plays in the El-Sayed household. We went to the Henry Ford museum or the River Rouge assembly plant. To be sure, I loved the exactitude that the sciences offered, a sharp contrast to the social sciences and humanities, which always seemed more the study of human aspiration and the conflict and failure that do it in.

And yet I felt called to the fluff. Science seemed too remote. What did the Pythagorean theorem or the Krebs cycle have to do with my cousins in Egypt or Ammu Othman's family? There was something about the imperative to do something about it all that called me back to the social sciences—the aspiration of it. I would split the difference. If I became a doctor, I reasoned, I could use my love for science to help heal the chasms in health and life expectancy I had traveled—whether the thousands of miles to Egypt or the twenty-six miles to Detroit. Even though my dad has always had an aversion to doctors, he didn't push back too much on my career choice.

I studied biology and political science in college. I'd use the doctor's tools to take aim at broader social and political injustices. I discovered the work of physician-reformers like Dr. Rudolf Virchow, a mid-nineteenth-century German polymath who put the final nail in the coffin of "humorism," the idea that disease was caused by the imbalance of the humors. Instead, by examining corpses and demonstrating how postmortem changes in different organs explained the illnesses that had led to death, Virchow founded the scientific study of disease that we now call pathology—literally the study of *pathos*, or illness. In all, Virchow published more than two thousand scientific writings and founded several journals in the areas of cell biology, physiology, pathology, and anthropology.

Much of Virchow's work, however, was in public health and politics, as he saw the two as intertwined. His argument was that "medicine is a social science and politics is nothing else but medicine on a large scale. Medicine . . . has the obligation to point out problems and to attempt their theoretical solution." Virchow would go on to help found Germany's liberal party, serving in the German Reichstag from 1880 to 1893. His vocal opposition to the financial policies of Otto von Bismarck so bothered the chancellor that he once challenged the good doctor to a duel. Virchow declined to duel the traditional way, believing it to be uncivilized. He responded with a counteroffer only a pathologist could have conjured: a "sausage duel." Rather than revolvers, they would duel by eating sausages, one of which would be loaded with roundworm larvae. Bismarck, irked, declined, citing the proposition as too risky.[1]

I read about trailblazing doctors from our own time, like Dr. Paul Farmer, whose organization, Partners in Health, revolutionized the way we think about global health delivery. I read about Dr. Denis Mukwege, who built a hospital in the Congo to support victims of rape. He was awarded a Nobel Peace Prize for his work in 2018. Then there was Dr. Mary Malahlela, South Africa's first Black woman to register as a doctor—and a leader in the anti-apartheid movement from her clinic.

I wanted to be a doctor like them. Surgery appealed to the athlete in me—the intellectual quest of the work coupled with the precision of the procedures, often under pressure. I got to watch surgeons work minor miracles every day. I shadowed Dr. Karin Muraszko, a pediatric neurosurgeon, and the first female chair of neurosurgery in the country. She operates on kids born with spina bifida, a serious birth defect affecting the development of the spine. No doctor could inspire more confidence in the face of unimaginable anxiety among the parents of her young patients. When she reassured them that their children could go on to live healthy, productive lives, she spoke with unmatched authority: she had been born with spina bifida herself.

I watched Dr. Rick Ohye perform the Norwood procedure, the first of three surgeries required to treat hypoplastic left heart syndrome, a congenital birth defect that leaves the left side of the heart, its workhorse, underdeveloped. Until a few decades ago it was a death sentence. But I got to see a toddler bounce into Dr. Ohye's clinic on a follow-up visit, bubbling with a joke his dad had just told him—the scars down his sternum the only marks of his brush with death.

I read about the unspeakable loss of life in places all over the world because of the dearth of trained surgeons. I would become a pediatric neurosurgeon, I thought, and work to alleviate that suffering.

I loved my college experience at the University of Michigan, built to provide an "uncommon education for the common [individual]." Like many institutions of higher education, it has struggled with diversity and inclusion—but it has also worked hard to be on the right side of history. The university led efforts to protect affirmative action, taking several cases to the Supreme Court to defend it.

Although the massive University of Michigan campus hosted nearly forty thousand students, it was easily divided into smaller communities. Between the lacrosse team, the Muslim Students' Association, and teaching organic chemistry lab courses, I found several niches that would frame my college experience.

Probably best of all, I lived with my grandparents about twenty minutes north of campus. Initially my parents had hatched the idea to save money on room and board—and I have to admit that I wasn't a fan of it at first. But I came to love it. Grandma and Grandpa were always eager to lend an ear and encouraging advice as I worked through events in my life. Their wisdom and hard-earned perspective helped put in context whatever it was I was sweating over that day. And living off campus forced me to be purposeful about my time on campus, building relationships with good friends and mentors alike.

The transition to medical school was harsh. Medical school happens in two phases, pre-clinical and clinical. During the first two pre-clinical years, I found my passion for people overwhelmed by an onslaught of facts I had to memorize off PowerPoint slides that hadn't always been updated.

But I found refuge in research. My senior year in college I had quit playing lacrosse, and I wanted to something more to occupy my time. I loved the sciences and I loved the social sciences, but I didn't realize that there was a set of disciplines that bridged the obvious gap between them. In fact, my friends and elders used to tease me: "How are you going to combine biology and political science?" I never really had a good answer.

Social epidemiology became that answer. When a mentor suggested that I learn more about public health, I reached out to a number of professors at my university's school of public health whose bios suggested some topics of shared interest. I sent twenty-three emails and got one response. Dr. Sandro Galea was the only one who got back to me. He remains a teacher, mentor, and friend today.

Dr. Galea invited me to meet him that next week. We spoke a little about my interests and about his research. After the interview, sensing a good fit, I asked if I could volunteer with his research group. While it was nice to have met, he said, he did not take volunteers, and there were no paid positions available.

"I'm not in it to pad my résumé; I really just want to learn. Give me a chance, and if I'm no good at this, then let me go," I pleaded. He'd email me if something came up.

I showed up again the next day anyway. "I'm ready to work," I said. He was clearly too busy to meet with me again but took the hint that I wasn't going to go away so easily. He introduced me to one of the directors of his research team—"This is Abdul; he'll be working on our disasters project"—then got back to his meeting, a puzzled look on his face the whole time. *It was already the disasters project,* I thought. *How bad could I screw it up?*

I would work with a team doing research for a book on the ways that context—things like poor governance, poor infrastructure, and deep social inequality—turned hazards like hurricanes, fires, and terrorist attacks into true disasters in which lives were lost, homes destroyed, and economies turned upside down. My job was to research historical archives about various disasters, combing through old newspaper clippings and municipal filings about each one.

I got to know a few more members of the research team; one of them, Dr. Craig Hadley, a social anthropologist, sent me a research paper that he said I might find interesting. Using a public dataset of birth statistics collected by California's health department, Dr. Diane Lauderdale, a researcher at the University of Chicago, studied whether birth outcomes among women with Arab names had worsened after 9/11.[2] Because information about Arab ethnicity was not collected by the State of California, she used ethnically distinctive names as a proxy for ethnicity.

Dr. Lauderdale's results were stunning. She found that the probability of low birth weight among newborns to women with ethnically distinctive surnames was 34 percent higher after 9/11 than the same six-month period in the year prior, and that that probability jumped to 125 percent higher if an infant's first name was also ethnically distinctive. Dr. Lauderdale reasoned that the experiences of 9/11 increased stress in Arab women, which elevated levels of cortisol, the hormone that mediates the long-term stress response and strong evidence suggests may also shorten gestation in pregnant mothers.

In that paper, science, social science, and my own life experiences collided in a way I had never known was possible. It was exhilarating and devastating at the same time. I had known the profound impact of 9/11 on my family, but to recognize that it might have set a generation of babies' health behind before they were even born was bloodcurdling. What more was there to know about how this event had shaped our health? What more was there to know about how poverty or race or opportunity affected the health of people like Ammu Othman's little girl or my cousins in Egypt? I had found social epidemiology, the discipline that would shape my work for years to come.

Understanding these mechanisms—the ways that social factors molded health—became my passion. I would spend hours analyzing huge datasets to unlock their secrets. I immediately set out to replicate Dr. Lauderdale's study, using data from Michigan instead of California. I hypothesized that the size and concentration of Michigan's Arab-American community would blunt the consequences of 9/11 on Arab-American birth outcomes that Lauderdale identified, as Arab-Americans in Michigan benefited from both a stronger Arab-American community and potentially less discrimination, given their ubiquity.[3]

Dr. Galea heard about the side project I had taken on and called me into his office one afternoon. I thought I was going to be sent packing. Instead, he prodded me on what data I was using and how I was performing the analysis. I explained that a few of the folks in the lab had given me a crash course in SAS—Statistical Analysis System software—and that I was learning it through the work. Dr. Galea then offered me a paid opportunity to pursue the project over the summer. No more researching obscure disasters; I would be focusing instead on this notorious one with such profound consequences for my community.

After we completed the daunting task of collecting and "cleaning" the data—the tedious work of identifying and correcting incomplete or corrupted data points—we began analyzing it. We found support for my hypothesis: Arab-Americans in Michigan had not suffered higher rates of low birth weight or preterm birth after 9/11, as their counterparts in California had. In the process, I also found that Arab-American infants had a lower risk of prematurity and low birth weight than their non-Arab white counterparts in the first place.[4] Digging deeper into this, we found that the advantage was more profound in Arab enclaves, like Dearborn, and faded away among second- and third-generation Arab-Americans.[5] We reasoned that it was probably because both immigrants and those living in enclaves were more likely to live among fellow Arab-Americans, empowering and supporting them while also shielding them from prejudice.

Each of these findings became another research paper. I loved the thrill of discovering a small piece of knowledge and then sharing it with the world—a stark contrast to the tedium of memorizing PowerPoint slides. By the end of the summer, Dr. Galea invited me to do a PhD with him alongside my medical degree.

That might be fun, I thought.

CHAPTER 5

Complex causes.

John Graunt made his observations on the Bills of Mortality to understand the plague, and John Snow made his observations to understand cholera. Those problems led them to think empirically about how and why the diseases occurred. Both wanted to understand the cause of a particular disease. That's how epidemiology progressed for a very long time: with researchers asking basic questions about the causes of a given disease.

Social epidemiology—the kind of research Dr. Galea and I were doing— turns that equation on its head: it asks questions about diseases that may result from a given social factor, like racism, poverty, or neighborhoods. This might seem like an odd way of asking a question. But it is based on one of the most consistent and profound observations of epidemiology: that the poor and most marginalized in society nearly always suffer more.

This fact scales globally: the highest national life expectancy in the world is in Japan, at eighty-four years (an astounding five years longer than America's).[1] In India it's sixty-nine years. And in Sierra Leone it's fifty-two years. Japan is a high-income country, India a middle-income country, and Sierra Leone one of the world's poorest countries. Countries with high life expectancies are more likely to be predominantly white, without a national history of having been colonized, whereas those with lower life expectancies are more likely to be predominantly people of color with a history of being colonized.

It's true within a country, too. The average life expectancy in the United States is seventy-nine years.[2] Mississippi, the poorest state,[3] has the nation's lowest life expectancy: seventy-five years. Hawaii has the country's highest life expectancy at eighty-two years, and it's also the third-richest state.

In Michigan, with a life expectancy of seventy-eight years, the county with the highest life expectancy is Leelanau, at eighty-three years.[4] Leelanau is Michigan's second-richest county. Wayne County is Michigan's poorest and home to Detroit. Here, life expectancy is a full eight years shorter, at seventy-five years. Wayne County is also home to more than half of Michigan's Black population. The life expectancy of Black male Michiganders in 2017 was six and a half years shorter than that of white male Michiganders.[5]

Social circumstances affect not just how long we live but also how often children—the most vulnerable people—die. Life expectancy is an average, not an absolute. People in Sierra Leone don't all just drop dead at fifty-two while folks in Japan all live until eighty-four. Instead, the life expectancy is basically the average age at death, calculated by adding up the ages of death for everyone who died that year and then dividing by the number of people who died. If you think about that formula, you'll appreciate how impactful an infant's death might be to the overall life expectancy: each baby who dies adds zero years to the overall years of life lived but adds to the number of people who died.

That's why the infant mortality rate is such an important predictor of a country's life expectancy. Thankfully, most of us living in high-income countries like the United States aren't used to the tragedy of childhood death. And the massive drop in infant mortality since 1900 is an important reason why life expectancy in our society has risen from forty-seven to nearly eighty years. The national infant mortality rate is 6 per 1,000 births,[6] but infant death is all too common in poorer countries around the world. It's also all too common in poor communities in the United States. Infant mortality is more than twice as high among Black Detroiters, at 15 per 1,000 births.[7]

Why is life expectancy nearly as low in Sierra Leone today as it was in the United States in 1900? And why is infant mortality so high? The answer is something called the epidemiologic transition. Societies undergo an epidemiologic transition and sustain a period of rapid increases in life expectancy as children stop dying in high numbers. The United States underwent an epidemiologic transition near the turn of the twentieth century. Sierra Leone still has not.

During an epidemiologic transition, not only does life expectancy change because babies live through their infancy, but the very nature of the diseases that people suffer from in that society also changes. Epidemiologic transitions happen when a society takes on the ability to control and vastly reduce the burden of infectious diseases—usually caused by bacteria, viruses, or parasites that can be transmitted from one person to another, sometimes directly, sometimes by way of a vector, like a mosquito, flea, or mouse. Infectious diseases are the worst murderers in human history; they include mass killers like malaria, tuberculosis, pneumonia, cholera, the plague, and HIV. Because their immune systems are so poorly developed, infectious diseases are particularly harmful to babies, killing countless millions throughout history.

But controlling infectious diseases is both simple and complex. Most assume that the advent of vaccinations or antibiotics are what ultimately protected people from infectious diseases. Not exactly. Although vaccinations are an extremely important innovation in public health history—and unless a credible doctor has specifically told you otherwise, *everyone* should vaccinate their kids—they don't account for the greatest reductions in infectious diseases in human history. Neither do antibiotics. The first widely available antibiotic was penicillin, first used in the early 1940s and only after infectious disease mortality had dropped to a quarter of what it was in 1900.[8] Nevertheless, vaccines and antibiotics combined for huge proportional reductions in infectious disease mortalities after they were introduced.

So what does it take to control infectious diseases, save babies, and initiate an epidemiologic transition if it isn't vaccinations or antibiotics? Far more basic solutions: sanitation systems that hold water to safe drinking standards; laws that support tenants and reduce overcrowding; and large-scale extermination efforts that eliminate rats and mosquitoes. These and so many other public health efforts heralded our epidemiologic transition, saving babies and prolonging and improving the lives of children and adults alike.

Sanitation, zoning and housing regulations, and mass vector control are all collective public actions. As simple as they sound, they remain devilishly hard to do well. They require a competent government that is well funded and empowered to act for the benefit of all. In the grand scheme of history, that's a relatively new thing, something many countries in the world still don't have—and something many (like our own) are at risk of losing.

But if people living in countries that have gone through an epidemiologic transition are much less likely to die of infectious diseases, what do they die of? Usually, diseases of excess. First comes body weight. Some 30 percent of Americans between the ages of twenty and thirty-nine are obese. Moreover, projections suggest that within the next two decades an additional 10 percent will become obese. With obesity comes high blood pressure and high cholesterol. Then comes diabetes, with excess sugar in the blood wreaking havoc on some of the body's most important tissues. Then heart failure, or a stroke, or cancer, or dementia. And finally the end.

Public health has been far less effective here. Overeating and conserving energy were hardwired into our DNA over millennia as we roamed about in hunter-gatherer tribes. Eating one more ripened fig or strip of cured meat might mean survival through the desolate winter—although that extra scoop of ice cream today decidedly does not. In fact, it becomes deadly when calorie-dense food products are so plentiful and our dependence on cars and highways has reduced any unintentional exercise. We have all but failed to stand up to the corporations that exploit these hunter-gatherer calorie-maximizing preferences to feed us excess sugars and fats. Rather, the fight against obesity, too, has been consumerized through spin classes and protein smoothies. I wonder what a Lower Paleolithic–era hunter-gatherer transported to a modern-day gym would make of the neat rows of us pedaling as hard as we can to shed excess energy on stationary bikes.

During my summers in Egypt, I used to be chided by my grandparents if I left even a grain of rice on my plate. My grandparents came of age in a pre–epidemiologic transition Egypt. Indeed, they lost two of their children in infancy, one to whooping cough, another to a diarrheal illness. So, for my grandparents, eating all of your food made sense: food nourished the immune system, and was critical to protecting against infectious diseases.

Yet, even in high-income, post–epidemiologic transition societies, the poor still die earlier and suffer more—from diseases of overconsumption. Conventional logic would dictate that if overconsumption is what causes premature death in high-income societies, then the poorest can just stop consuming so much, which would save them money and add years to their lives. But remember, one of the abiding truisms in epidemiology is that the poor will *always* suffer more and worse.

While it may not make immediate sense, there are some good explanations for this. First, while a bag of spinach may be cheaper than a Big Mac, that spinach is far more expensive *per calorie*. Second, that bag of spinach is much harder to come by in lower-income communities, particularly in the food swamps of urban communities like Detroit, places where the ubiquitous fried food sold at liquor stores or fast-food joints is, in fact, plentiful, but of poor quality. The profit margin on that Big Mac is much higher than on that bag of spinach, and so McDonald's has a much bigger profit motive to move it. Third, preparing that bag of spinach to eat is time intensive, and it's not a complete meal on its own. Because many low-income Americans are working multiple jobs, the time-cost of serving up spinach is prohibitive compared to buying a Big Mac.

Then there's food insecurity. To understand how it works, consider this: if you don't know where your next meal is coming from, what do you do with the meal in front of you? You eat it all. If you get another meal in a few hours, what do you do? Same thing. And so on. For too many Americans who don't know where their next meals are coming from, this food insecurity paradoxically causes obesity.

* * *

Chronic diseases, like obesity and diabetes, are a lot more complex than the infectious diseases epidemiology was invented to understand, and our tools haven't always caught up. Again, causation is hard to disentangle from correlation, particularly when you're talking about the social mechanisms of diseases like the ones I was focusing on. Although we were building complex statistical models to try to control for confounders like differences in age and smoking status in our studies of birth outcomes, it was hard to isolate social *causes*: we were really just identifying interesting correlations.

In fact, the very idea of "cause" in epidemiology just may not be nuanced enough for studying complex social interactions that might be really important to understanding chronic diseases. For example, people usually eat together . . . but what happens when they don't? Throughout our early history, we would exercise together, too. What happens to exercise habits when families and communities fragment as members move away?

This has led the field to think more deeply about what it actually means to *cause* something. Lawyers, who spend a lot of time trying to prove or disprove causes, define a cause specifically as that thing that most directly results in an outcome. To understand what that means, consider this example: Imagine it snows in April. Someone, sick of a long, snowy winter, neglects to shovel the sidewalk. Within a few days the snow turns into a patch of slick ice, and you slip and fall on that ice one night on your way home from work, slipping a disk and requiring back surgery. You might contact an injury attorney, who might try to prove that failure to shovel the sidewalk caused your slip and fall—and you might win the lawsuit.

But this is a limited notion of a cause. To understand why, ask yourself this: Is that the *only* cause? What about the snow itself, which is uncommon in April but more common now because of climate change? What about the fact that you chose your dress shoes with bad treads because you had to give a presentation at work that day? What about the fact that it was dark, and the bulb in the streetlamp that was supposed to light the area had gone out and hadn't been replaced yet?

In fact, all of these things conspired against you. Individually, perhaps none of them would have caused your fall, but what we know for sure is that this particular combination of factors led to your fall, even though the personal injury attorneys will focus on just one (that they can blame on someone for a payday).

If we wanted to prevent your slip and fall, rather than just attribute blame for it after the fact, we might take a much more comprehensive view of a cause than the lawyers. First, we would have to appreciate that causation isn't fully attributable to one thing or another but is rather a complicated web of interrelated "chains" of causes. Within these chains of causes are some that cause others. Epidemiologists distinguish between these as "proximal" ("near," or direct) causes—for example, the slip was caused by the wrong shoes—and "distal" ("far," or indirect) causes—the presentation at work and climate change.

And then we want to consider how we interrupt any given cause. For example, to make sure that the walk is safe, we might make sure that there is an enforced law in place that compels that public sidewalks to be shoveled, or we might employ a public agency to salt the walks. We might have a backup lighting system to make sure that faulty lightbulbs don't leave people in the dark. We might put hazard signs up in places where ice tends to form after a snow. We might even focus on addressing climate change so that it doesn't keep snowing in April. It is with interventions like these in mind that we epidemiologists approach the question of cause.

Now think back to the hypothetical time-traveling experiment I proposed earlier that considered the effects of smoking on prematurity. Consider this:

What if smoking *were to have an effect* on prematurity, but that effect differed based on other factors, like living in a polluted environment or taking prenatal vitamins? The polluted environment might exacerbate the impact of smoking, while the vitamins might mitigate it.

Also, what if there's a feedback loop? For example, if, after smoking, our subject starts coughing regularly and, fearing the worst for her baby, moves to a new neighborhood and starts exercising, thanks to the encouragement of a support group of pregnant mothers? Our experiment—and the intellectual infrastructure around it that relies on direct, controlled comparisons—has no way of dealing with those kinds of scenarios, which are common when you're thinking about how the real world shapes our health. They introduce a complexity with which our traditional approach to thinking about causes just isn't equipped to deal.

That critique—not just on epidemiology but on science as a whole—is the basis for complex systems science, an epistemological approach that argues that things like feedback loops and interactions between people matter for understanding the sum of the parts. Although the traditional approach has gotten us pretty far, perhaps it's time for us to think about how much further we can go. That's particularly true in social epidemiology.

I wrote my doctoral dissertation on using more complex analysis tools to understand these complex relationships in epidemiology. I used a relatively new approach called agent-based modeling. It's like playing the epidemiological version of the popular 1990s video game *SimCity*. In case you've never played it, you start with a group of simulated people in a barren plot of simulated land. You act as the master planner, making decisions about where and how you might build the foundations of a city. You invest in a market here, a school there, and you judge your outcome based on how well your simulated people thrive and how well your city performs across a series of measures of economic, social, and communal wellbeing.

Graunt and Snow's epidemiology starts with collecting a dataset about individuals, some of whom suffer from the disease you're studying. Using that data, you try to replicate the experiment you wish you could have carried out, employing complicated statistical models to understand the relationships between factors you hypothesize may be causing the disease and the likelihood of disease itself.

In agent-based modeling, we do the opposite. As with *SimCity*, we start with a simulated group of people in a simulated environment. Then we use empirical data to program the individuals and the environment to change and interact with each other, each interaction shaping the future that those individuals and environments experience. Every time we let the simulation run, we're effectively conducting a simulated trial. We program each simulation to differ from the others based on changes that are programmed into the model—like how segregated people might be, or the impact the environment has on the likelihood of the outcome. Then we compare these simulated trials to each other and to what we observe in real life. By isolating variables in our models and comparing them to each other and to what we observe in real life, we attempt to approach an understanding that takes us beyond the factors—to the mechanisms—that cause disease.

CHAPTER 6
Ideals and institutions.

I watched the Egyptian revolution to oust President Hosni Mubarak from the fifth floor of my three-century-old college quarters in Oxford. I had just come back from Egypt, where I had spent the better part of the winter holiday visiting family and touring with some of my classmates. Not two weeks had passed before what history would name the Arab Spring erupted. And perhaps it's just hindsight bias, but I swear something was different that December of 2010: everyday people were more considerate of each other, and the authorities were just a bit jumpier. Egypt's protests came on the heels of massive Tunisian uprisings that had deposed the dictator of that country. When reports started to surface of camp cities being erected in Tahrir Square, the possibility of real change seemed imminent.

I had walked through Tahrir Square—roughly equivalent to New York's Times Square—so many times. I could almost imagine the combination of excitement, fear, and anticipation on the ground. And I knew the risks those young women and men were taking to reshape Egypt's future in the shadow of the museum housing the relics of its millennia-long history.

As I watched history write itself in real time, I just knew President Obama would stand up and support the protestors. After all, he had run in opposition to the war in Iraq specifically and America's wayward wars in the region more broadly. In 2009 he chose Cairo to make a policy-defining speech, opening a new conversation with the Muslim world. "I do have an unyielding belief that all people yearn for certain things: the ability to speak your mind and have a say in how you are governed; confidence in the rule of law and the equal administration of justice; government that is transparent and doesn't steal from the people; the freedom to live as you choose,"[1] he said. Less than two years later the Egyptian people were rising up in hopes of tasting those very freedoms.

But yet, my hopes for change had started to ebb by then. I had been watching Barack Hussein Obama since 2004, when—as a state senator—he showed me for the first time that politics could look even remotely like me. Obama's father emigrated from eastern Africa; my father emigrated from northeastern Africa. He was a child of a mixed family; I was a child of a mixed family. People thought he was Muslim; I'm actually Muslim.

I was washing dishes when he delivered his 2004 keynote address at the Democratic National Committee. As he began to speak, I just stopped and watched, dumfounded, suds still dripping off my hands.

Four years later I learned that that skinny Black man with a funny name would be the forty-fourth president of the United States of America. As I watched the election returns on a laptop in Ann Arbor, while studying for a medical school exam, my eyes welled up at the profundity of that moment.

Obama changed what I thought was even possible—especially for me. In fact, when I graduated from college, I had actually told another former president that there was no way I could even consider a career in politics.

I had been selected to give the student commencement speech. Knowing I would have to speak from the same lectern as President Bill Clinton, who was giving the keynote address, I practiced my speech over and over again.

After being introduced by the dean of my college, I approached the lectern and looked out over a sea of faces. There were *a lot* of people—sixty thousand, I would learn later. Was I ready for this? I began to speak. "Thank you, Dean McDonald." My voice reverberated off the grandstands and ricocheted back to me a microsecond later, just long enough to be noticeable. At our dress rehearsal they had told me to expect this distracting echo, but it was the first time I really felt it. I had made the decision to jettison my notes that morning, realizing that I was smoother in my delivery when I wasn't checking what I had written.

But I was starting to regret that decision. What if I forgot my words? I was starting to panic. I could feel the blood pulsating through my arteries with every heartbeat. Were the jokes even funny? Would people get my references? I wished the damn echo would stop.

Keep speaking, a calm voice from inside said, overriding the panic. *All you can do now is speak!* After my first joke, about a local burrito joint being open until 4:00 a.m., I felt the laughter of the crowd hit me. It carried me through the rest of my delivery, silencing the panic inside.

When I stepped off the dais, I could still hear the applause. I knew I had nailed it. You can always tell if you've connected to an audience. It's the look in their faces that registers the emotions that were, seconds ago, in your heart alone. Thousands of speeches later, it remains one of the most unique, most exhilarating experiences for me, knowing what the audience is about to hear—a secret you get to share—and moments later seeing it register on their faces.

President Clinton talked about inclusivity, diversity, and engagement—the usual post-presidential college commencement fare. But he added a little extra in the middle of his speech—a gift to my parents, perhaps. "I don't mean to embarrass your senior speaker . . . ," he said with a tilt of his head to look back at me.

Wait—that's me! I thought to myself, embarrassed. I saw my face on the giant scoreboard as the camera moved to catch me. I looked down immediately, not knowing what else to do—half-embarrassed, half-frightened by the twenty-five-foot image of my own face.

". . . but I wish every person who believes that we are slated to have a clash of civilizations and cannot reach across the religious divide could have heard you speak today . . . I just wish every person in the world could have heard you speak today."

In that instant, three feelings did battle in my mind. The first was the kind of embarrassment you get when, as a little kid, your parents talk about some dumb thing you did at school as if it were the second coming. Second, had my parents heard that? They'd better have. Third, a sense of profound responsibility, the sense that, in that moment, you represent every Mohamed or Aisha—every Juan or Maria, even—to everyone there.

After the processional, we went back to the locker room to change out of our regalia. After I had finished, I was getting ready to meet my parents and Sarah outside. I had wanted to say goodbye and thank President Clinton, who was still at his locker in the corner, but a horde of university higher-ups surrounded him, each trying to impress him with an elevator pitch about their research or an anecdote about their recollections of his time as president.

I'm a good Midwestern boy and didn't want to bother the man, so I figured that it wasn't meant to be, and packed the rest of my things. I started toward the exit when I felt a tap at my shoulder. It was President Clinton. His face was concerned—the kind of look your parents put on when they hear from your teacher that you had a bad day at school.

Among his political gifts is his incredible ability to look *through* you—as if he's put your soul in an emotional half nelson even as his hand offers itself to yours in a sign of warmth. There was no breaking free.

"Son, why are you going to medical school?" he asked.

The first thing that popped into my mind was *Well, I'm Brown and Muslim—that's just what we do.* Thankfully, I caught it just before it came out of my mouth.

"I love people and I love science," I told him. "And that's how I hope to serve."

"Well, you've got a natural gift for speaking. Maybe someday you'll run for office," he replied matter-of-factly.

It was six years after 9/11. My name, in all its glory, is Abdulrahman Mohamed El-Sayed.

"Mr. President," I said, "I really appreciate you saying that, but I don't know if you saw my name. There are eleven letters in my first name—and that's *just* my first name. People like me don't get to run for office."

We both chuckled, uncomfortable because of the unbearable, un-PC truth of what I had just said.

Consider the irony: I had just graduated at the top of my class, Phi Beta Kappa, with highest distinction from one of the finest universities in the world. I had just delivered the student commencement speech to sixty thousand people, in which I told them that we had "the audacity to believe that we could change the world." And then I had proceeded to tell a former president of the United States that I could not imagine ever being elected to public office in the country of my birth because of my name. So much for having the audacity to believe . . . anything.

But President Obama's was the audacity of hope: the idea that someone whose father had immigrated from eastern Africa—someone who was marked by a funny name and dark skin—with a lot of perseverance *could* change the world. And I adored him for it. Of course he was going to fix healthcare, bring peace to the Middle East, solve our immigration crisis, and finally do something about gun control. How couldn't he with *all that hope?*

From my perch in Oxford, I watched the healthcare debates unfold in the windup to the Affordable Care Act, the important if tepid healthcare reform that would come to be better known as Obamacare. While it was clear that

President Obama wasn't as interested in pushing a structural reform to fundamentally change the way that healthcare is accessed and paid for, the way Medicare for All might, there were still important reforms in his plan.

Yet I watched so many of them get stripped in the spirit of compromise and bipartisanship. The Republicans were *never* going to give Obama a win, no matter what. He seemed so stuck on hope that he couldn't see that. Overboard went measures meant to curb the greed of the pharmaceutical industry, which could vastly reduce the cost of prescription drugs, which were higher in the United States than in any other country in the world. Then there was the "public option," a government-operated alternative to private health insurance. Gone. And for all that compromise, in the end, the ACA passed entirely on partisan lines—as almost anyone watching could have predicted.

Although my hopes for Egypt were measured—as my expectations generally from this president had become—I remained confident that President Obama would do the right thing and stand with the Egyptian people, who were throwing off the yoke of tyranny. Of all people, surely this president, whose father had come from a country more like Egypt than America, would understand what this would mean for Egypt, for the Middle East, and for the world.

But that voice that had seemed so resonant and so sure just a few years earlier was deafeningly silent now. For too long, American foreign policy had appeased strongman dictators in the region—Hosni Mubarak chief among them. It seemed little was changing.

I had started to write op-eds and commentaries—mostly about public health and healthcare—but this time I felt I needed to pipe up on something so close to my own experiences as an Egyptian-American. In a column in the *Guardian*, I implored the president to stand unqualifiedly with the people of Egypt. Given my own firsthand experiences with the brutal Mubarak regime in stark contrast to the freedoms I enjoyed as an American, I knew that history was presenting us with a unique opportunity to stand for our values as Americans by protecting them abroad. And yet, only after many anxious days did President Obama join the chorus of world leaders calling on Mubarak to resign—and only with lukewarm words calculated to appease other strongmen waiting in the wings.

And so it was with many of the outcomes of Obama's presidency: inspiring intentions unfulfilled or reversed. President Obama oversaw the expansion of

America's drone war, inaction on immigration reform, and the failure to close down the prison detention camp at Guantánamo Bay.

Still, there was *so much* to admire in the man, and I will always remain deeply grateful for what President Obama and his family did—for America and for me. He showed us the power of dreaming that impossible dream. I never would have considered running for office if he had not shown me that I could. I know only a small taste of the kind of hate and criticism he took, simply for being a Black man who dared to aspire to lead in our country.

However, I am also grateful that he taught me about the limits of people and institutions. I had believed that if only we could come up with the right answers, the politics would work themselves out. *What's politics in the face of truth?* I had thought. Watching President Obama struggle to advance public policies that often lost much of their bite before they ever got to the negotiation table demonstrated that advancing truth isn't just about discovering and understanding what that truth is. It's also about having the will to stand unabashedly for it—and against the people and institutions who oppose it.

* * *

I learned that I had won the Rhodes scholarship and would travel to Oxford just three weeks after then-senator Obama was elected president. The emotional trajectory of my time in Oxford mirrored the first few years of Obama's presidency in many ways.

When the chair of the Rhodes selection committee, a judge, announced my name, I couldn't believe it: "You're kidding, right? Show me that piece of paper!" I'll admit it wasn't the most couth response. I just couldn't believe it: *People like me don't win awards like that,* I thought. I could have named ten reasons why every other candidate at my interview was better-qualified than I was, not to mention smarter, nicer, and generally more erudite.

I thought back to Teta: she had never had the opportunity to step foot inside a classroom. Two generations later I would study at Oxford University on an all-expenses-paid scholarship. She had passed away ten years earlier, the victim of pancreatic cancer. I wondered what she might have thought, and I wished I could have shared it with her.

* * *

Oxford truly is an incredible place, its hallowed history etched into the age-old stones of its ornate colleges. And yet, too few have had access to it. Though it is one of the UK's most important passageways to social mobility, young people of color have found it far too hard to traverse. While I was a student there in 2010, two-thirds of the university's thirty-two colleges—think residential and educational units much like Hogwarts's fabled houses from Harry Potter—failed to admit even one Black student.[2]

My experience was not without hiccups. After finishing my first two years of medical school, I had applied to do a master's in global health sciences, a program focused on international health research and delivery. Given my previous work in epidemiology and my goal to practice abroad, this program seemed tailor-made. The plan was to finish my master's, head back home to do my PhD in epidemiology, and finish medical school—then I'd be off and running.

The course was small, with just under thirty students, intended to offer an intimate engagement with the instructors. But by then I had already done two years of research in epidemiology with Dr. Galea, learning by doing—which meant that I had covered much of the material already. By the end of the first term it was clear that the course was a poor fit. In a candid conversation with the course director, we agreed that I should find an alternative. But a full term into the school year, there were few options left to transfer into.

I was frustrated. Two weeks before the term ended, I left Oxford for home, just before Thanksgiving—much to the chagrin of the scholarship administrators.

* * *

Truth be told, frustration was only a small part of what brought me home. It was something deeper, part homesickness, part need for re-centering. But mostly I missed Sarah. We had been married for three years by then. Having decided late in college to pursue a career in medicine herself, she chose to take a fifth year to finish up her premed requirements and stay back in Ann Arbor while I was abroad. Rhodes scholarships are nondeferrable, so I had to go then or lose my scholarship.

Sarah and I had met in the fall of 2005, at "Festifall," the University of Michigan's annual fair to connect new freshman to student organizations. Although she was one of those freshmen Festifall was intended for, she had somehow found her way into helping staff the Muslim Students' Association (MSA) table, next door to the Baha'i student table and across from Ultimate Frisbee. When I approached the table, she earnestly began to hand me some literature about the MSA, a home away from home for Muslim students. With a bemused grin on my face, I kindly declined: I had already been an active member of the organization for several years.

What struck me was her huge smile, with which she was so generous. So did her big, twinkling mahogany eyes. She was tiny—five foot one, I later learned—but her confidence was gargantuan, this freshman who had invited me to learn more about a club I was already part of. Sarah had the quiet confidence of someone who had known love unconditionally. She didn't need to explain, prove, or justify herself. To be sure, she had insecurities, but she was secure with them. And it radiated. I'd come to love her for it.

Sarah is the fourth of five children of two loving parents. Her father, Tayeb, adores spending time with his family and works hard to earn his living as a kidney doctor—just to give it away to one charitable cause or another. Her mother, a homemaker who raised five kids almost entirely alone while her husband was still training, is a source of quiet strength. They have become an important, stable extension of my ever-diverse family.

Sarah's parents emigrated from a tiny coastal village in Karnataka, India, where they speak an unwritten dialect and every recipe starts or ends with rice, coconut, or chili paste. Sarah and her siblings spent the better part of every summer in that village, where they would float from house to house, eating and chatting with distant cousins, growing their roots.

Sarah's quiet confidence was a stark contrast to my own. I've never been told I lacked for confidence, but—particularly as a young man trying to get a clear sense of myself—mine was not the quiet sort. I struggled to learn who I was. Sarah did not. She danced with her emotions. I wrestled with mine. And in time she would teach me to dance, if awkwardly, with mine too.

In May 2006, less than a year after we met, we married in a small ceremony at our local *masjid* and had a reception in my family's backyard. We were building a life together—she nineteen, me twenty-one. We were young and dumb—and totally and resolutely in love. To be sure, both of our parents were uncertain about the prospects of our getting married so young. My parents knew me well enough to know that once I had made a big decision like that, there was no opposing it. Sarah's parents made us promise that we would finish our education before having a child. They came to regret how long we would make them wait for Emmalee. Sarah finished her undergraduate degree, then a master's in comparative social policy from Oxford, a medical degree at Columbia, and half of her four-year psychiatry residency before our little one was born in 2017.

It makes sense that Sarah would eventually become a psychiatrist, mainlining that quiet security into people struggling through some of the vilest experiences life can offer. After all, I admit that our life partnership prepared her well for this work.

As a young man growing up between worlds, one of the few consensus lessons that I was taught from every side of my diverse background was that I was not allowed to feel sad—and certainly not allowed to cry. Stoicism? Fine. Anger? Certainly. Sadness? *What are you, a sissy?* Among the greatest gifts Sarah has given me is the assurance that it is okay to feel sad. I came to appreciate the meaning of this gift only while I was in Oxford. During my first term there, I met some of the world's most brilliant people, folks whom I know will change the world, if they haven't already. And yet the thing they—we—all had in common was the uncommon will to achieve. Behind the conversational wit, big ideas, and immaculate grades was a drive to work harder, to push beyond the limits of pain, tedium, and sleep.

But ambition born of insecurity can poison you. You constantly feel inadequate—never smart or worthy enough. You try to knock that ubiquitous chip off your shoulder with achievement and the validation it offers, rather than the fruit of the work itself.

When you ask folks what they want in this world, most of them will say something about happiness. But that word, "happiness," is too imprecise a term. It stands in for a diverse mix of emotions that range from euphoria, to joy, to contentment, to fulfillment. Euphoria is intense but short-lived—the stuff of addictions. Joy is less transient, more wholesome—but just as fleeting. Contentment and fulfillment are much harder to come by, but more enduring, requiring balance and delayed gratification. When they talk about happiness, I think what most people pine for is contentment and fulfillment with some joy interspersed—and perhaps a few good moments of euphoria. But it takes security to commit to the future, to delay gratification and believe in the returns on your emotional investments.

I needed to come home because I needed Sarah. I was discontented and unfulfilled. She was honest with me; it was all she knew how to be. Over years of introspection, and the loving support and guidance from her and so many others, I have come to appreciate where the chip on my shoulder comes from, and why.

Divorce is a hard thing. And I had never fully grieved my parents' divorce. As a younger man, I dealt with it by rebelling. As I grew older, I channeled it into a more disciplined drive. Yet it held power over me. And it wasn't until I could learn to mourn it that I could take away its power. Sarah taught me how to mourn it—to just sit with the sadness of it without reacting, or numbing, or running away. And sometimes to cry.

Becoming a parent has reframed my own parents for me. When I was gifted with my daughter, I was exactly the same age my father was when he had me. I think about who I am as a father: flawed, imperfect. I will face hard choices and inevitably make mistakes. In seeing that in myself, I realized that my parents, all those years ago, were nowhere near perfect either, contending with challenging decisions in imperfect circumstances—all while feeling the overwhelming love a parent has for a child for the first time, and trying to do the impossible work of attempting to glimpse that child's future and ask how that path will unwind. All of this has taught me a profound mercy for my own parents—something I hope I can earn from my own child.

Connecting with my own grief, insecurity, and sadness also opened up a latent empathy in me. It had always been there—but I couldn't access it because I didn't know how to identify it. Facing my own grief and sadness allowed me to connect with those same emotions in others. And recognizing that I had, for so long, sublimated my grief into so many other emotions—anger, frustration, resolve—helped me identify the real emotions underlying the complex reactions so many of us put out in the world to hide the ones we are really feeling. In finding myself in what I had been avoiding, I found others, too. I learned to listen, not just to the words being spoken, but to the *feelings* being spoken.

* * *

Back home, I spoke with Dr. Galea and some of my other mentors and decided that, although I was already planning on doing a PhD when I returned to Michigan, that I should use my time to do a doctorate in Oxford. Oxford's approach is different from American PhDs (besides being abbreviated "DPhil"): there is no course work, only a dissertation, with students left to pick up the skills they needed to complete it on their own.

On the plus side, I thought, doing an independent dissertation would also allow me to invest more of my time in the other education I was getting—ad hoc, in lessons from my classmates over lunch. The truth was that, regardless my course of study, my classmates in Oxford taught me more than I could learn in any classroom.

We would meet regularly for sandwiches at Ricardo's, my favorite spot in Oxford's Covered Market. With Noelle, a moral philosopher, I would dissect Plato, while with Rakim, a political philosopher, I would debate the philosophy of public health and public goods, refining my understanding of why I even believed what I did about public health and healthcare. With Aisha—a political geographer and the other Egyptian-American in my Rhodes class—I debated the developments in Egypt and how they related to our experiences as Egyptian- and Muslim-Americans. With Jisung, an environmental and labor economist, I reviewed the basics of economic theory and debated the finer points of environmentalism. With Oussama, an Algerian-English law student, Liban, a Somali-English chemist, and Imran, a medical student, I would learn more about what it was like to be Muslim in the U.K.

Although our lunch conversations varied from the cellular physiology of DNA silencing to Plato's musings on love, my lunch fare at Ricardo's was always the same: Coronation Chicken (a curried chicken salad created for the coronation of Queen Elizabeth) on a fresh-baked olive ciabatta topped with sharp cheddar cheese, banana peppers, and red onions, grilled and topped with lettuce and tomato, salt and pepper.

I had heard about the shop from a mentor at Michigan and immediately fell in love: the food was delicious, and hearing Ricardo and his partner, Anita, bicker as they worked reminded me of home. Since I extolled the shop and the sandwich, my friends would often let me order for them. Soon they'd come with their friends, asking for the sandwich they got "with Abdul." By the time I left Oxford, Ricardo and Anita christened the sandwich "the Abdul" after I bound and printed them a copy of my doctoral thesis—with a full paragraph acknowledging their contribution to the project by nourishing my stomach and my soul.

My classmates and I even organized a philosophy discussion group on Sunday afternoons that we lovingly called "Phight Club," where we'd debate fundamental questions like "What is love?" or "How do we value the environment?" Usually the least informed and least intelligent person in those rooms, I learned so much. Discomfort, I have come to appreciate, is the optimal learning environment.

Early in the next term, returning to Oxford, I met Dr. Peter Scarborough, a prolific young academic who was always interested in applying new approaches to old epidemiologic questions. When I told him that I wanted to take a nontraditional view to understanding social inequalities in obesity in England, he didn't even flinch. When I said I wanted to finish the project in two years, he flinched a little. Yet he proved a fantastic mentor and a good friend.

I completed my dissertation in April 2011. Sarah had joined me for my second year in Oxford to pursue her master's. After completing our degrees, we moved to New York, where Dr. Galea had been appointed chair of the department of epidemiology at Columbia University Mailman School of Public Health. Although I would miss Michigan, I wanted to continue my work with him. Columbia facilitated the transition by accepting Sarah to medical school—on the day of her interview, a nod to her incredible talent.

Despite having just finished a doctorate at Oxford, to catch up on the doctoral coursework that wasn't included in my Oxford education I enrolled in the PhD program in epidemiology at Columbia. After about eighteen months, and having gotten my fill of coursework—nearly six years after starting graduate school—I decided to forgo writing a second dissertation and go back to medical school.

CHAPTER 7

Not that kind of doctor.

Nearly four years as a graduate student had immersed me in the world of ideas. The transition back to the applied, tactile world of medical school would be jarring. I'd be a third-year medical student entering the clinical phase of my medical training—on the lowest rung of the medical hierarchy. Nevertheless, the third year would be a welcome shift from the rote memorization that characterizes the first two years of medical school. I would be fully engaged in the day-to-day care of patients, which was, after all, the reason I was pursuing a medical degree.

But doubts about my ultimate vocation had already started to creep in. My time as a public health researcher had impressed upon me just how much the world around us shapes our wellbeing—and what could any one doctor do about the profound structural forces that affect patients' lives for the 99 percent of the time they live outside of your care?

As a medical student in one of the country's biggest and busiest hospitals, I was immersed in the day-to-day of providing medical care. I was awestruck at both how complex and how broken our healthcare system really is. Nearly twenty cents of every dollar spent in our economy is spent on healthcare—for mediocre health outcomes. Our counterparts in Japan outlive us by more than five years, and our infant mortality rate is higher than average among our peer countries. Worse, our health outcomes are disproportionate: far worse among people of color, the poor, and marginalized people across the country. Because of doctors like Karin Muraszko and Rick Ohye, the system performs miracles for individual patients every day, but it fails our country as a whole.

* * *

There is a shameful political history that stains our white coats: the fact that the American Medical Association, the largest physician organization in the country, has been on the wrong side of every effort at real American health reform since World War II. That includes, most recently, helping gut the public option in the Affordable Care Act debates. And, to be clear, their advocacy wasn't for fear of what those reforms would do for patients. No: it was self-interest that led to their shameful opposition to universal healthcare reforms. The AMA was one of the founding member organizations of a coalition calling themselves the Partnership for America's Health Care Future, a junta of industry corporations and their lobbyists united for the soul purpose of crushing Medicare for All, though it has since dropped out of the coalition after it expanded its opposition to other types of reforms. So much for the "First, do no harm" oath we took when we got our medical degrees.

As the hospital and insurance industries have grown through healthcare consolidation and massive buyouts, industry executives—increasingly with MBAs rather than MDs after their names—have stripped doctors of much of their political power. They've hijacked a wayward health system, exploiting its complexities to create massive sums of wealth for their officers.

On the wards, I fought for a small modicum of control of this system for my patients every day, hoping to steer it, even if for just one or two of them, in the right direction. Massive hospital bureaucracies exist to maximize how much the hospital can bill for every patient. Meanwhile, critical healthcare functions like the labs that analyze blood samples remain underfunded. Trying to be helpful for my team, I became a master at expediting my patients' lab tests by getting to know the small team of administrators at the lab—and what candy they liked best. When my residents would order a test, I would see to it that blood was drawn quickly, often doing it myself; then I'd personally deliver the blood samples, navigating the labyrinthine hospitals to the dungeon that was the lab, making sure to pick up en route the Kit Kat or Milky Way that I knew would move my patient's sample up the list. I got to know the right folks to talk to on any given service—surgery to dermatology—to get our consults done faster. And I learned exactly the right thing to say when I was trying to get a patient's charts faxed over from another hospital—something that shouldn't require a phone call to begin with in the age of the Internet.

I learned always to listen to the nursing and support staff: they could make or break you as a medical student. And their hearts were almost always in the right place. A painful truth in our healthcare system is that as executive profits have gone up, respect for and relative pay to nurses and support staff have gone in the other direction. Yet they deserve so much of the credit for the good things that happen for patients in our clinics and hospitals every day.

I won some fights with the system, but I usually lost. The financial incentives of huge corporations—hospital chains, insurance companies, pharmaceutical companies—usually trump the best interests of patients and the providers who take care of them. That financial motive, more than anything else, is why we pay more for worse healthcare than any other country in the world.

* * *

And yet, I had set out on this path and I was almost there. Perhaps I could work within the system to help reshape some of those incentives. I could also continue to do my public health research, which would allow me a role beyond the clinic doors in helping to shape the communities in which people live—and get sick.

I revised my goals. Perhaps, rather than being a surgeon, I would pursue my training in internal medicine. "IM," as it's called in by most doctors, wasn't the most awe-inspiring subject to me, but it was a reliable, practical, useful career that could give me time for the research that had become my passion. And I loved the human aspect of the work. You see more patients as an internist than you do in most other specialties.

Training in IM would be a sort of truce, admitting the limits of medicine in order to solve the bigger-picture problems I wanted to take on, while not giving up on a clinical career entirely. I could see patients two to three days a week and spend the rest of my week as a researcher. I had already been offered a faculty position at Columbia and had even identified a few IM residency programs that would allow me to be a professor part-time while I completed residency. The fact that IM required fewer years as a resident than surgery was a good thing for me, too, since I was already getting antsy to get into the real world.

With my new, revised goals locked in, I began my subinternship in internal medicine at a small hospital. I was assigned to work under Dr. L, a spritely, whip-smart young doctor from the South. From the first day we met, I knew we were going to get along. Beneath her charisma was a genuine love for her craft. And she was kind to me, which is uncommon among medical higher-ups. Dr. L's respect and appreciation for my work as a researcher were refreshing. Not to mention the fact that she made her expectations clear.

"You're here to take care of our patients," she told me on our first day of work together. "And I expect that you're going to work hard. We'll work together as partners so long as I know my partner cares as much about our patients as I do."

Dr. L was true to her word. She let me take on most of the decision-making, although she also double- and triple-checked my conclusions. When I miscalculated, she helped me get to the right decisions through my own logic rather than the usual condescension or berating I had come to expect. It made 6:00 a.m. starts and being on call every third night a lot more enjoyable.

A patient I'll call Martha came in on a particularly cold and wet day. In a city where most people get around on the subway, the stairs going up and down can make for a treacherous journey. As hard as they try, the workers can't clear off all the snow. After a few minutes of cold wind and hundreds of wayward bootsteps, it turns into ice. I've slipped on subway stairs myself on days like that many times before.

That morning Martha was the one who slipped. A homeless woman, she had been drinking, which didn't help. She hit her head and was found writhing in pain by a passerby, who called 911.

I met Martha in our emergency room. In her mid-sixties, she was a large woman, about 250 pounds, with a booming baritone voice. Had life turned out differently for her, I might have heard that voice on stage or over the radio, but instead it was yelling at everyone in the ER: "What you all got me here for? Let me go!"

I was the subintern on the "floor," a shorthand for the hospital ward where patients who were admitted would stay. I was supposed to clear Martha for discharge. Her eyes found me across the room as I approached her, and she asked again: "What you all got me here for? I'm good. Just let me go."

I introduced myself and asked what happened. "Nothing happened. I'm good. See, I'm good!" She showed me what was a clearly developing welt on her head.

"Looks like you hit your head pretty bad."

"She's fine. We looked at it. Think we should probably let her go," interjected the emergency room doctor—a young resident, just a year or two ahead of me in his training. He looked the part of someone who was in the middle of an eighty-plus-hour workweek and desperate to sleep.

"What'd the CT show?" I asked.

"We didn't do one. She barely hit her head."

If you or I had hit our head—even barely—falling down the subway stairs, the first thing we would get is a CT scan. It's standard care for anyone who doesn't present as drunk or homeless. It's a bill the hospital would have been happy to file with an insured patient's insurance company. It's also the standard of care for a reason: you do a CT to rule out a brain bleed, which can be deadly.

However, people like Martha, indigent and without insurance, are a different matter. The only reason she wound up in our emergency room at all was because of a law called EMTALA, the Emergency Medical Treatment and Active Labor Act. It mandated that patients suffering emergencies got the care they needed. But what was a "need"? That was up to a doctor's interpretation, and in the case of indigent people doctors can often "interpret" those needs right down to zero.

What's more, Martha had come into our emergency room drunk nearly three hours earlier. Almost nobody gets drunk on a random weekday morning unless they suffer from serious alcoholism, and serious alcoholics need a baseline level of alcohol to function. Without it, they start to withdraw—violently, sometimes fatally. And I could see that Martha was starting to get agitated. Had she been outside the hospital, she would have found her way to another bottle. But she was here, and she couldn't. And that was about to create another urgent medical situation for her.

I was so frustrated with the poor level of care that she had gotten: I knew that we hadn't done justice by her and that she deserved a full workup and, at minimum, that head CT. But she wasn't going to get either if we let go of her now. So instead of getting the sign off on her premature discharge immediately, like the resident wanted, I went to see Dr. L to make my case in person. By the time I got to her, the emergency room had paged her directly, complaining that we hadn't signed off. When I told her what had happened—that

Martha needed a head CT, not to mention a full workup—she agreed that we should admit her.

Now I was going to have to put my money—and my limited medical knowledge—where my mouth was. Martha was admitted and given a room at the end of the hall. We immediately started her on a benzodiazepine taper to ease her creeping withdrawal and soothe the chemical dependency.

And then I got to talking to her. We had all day, after all. I learned that she was HIV positive, diabetic, and bleeding from her vagina despite having gone through menopause years ago—all facts that the ED doctor had missed.

We took labs to measure her HIV viral load and white blood cell count and to look at her kidney function. We consulted the infectious disease service and the gynecology service and put the nephrology service on notice. Martha's blood pressure was low, despite the fact that she said that she had always had *high* blood pressure. One of the things that HIV can do is infest the adrenal glands, the hormone centers that regulate blood pressure. We ran a test to see whether or not this had happened—and, sure enough, she had been untreated for HIV for so long that her adrenal glands were shot. Her viral load was so high, and her white cell count so low, that she met criteria for full-blown AIDS.

I asked why she didn't tell anyone she had HIV or diabetes. "Because no one asked," she said. In short, that had been her experience with doctors her whole life. No one asked. No one cared.

"You people just want your money. You don't care about people like me, so I don't care about people like you," Martha said. She wasn't wrong.

That doctor in the ED who just wanted to go to sleep probably wasn't overtly discriminating against Martha. He was doing something subtler: reinforcing a discriminatory culture that had overlooked and dismissed people like Martha because of their poverty, their indigence, and their substance dependency.

He'd probably seen many other patients like her. And he had learned the drill. Any effort to admit her was going to be met with pushback—not overt, but subtle. She'd be a "social" admit, they'd say. The hospital lost money on patients like her.

For her part, Martha had learned the drill, too. She didn't *want* to be admitted. She wanted to go back to her day as usual, not sit down with me and get poked, prodded, and put on medications. But she was sick and needed the care.

This ends with me, I thought. The cycle of Martha's pain and cynicism was going to end there. I, subintern and soon-to-be Dr. El-Sayed, was going to break the cycle. I was so full of myself.

Martha was the kind of person I got into medicine for—the kind of person whose life I wanted to dedicate my life to changing. I was going to be the doctor she'd never had: I would ask about and listen to every concern and make sure it was treated. I was going to make certain she was placed into a rehab facility that could treat her alcoholism and then placed back in a public housing program for people with HIV. I was going to be the doctor I had always idealized.

I worked my butt off for Martha. For two weeks I would start and end my days in her room. We got her that CT, which was negative. We had her pelvic bleeding checked out. We saw to it that her diabetes was controlled and her blood pressure medications titrated. We made sure that she was started back on antiretrovirals for her HIV. I tracked every consult myself and saw to it that my colleagues were treating her with respect and diligence. I prodded the social work team to make sure her discharge was all set up, calling the facilities myself. She would spend two weeks at the only rehab facility we could find that took patients with HIV, and after that her old apartment would be waiting for her.

On the day of discharge, she was all ready to go. We had gone through her plan together every day for a week. And she had agreed every single time. I had called each of the facilities myself that morning to make sure they were all lined up.

The very last time I confirmed the plan with her, on the morning of her planned discharge, was when she dropped the bomb: "Doc, I'm not going there," she told me.

"Wait . . . What?"

"I'm going home with my daughter. She's coming to pick me up."

"Martha, I didn't know you had a daughter. You never told me."

"I know. I just called her yesterday, and she said I can come live with her."

"Martha, when was the last time you spoke with her?"

"About two years ago."

"And what happened that made it so that you didn't speak again for two years?"

"I started drinking and, you know, did some things, and . . ."

"Okay, what makes you think you're not going to do that again?"

"You all fixed me. I don't gotta drink no more. I ain't had a drink for two weeks!"

"Unfortunately, this is something you're going to have to deal with your whole life. It's not gone. But the rehab we've got lined up for you will help. I really think it's a better idea for you to do rehab, then get all set up in your new house, and then—"

"I told you *I'm not going*. I'm going with my daughter! You can't tell me what to do. It's my life. You're all the same, trying to take away my rights and tell me how to live. You're not better than me!" She was right.

Her daughter was three hours late picking her up. Then she was gone. And that was it.

* * *

Martha had become a stand-in for all the things I wanted to fix about medicine. But people are fickle. They fail sometimes, and you fail them. I couldn't help but keep reviewing the case. Where had I failed her? Was there something I should have done differently?

I thought about Dr. Sleepy, the emergency room doctor whose cynicism had been validated. He was the system embodied: a jaded, once-optimistic young doctor who'd probably been in my shoes a few times before. I hated him—because I never wanted to *be* him.

I had come to really like Martha. She was funny, warm, and strong. It takes so much strength to persist, to survive, when you're so sick and you've been neglected so profoundly your entire life. But in refusing to go to rehab, she was betraying that strength—mirroring the betrayal our system had perpetrated on her for so long.

I spent the better part of the next two weeks reflecting on her, on her case, and what it meant for what I wanted to do. Although this was a reminder of just how hard real change would be, I *was* going to change the system from the inside, I concluded. I didn't succeed this time, but there'd be a next time.

I thought I'd never see Martha again. Two weeks later I was jumping on the subway to meet a friend for dinner downtown at a Turkish restaurant. As I stepped onto the train, I saw a woman lying facedown on the subway seats. Slowly, she turned over: it was Martha.

As she turned her head, the lights went out on my clinical career. When I got home that evening, I pulled my residency application. Any hopes I had had of working within the system had been extinguished. Practicing medicine wasn't the path to solving the problems I cared about, as scared as I was to admit it after so many years of training to be a doctor. I knew I could never be a practicing doctor now. I didn't want to get beaten down by cynicism. I didn't ever want to think that the forces of poverty, racism, and marginalization were insurmountable.

I had failed Martha—but I wasn't the first, and I wouldn't be the last. Because *we* have failed—and are failing—her and so many others like her every day. We failed her when the schools she went to spit her out in the eighth grade because she was a "problem" child. We failed her when her mom couldn't make enough to support her on a minimum-wage job, forcing her family to bounce around from one boyfriend's house to another. We failed her when we couldn't protect her from the abuse she suffered as a teenager at the hands of one of those boyfriends when her mom was at work. We failed her when welfare reform undercut her just as she was starting to get things right for herself and her five kids in the 1990s. We failed her over and over and over. And our failure has been imprinted on her, shaping her every interaction with the system.

There was no way, I realized, that I could be an internist. What I wanted to do was turn back time and save Martha decades ago, before we all lost hope. Or, if I couldn't do that, I wanted to take the elevator down to the ground floor of failure—to the beginning of the poverty cycle, where I could make a difference in the lives of other people who might otherwise suffer her fate.

I wasn't going to practice medicine after all.

CHAPTER 8

Contagion and miasma.

John Snow, who built on John Graunt's technique of counting and analysis, is famous for trying to understand the cause and spread of cholera in the mid-nineteenth century. Cholera is a severe diarrheal illness. It is among the worst killers in human history, killing hundreds—even thousands—at a time. Although it was much more common in Snow's time, it still ravages low-income communities with poor water infrastructure today. In fact, during the vicious Saudi-led, U.S.-backed civil war in Yemen, an epidemic of cholera took thousands of lives. Tragically, it has a predilection for children—as most infectious diseases do.

In John Snow's time, the dominant theory about the transmission of cholera was that it was transmitted by "miasma," a catchall term for some combination of gases that emanated from the fetid open cesspools, garbage pits, graveyards, and sewers ubiquitous in nineteenth-century European cities before proper sewers and sanitation were installed.

To some degree the hypothesis was based in truth. Infectious diseases like cholera, and its upper respiratory cousins tuberculosis and pneumonia, afflicted people who generally had a few things in common: they were poor and likely to be urban dwellers inhabiting dark, damp, cramped living quarters. We know now that these circumstances create optimal environments for the transmission of infectious pathogens. But without the insights afforded by modern microbiology, it was not a far stretch to assume that there was something particular about those places themselves that caused disease.

Snow disagreed with the miasmatists, arguing instead that cholera was a contagion—that there was some "poison" that was spread from one victim to the next. First, it's worth noting that Snow knew a thing or two about gases: he was one of the pioneers of anesthesiology and he was chosen to personally administer chloroform to Queen Victoria during childbirth. Snow didn't believe that the natural properties of gases would allow them to concentrate in one place long enough to cause disease.

Second, Snow had treated victims of a series of cholera epidemics in the 1830s and '40s, and his experiences led him to several observations that were at odds with the miasma theory. For example, he observed one row of houses with many victims, while another, directly facing it, had only one. Yet, if cholera were transmitted in a miasma, both rows should have a similar number of patients.

Snow began to painstakingly trace individuals who had suffered the disease, collecting information about their eating and drinking sources, living quarters, and shared contacts. He also traced the flow of human waste through cesspools and channels and ultimately back through water pumps and into future patients. He identified the various people who might have come in contact with water from different sources and calculated their probabilities of becoming ill. In doing so, Snow was able to trace their common exposures, painting a picture of the experiences common to those who got sick.

Snow published his findings in two editions of *On the Mode of Communication of Cholera*, linking the likelihood of disease with exposure to various water supplies, all pointing to one likely culprit: the ingestion of water that had been contaminated by the excrement of a previous patient. During an outbreak in 1853, for example, Snow identified that water in the affected district was provided by two companies: one of them with an intake facility located in a part of the Thames known to be contaminated with sewage.[1] By starting with cholera patients who had died and tracing their water consumption back to its source, he found that those who took ill were fourteen times more likely to have consumed water from the contaminated source.

During an 1854 outbreak near his home, Snow used the same technique to trace the source back to a local pump on Broad Street. Petitioning the Board of Guardians, he had the handle of the pump removed. The outbreak quickly subsided.

Nevertheless, the idea that cholera was contagious and spread from person to person by a poison found in water was ridiculed during his time. Snow could never find the smoking gun: proof that a microorganism was the culprit. He even had water samples from the Broad Street pump examined by a microscopist. But nearly all drinking water at that time contained microorganisms, and without knowledge of which specific microorganism caused cholera, the effort was inconclusive.

Tragically, Snow died before learning that in the same year that he had had the Broad Street pump handle removed, an anatomist in Italy had identified *Vibrio cholerae*, a comma-shaped bacterium that was ubiquitous in the intestinal walls of victims of the disease. In the next decades Louis Pasteur would demonstrate conclusively that microorganisms caused infectious diseases, and Robert Koch would identify a rubric for identifying which diseases were caused by bacteria, connecting various microorganisms to the diseases they caused. Today, we consider Snow's work conclusive: cholera is contagious, spread by the transmission of *V. cholerae* from one person to the next.

His work—alongside Pasteur's and Koch's and that of many others—is critical to our understanding of infectious diseases and their treatment today. Every time you vaccinate your child or take an antibiotic, you're targeting one of those infectious agents, training the immune system to recognize its outer coating or sending a chemical in that will destroy it. It's why we wash our hands after we go to the bathroom (in fact, I think this a good moment to ask you all to wash your hands after you go to the bathroom).

* * *

But that's not the whole story. While the science is clear that infectious agents transmit these diseases, the miasmatists were not, in fact, too far off. If infectious agents were the only explanation, then each of us should have equal probability to incur the illnesses they cause. And yet this is patently false. When scientists like Snow isolated and discovered the infectious agents that cause diseases like cholera, they were answering the question of *how* people get sick but perhaps missing the question of *why* they do.

The miasmatists, after all, were arguing that there was something about the environments within which the poor lived that might be transmitting disease. They were responding to the observation that the poor suffered more. After all, who was forced to drink contaminated water carrying the disease-causing bacteria? Who was forced to live in overcrowded circumstances, virtually guaranteeing that every member of a household would be exposed to cholera? Although the agents that cause these diseases may move from one person to another, the circumstances of contagion aren't simply a matter of individual infection. Rather, the forces of poverty and marginalization predict who suffers them; *those forces are the miasma.* And those forces persist today, as the cholera epidemic raging in Yemen—a war-torn country without the basic infrastructure to protect people from this preventable disease—demonstrates.

Epidemiologists who study infectious diseases today are keen to admit that while the agent—a virus, bacteria, fungus, or parasite—that spreads an infectious disease matters, it's not the only thing. They also discuss characteristics of the "host" (one of those odd science terms that's not quite right, given that nobody actually invites a disease-causing agent into her body) and the environment that can lead to infectious disease spreading.

Recent outbreaks of previously rare diseases demonstrate why this is so important. In the past several years, outbreaks of measles and whooping cough have alarmed public health officials. After all, with extremely effective vaccinations available for these diseases, we thought they had been relegated to the history books.

Their near disappearance—and resurgence—has nothing to do with changes to the virus that causes measles or the bacterium that causes whooping cough. Rather, they have everything to do with changes to hosts and environments. The choice not to vaccinate, fueled by fabricated claims of severe side effects like autism, also means choosing to expose children to diseases we nearly eradicated just a generation ago.

While the implications of the host characteristics are obvious, the environment here matters too. Even if she was unvaccinated, to be infected, a child would have to contract the disease from a carrier, who, presumably, would have to be unvaccinated herself. It follows that the fewer unvaccinated children the child interacts with—the only ones who could even carry the disease—the lower the probability that an unvaccinated child will contract the disease. This concept is called "herd immunity": the idea that even if every single individual in a group—a "herd"—may not be immune, if enough of them are, the probability that the disease will spread among them is low.

But here's the problem: the choice not to vaccinate doesn't happen at random. Rather, anti-vaxxers have clustered in upper-middle-income, (ironically) highly educated communities. Because they do, they create pockets of non-immunity that allow these previously uncommon diseases to spread and multiply.

In Michigan, Detroit routinely has the lowest vaccination rates in the state—largely because of poverty, which leaves too many families without access to vaccination services. Ironically, the community with the next lowest likelihood of vaccinations isn't the next poorest public health jurisdiction; it's one of the richest. Washtenaw County, home to the University of Michigan, is one of the richest and most highly educated communities in Michigan, but they struggle to keep their vaccination numbers up as well.

The choice not to vaccinate, though an ideology, acts like a virus: it spreads from person to person—not only directly, but also over the Internet. And when it spreads, it attacks a host's immunity, rendering that person susceptible to potentially deadly disease. Indeed, anti-vaxxer ideology has gone "viral." The Internet has become a repository of this ideological virus, a place that exposes susceptible people, infecting them en masse . . . a miasma, if you will.

CHAPTER 9

Home again.

On my first day as public health director for the city of Detroit, I resolved to look extra-professional. I had grown my (admittedly scraggly) beard out a little thicker. I put on my big-boy suit and my big-boy tie. I was thirty years old but I felt all of twenty-two; it was my first job outside of the "anything goes" ivory tower of academia. I was walking into a department with five city employees and eighty-five contractors, stuffed into the back of the building where people paid parking tickets. I wasn't just the youngest big-city health official in America; I was one of the youngest people in my own department.

On my way in, I was getting into the right mind-set, psyching myself up for my first day. *You're the commissioner. You're going to commission. I don't know what that even means . . . but I'm going to do it.*

A gentleman, clearly on his way to something more important, called to me. "Hey, you! You work here?"

I did! I was the director! I turned around and in my most confident manner told him, "Why, yes . . . yes, sir, I *do* work here."

"Great, can you take my parking ticket in for me?"

"Sir, I'm the health director."

"Then why are you walking into the parking building?"

I thought for a second. It was a good question. I took his parking ticket in for him—my first good act. This would be easy, right?

I had spent the last year as a professor in the department of epidemiology at Columbia University Mailman School of Public Health. I was thriving as a professor, one of the youngest in the school. We had just put the finishing touches on a textbook I coedited with Dr. Galea, *Systems Science and Population Health*, published by Oxford University Press. The book emerged out of a course I had developed at Columbia, which had emerged out of my doctoral thesis at Oxford. My research team was growing, and I was co-leading several school- and university-wide initiatives.

Sarah and I had fallen in love with New York, learning how to adapt to the city rather than trying to live a suburban lifestyle there. We loved Friday and Saturday nights on the town, trying this or that new cuisine, and going on Sunday morning runs through Central Park to burn it all off. But I only really had to be in New York one day a week to teach. Most of the time I was traveling, speaking at conferences, and meeting with or advising public officials from Beijing to Cape Town, from Delhi to LA. I've always done my best thinking and writing in transit, in the backs of cabs or on trains or planes, so I got really good at writing research articles en route between one place and another.

Universities are essential institutions that have done—and must continue to do—great good. But as an assistant professor, I could never draw a straight line between what I was working on and what I had set out to do. I went into medicine to heal people. I left it because I came to realize that our healthcare system had become part of the illness. But in my current role, I was, at best, critiquing the system. At worst, I was publishing paper after paper about more and more minute mechanistic details in esoteric journals that were usually read by people who already agreed with the general point I was trying to make. The basic gist of almost every paper I wrote was this: social factors matter for health. Marginalized people are less healthy because of this. We really should do something about it.

Scientific research matters, but we have to be willing to disseminate it in the world, to empower people through it to demand solutions to the problems we're identifying. I thought that perhaps I could help unlock this critical trove of knowledge. But anytime I'd write an op-ed trying to translate our research for the general public or volunteer to serve on a panel actually trying to fix something, my academic colleagues would look at me askance. "That's not going to get you tenure."

Then who gives a damn about tenure. But my mouth would save me, saying instead, politely, "I know. You're probably right. But then what are we doing this for?" I can understand academics engaging in other subjects for purely theoretical purposes, but not epidemiologists. Ours is the basic science of public health. And public health is fundamentally an applied subject. Epidemiology exists specifically to change policy to improve and extend real people's lives. And often the incentives of our academic institutions are keeping us from achieving that purpose. Rather than write about the fact that something needed to be done, I wanted to be doing it.

My existential crisis hit a rolling boil at what should have been a point of triumph. Our complex systems approach to epidemiology was by no means accepted logic, so it had become a contentious topic among theoretical purists. I had organized a symposium on the topic at our annual conference, inviting a panel of experts to participate. Mine was the final presentation. I had worked hard on it. I would reframe the debate around the idea of interventions in public health—again, that our science should be about figuring out how to solve actual problems rather than publishing papers about it.

As I spoke, I noticed some of the sharpest minds in epidemiology nodding in agreement. One of them, a titan in the field whom I had come up reading and rereading as a graduate student—approached me afterward at the wine-and-cheese reception. I was chewing a slice of Comté on a slice of toasted baguette. "Your work is really on to something; it could really change everything."

And that's when I realized the problem: I simply didn't believe that. But the cheese *was* nice.

Later that day I sat down with Dr. Galea, an advocate for what he calls a "consequential epidemiology," who insisted on translating our work to the world. He had just left Columbia to become, at just forty-three, dean of public health at Boston University.

"You were never long for this world, Abdul." He had seen my frustration coming miles away, but he had also seen how valuable time in the academy might be for me.

Although I had learned to really listen in medical school, I learned to communicate in the academy. My first speaking experiences, before my commencement speech in 2007, were preaching sermons at campus Friday prayer services in college. I had always been told that I had a knack for connecting with my audience, and after the commencement address, the praise came thick and fast. I was confident—in fact, overconfident.

During the summer when I had first started working in Dr. Galea's research group, I was asked to give a presentation on my work about adverse birth outcomes at a department-wide seminar for social epidemiologists. *I got this*, I thought. I threw together a few slides the night before the seminar and gave a sloppy presentation the next day. As a shark senses blood in the water, one of the senior professors in the department saw the contrast between my overconfidence and my underpreparedness and began a line of questioning that ultimately left me in a crumpled heap as she asked question after question I couldn't answer. Plain and simple, I got torn apart.

Embarrassed, Dr. Galea made me present a dry run of my next talk to him first. After another night-before performance, he asked, "Abdul, you're pretty used to skating by on pure charm, aren't you?"

"No, I prepared for this, and I really thought about it," I insisted. I hadn't. That much was obvious.

"Bullshit. I want you to strip yourself out of this presentation. Nobody cares what you have to say; they care about your evidence. Get your personality out of the way. 'Just the facts, ma'am,'" he said. "You're an athlete, aren't you? Would you ever go to the game without practice?"

I had never heard it put like that. As I said, I was never a great athlete, so to compensate, I had to master the fundamentals; that meant more reps, watching more tape, and putting in more time. With sports, I wanted it bad enough, so I put in the work. What might happen if I put that kind of work into something that I actually had some talent for?

After dozens of presentations over the next several years, Dr. Galea pulled me aside at the end of one. "That was really boring. Maybe spice it up a bit?" It was his way of telling me I had graduated from his academic version of "wax on, wax off" Mr. Miyagi training. I had learned a lot as an academic: linear thinking, disciplined and evidence-based inquiry, and the patience of wading through complex datasets—not to mention putting substance over style in the way that I communicated complex ideas. But my training was over.

Rich, a friend of mine from the Paul & Daisy Soros Fellowships for New Americans program—founded through the generosity of the famous financier's brother, Paul, and his wife, Daisy—had just graduated from Yale Law School. Like me, he had grown up in suburban Detroit in an immigrant household. A multitalented wunderkind, he had worked for a finance shop in Hong Kong while doubling as a Yale Law student. He'd been offered clerkships with federal court judges and his pick of jobs at prestigious white-shoe law firms, or a full-time gig at the finance shop on the other side of the world. But instead of high finance or a court clerkship, he chose to take a role with Detroit's new mayor, Mike Duggan—an unlikely choice, to be sure.

Rich had interned with the mayor's office the summer before and fallen in love with the work. The city was just emerging from bankruptcy and had an all-hands-on-deck approach, the closest thing to a municipal start-up in the shell of a centuries-old city. Committed to our hometown, he decided to sign on when he got a full-time offer, taking hundreds of thousands of dollars less than he could be making as a hotshot in high finance.

I had been in touch in hopes of learning more about his decision. We had agreed to have lunch a week after my conversation with Dr. Galea in June. I brought some CVs for the hell of it and peppered my friend with questions about City Hall in Detroit. "What are you guys doing on public health?" I asked. Although he didn't know, his focus being education reform, he introduced me to a few folks involved in the work before hustling off to his next meeting. I left them my CV and thought nothing more of it.

The next week I got a call from a number with a 313 area code. The gruff voice on the other end of the line was Mayor Duggan, asking if I'd like to come back to Detroit and have lunch with him to talk about a "public health job." Somehow my CV had made it to his desk. "I would be happy to, but—"

"Great. I'll hand you over to my scheduler to set it up," the mayor said.

The truth is I didn't know what the "public health job" was, but I spent the next two weeks reading everything I could about the history and current state of public health in Detroit. I learned that in 2012, when the city was facing bankruptcy, it made the disastrous decision to privatize its health department—a department that had existed in some form since 1827. One of the least healthy cities in the country had *shut down* its health department!

Why? Emergency management. Three years later, we would all learn just how devastating Governor Rick Snyder's emergency management policies would be for public health as we saw story after story out of Flint, Michigan: children breaking out with rashes, parents struggling to provide them water after one of the biggest municipal water disasters in recent history . . . Snyder's government was responsible for exposing more than a hundred thousand people—nearly ten thousand kids—to lead when they decided to change Flint's water source from Lake Huron to the Flint River, setting off a chain reaction that leached lead from Flint's lead pipes into the drinking water and into the arteries of young children.

That decision had been initiated and signed off on by Flint's emergency manager, an autocratic czar who had been appointed to run the city government after serious financial difficulties and was answerable only to Governor Snyder. Snyder's controversial first piece of emergency management legislation, Public Act 4, granted him the power to appoint emergency managers over financially struggling municipalities. It was so unpopular that it was repealed in a statewide referendum vote—only to be replaced by a second law anyway. This time Governor Snyder made sure to shield his law through a legislative trick, tying it to an appropriation so it couldn't be repealed.

Under these draconian policies, democratically elected municipal governments were reduced to ceremonial duties, with all real governing power concentrated in the emergency manager. Worse, the emergency managers' mandates weren't to ensure the effective and efficient operation of the governments they had taken over but to see that their debt obligations were fulfilled. This led to wanton cuts in mission-critical services, like water management. In Flint, basic corrosion controls costing less than $150 a day could have prevented the mass lead poisoning disaster.[1]

Sadly but predictably, the brunt of emergency management was not borne equitably. Fourteen percent of Michiganders are Black—but nearly half of them lived under an emergency manager at one point,[2] their democratic right to municipal self-determination obliterated.

This was the context for Detroit's public health shutdown. In 2012 the mayor and city council were throwing everything they could overboard to try to stay out of emergency management—and that included the health department. A nonprofit was created to administer key programs, like vaccinations, food inspections, and lead elimination, but its leadership seemed more interested in lavish offices with plush carpets than in kids with asthma. Other nonprofits sprang up to compete for their lucrative grants. Services dwindled, leaving people in Michigan's biggest city largely without access to basic public health services.

After a two-hour lunch, I was offered the "public health job"—which I came to learn that day was that of health director. Offer in hand, I went back to New York for an even more important conversation: Sarah had just started a residency in New York. But she saw the meaning in the work in Detroit and was willing to transfer to Michigan after her first year as a resident to allow me to do it. But that meant that we'd have to spend another year apart. Almost every weekend for my first year in Detroit, I would catch the 7:20 flight out of DTW to LGA on Friday evenings, only to catch the 1:30 flight back to Detroit on Sunday afternoons.

I will always be deeply grateful to Sarah for her support in general, but in particular for this sacrifice. We both knew that our values dictated that we find opportunities to serve and seize them. But a long-distance marriage is hard, and transferring residencies is even harder.

* * *

During my first weeks on the job, I heard stories every day about the great good the department used to do and what it meant to residents of the city. One night during the first month, I had gotten out of the office around 9:00 p.m. Hungry, I made my way to a local barbecue joint. As I was getting out of my car, an older man emerged out of the shadows and asked me for a few bucks. I offered to buy him dinner instead.

As we waited for our food, Chuck told me his harrowing story: he was a veteran who had seen combat duty in Vietnam. But like too many of our veterans, he was homeless. He was in and out of drug and alcohol rehab programs and couldn't hold down a meaningful job. His daughter had just died, and that tragedy had thrown him into a tailspin from which he was still trying to recover.

As we tucked into our brisket and mashed potatoes, Chuck asked what I did. When I told him I worked for the Health Department, his eyes lit up. "When I was a boy, my mama used to leave a few bucks in my back pocket. She told me if anything happened, I should take a cab to Herman Kiefer; they'd take care of me." I had to break it to him that Herman Kiefer had shut down a few years back. "Well, damn, ain't nothing good lasts here."

Herman Kiefer was a mammoth hospital, synonymous with the Health Department to any Detroiter older than forty. It had been founded in 1893 as a smallpox hospital—more buildings were constructed in 1911, with pavilions designed by the famous architect Albert Kahn added in the 1920s—but it was variously a tuberculosis hospital, a general hospital, and a psychiatric hospital, its 1,200 beds constantly occupied. It was decommissioned for clinical use in the early 2000s and then housed the administrative offices of the Health Department until it was shut down and sold to an out-of-state developer for mixed-use redevelopment. At least, that's what we were told. It sits like an abandoned anchor in Detroit's North End, a hulking reminder of a bygone era.

On one of my first days at the department, a state official contacted me about Herman Kiefer. He told me that they suspected that there might still be some old medical files in the building. A clear liability, they needed to be destroyed.

A few days later, I set out with Dr. A, one of the few department employees who remembered what it was like to walk through those halls when they didn't seem haunted. With a few flashlights and accompanied by a security guard assigned to protect the building from copper scrappers (who had already picked the place clean), we explored the labyrinth of underground tunnels connecting the various wings of the hospital. The department had been decommissioned without warning: one day it was a hustling, bustling big-city health department, the next day a corpse. Books and papers piled on desks had been abandoned overnight, as if the workers who occupied the offices had just gone on a three-year bathroom break. After we had swept through the hospital, Dr. A led me to the old director's office, where framed portraits of all the past directors hung. In the center of the room was a beautiful large birch desk; Dr. A said that rumor held it to be original to the hospital at its founding.

This was our history, I thought. We didn't find any medical records to destroy, but we did find potent reminders of the department's past. If we were going to rebuild, I thought, we would rebuild on our history. We started to unhook the portraits, taking them to be hung in our new offices.

* * *

My new job involved overseeing basic public health operations for Detroit's seven hundred thousand residents, people who'd been systematically marginalized by every single level of government intended to serve them. On paper I was qualified. I'd just left a career as a professor of epidemiology, and I'd completed two doctorates in related fields. I knew quite a bit about the *theory* of public health.

But theory is one thing; applying it in Detroit was going to be another. Where do you even begin? How was I going to connect abstract knowledge to concrete policies and programs that would actually help people? What was the operational definition of "public health" that I could use in this new job to make a tangible difference in people's day-to-day lives?

A few weeks later, as I was touring a vaccination clinic, the answer to my questions walked through the door. He was a toddler named Marcus. The child of a young mom working two jobs to make ends meet for her four children, Marcus had met his incarcerated father just a couple of times. His primary caretaker was his grandmother, who cared for all four of her daughter's children despite regular trips to the hospital for her own poorly treated heart failure.

I've been introduced to my fair share of toddlers over the years, and I know the drill: they look at you just long enough to realize they don't know who you are, then they bury their faces into their parents' legs. Not Marcus. He had swagger and charisma: he looked right at me with his big brown eyes, shook my hand, flashed me a big, toothy grin, and walked back over to his mom.

At that moment I couldn't help but contrast his confidence with his circumstances. To make it past the age of one, Marcus had already cheated death. He was growing up in a place with an infant mortality rate nearly as high as that of my father's native Egypt. Children in Marcus's community were three times as likely to be hospitalized for asthma and four times likelier to be exposed to lead than the state average. And those were just the odds Marcus faced with regard to his health.

Watching this little boy walk back to his mother, I realized that, for me, the definition of "public health" that mattered most was this: whatever was necessary to sustain this kid's natural confidence into adulthood. This would be epidemiology applied: what could we—a team of ninety crammed into the back of the parking department—do to improve Marcus's shot at the dignified life he and every kid in the city deserved?

This realization crystalized into a specific goal: we would leverage public health to disrupt intergenerational poverty. Put simply, we wanted to break the barriers that prevented kids in our city from being able to learn and earn like children anywhere. We would concentrate on those health outcomes that were both a consequence and a cause of the cycle of intergenerational poverty.

We identified a set of critical outcomes that were part of the poverty cycle in our city. Teen pregnancy accounted for 16 percent of all births in the city—and statistics tell us that if a young woman has an unwanted pregnancy before she graduates high school, she's half as likely to graduate.[3] Infant mortality is a serious epidemic in Detroit—but even babies who live past their first birthday who were born prematurely suffer the consequences over decades; studies show that their long-term wealth is lower even decades after birth.[4] Lead, which competes with beneficial minerals in the body, poisons children's minds just as they're growing fastest. Vision deficits keep too many of our kids from seeing the blackboard, and if you can't see the board at the front of the classroom, you can't learn what's on it. Yet nearly 30 percent of the kids who have vision problems weren't going to get a pair of glasses in the next year. We also took on problems like asthma, which is one of the most common causes of school days missed, and childhood obesity, which is one of the strongest predictors of adult obesity, a precursor to heart disease and early death. And we worked to foster tighter community bonds by bringing kids and seniors together.

* * *

But before I could get to all that, I was handed another, more immediate task. I almost couldn't believe that, according to the city higher-ups, the most pressing issue—among all those that I just mentioned—was animal control. I had left my ivory tower academic job, and I was literally being thrown to the dogs. I soon came to understand why.

Daily, protestors were demonstrating against the extremely high kill rate in the animal shelter, a rotting facility built in 1927. Eighty-six out of every one hundred dogs that came into the facility would leave in a carcass bag, and dog bite rates in Detroit were among the highest in the country.

Although responsibility for animal control had traditionally belonged to the Health Department, after privatization it had fallen to the police department. Cash-strapped, overworked, and underpaid, the police wanted nothing to do with animal control; they stripped out its budget to pay for traditional police work, and left it to the quirky animal control director, who was well-meaning if underskilled.

My job was to fix it, and while the department remained under the administrative control of the police, I had to figure out how to engineer change as the director of health. The shelter was decidedly mismanaged, but much of the dysfunction was just a result of being under-resourced and neglected. Worse, suburbanites, frustrated with their ill-behaved dogs, made a habit of driving them to the city late at night and kicking them out of the car, dooming them to roam Detroit's streets. And dogfighting remains all too common in Detroit. Breeders select for aggression and violence, and when they have no more use for these poor dogs, they just let them go. Roaming packs of dogs terrorized local neighborhoods. Worse, many owners didn't properly care for their dogs, leaving them to terrorize neighbors. On one of my first weeks of work, a four-year-old boy named Xavier was tragically mauled and killed by a neighbor's dog on his way to school. It was the first of many times I would find myself sobbing alone at my desk late into the night.

Almost every day I would go out and meet the protestors myself, asking their demands and listening to their grievances. I will never shun a protest, knowing firsthand how important this right of ours is, given my experiences in Egypt. I wanted them to know that I wasn't going to ignore them: their voices would be taken seriously.

For the most part, they were suburban animal activists who wanted better for the animals in the shelter. I understood that; I believe that the way we treat animals is a measure of our humanity. Like the protestors, I was ashamed of the high kill rate at the facility and was determined to fix it. And yet they seemed oblivious to—even flippant about—the fact that kids were being mauled in the streets.

One day I got a call from the animal shelter: they needed me there STAT. A mob was growing outside. I jumped in my car and raced over. I could see the crowd as I pulled up. They were pounding on the shelter door, demanding to be let in. The staff had barricaded themselves inside, fearful of what the protestors might do. Local news cameras had arrived on the scene, tipped off to the protest by an activist.

As I got out of my car, the crowd forced open the door and streamed inside. I quickly maneuvered my way to the front of the lobby before the protestors could get to the door in back that led to where the animals were housed.

I tried to calm everyone down. "I am here to listen to your needs. I wish I could snap my fingers and fix this—but I can't. I assure you, changes will come soon."

I heard angry murmurs. "Yeah, right!" said someone in the corner.

"Look, I'm here now," I reasoned. "I'm missing a meeting about infant mortality in this city, and we can all agree that that's more important."

"You have your priorities and we have ours," someone shouted. I shot a glance in the direction of the voice and saw heads turning to face a woman at the back of the room.

"I'm sorry. Excuse me?" I retorted. "Ma'am, do you have kids?"

"Yeah."

"So how many dogs would you let die to save *your* kids?"

"That's not the point."

But that was *exactly* the point. In that moment her bias had been revealed. The suburban folks who had left their homes and workplaces to come to Detroit were raising their voices in defense of Detroit's dogs. I appreciated their passion for defenseless animals. Yet an obvious question remained unanswered: Where were they when it came to defenseless *people*? Why weren't they protesting the poverty, the disease, and the insecurity that afflicted so many of Detroit's children?

You couldn't miss the symbolism: a group of predominantly white, predominantly suburban protestors storming a door behind which were predominantly Black, predominantly urban workers making a measly $12.50 an hour to wrangle dangerous dogs off Detroit's streets. They couldn't see the humanity in people like those workers—or their kids. They were betraying the humanity they claimed to support.

As promised, within four months we were on the way to improvement. I had forged a strong relationship with the folks in the police department who held the purse strings and had managed to engineer a transfer for the shelter director. He would oversee the horse stables for the mounted police.

I had also worked out a way to appoint a new leader at Animal Control. Melissa Miller was one of the animal rights advocates whom I had met early on—but one who had worked in animal welfare professionally, setting up temporary shelters in disaster settings all over the country. She was committed, caring, and effective, and I invited her to take the position as an appointee.

But without an animal control budget, I needed to find the money to hire her. To be sure, I had to figure out how to grow our department's budget anyway. At that point the city's investment in the Health Department was a mere $1 million, or only $1.50 per resident. To put that in perspective, in 2015, New York City's budget allocated about $75 per person per year for public health.

I looked to the law. Under the state public health code, municipal health departments receiving grants from the state had to make investments in their departments from their own municipal funds relatively equal to the amount that the state invested. At that point the state was investing about $14 million a year in public health in Detroit—meaning the city of Detroit should have been investing $14 million in public health as well. But because of Detroit's recent budget difficulties, the state wasn't enforcing the law. If I could just get the state to do so, rather than give Detroit a pass, which helped no one, we might get the resources we needed to start tackling our challenges.

I called my liaison at the state and asked if he'd be interested in helping me grow the city's public health budget. I knew there was no way we could manage fourteenfold growth that fast. Perhaps we could jump the city public health budget to $5 million that year and $10 million the next?

"It'd be a minor miracle," my liaison said.

I had a plan. But I needed a sharply worded letter from him that cited the public health code, stating that if Detroit could not meet the public health code requirements and make good on the full $14 million it was required to budget for public health, we'd be at risk of losing our state funding. I took the letter to the mayor's staff. Could I negotiate on the city's behalf? They agreed.

Within two years our budget climbed to $10 million—money we used to fix animal control and to invest in our broad goals of disrupting intergenerational poverty for kids like Marcus.

First, at Animal Control, Melissa, her staff, and I worked ourselves to the bone. In the face of shelter-wide disease outbreaks, temporary funding lapses that threatened the supply of basic things like dog food, and staffing challenges, we made real improvements. We moved into a newer facility that had been vacated by the Michigan Humane Society. We negotiated a raise for our animal control officers with the Teamsters Union local that represented them, taking them to $15 an hour—their first raise in more than ten years. We increased our live release rate—the number of dogs that left our facility alive—from 14 percent to 70 percent. More importantly, we reduced our city-wide dog bite rate by nearly 30 percent.

Unfortunately, maintaining change is sometimes as hard as making it in the first place. After Melissa and I had left the city, Animal Control was largely neglected again. In the summer of 2019 a nine-year-old girl, Emma, was mauled and killed by three dogs owned by a neighbor likely training them for dogfighting. It's a devastating reminder that in fact animal control *is* public health, and when we mistreat innocent animals, innocent people suffer, too.

CHAPTER 10
Doctoring Detroit.

Our budget growth gave us the space to build out programs with real consequences for Detroit kids. That meant building the infrastructure to support the stalwarts who had stuck it out and building the team we needed to be bold and effective, empathetic, yet muscular with our vision.

My first hire was Leseliey Welch as deputy director. An expert on infant mortality, Leseliey had worked at the department in the past, where she led efforts to address the terrible epidemic of infant death in Detroit. With dual training in public health and business, she was exactly the kind of expert I needed alongside me as we developed. What's more, her temperament reminded me of my grandmother's: grit and kindness combined in a jovial, uplifting soul. Dave Yeh left a lucrative job in corporate consulting to lead our special projects division, charged with executing key initiatives that would challenge the city's bureaucracy while managing the details that can stymie endeavors like these. His work ethic and leadership were critical to advancing so many of the most impactful projects we kicked off. They joined a team of incredible people like Mildred, the kindly and empathetic leader of our infant mortality review team, and our gritty lead, vision testing, and food safety teams, who had stuck it out through the toughest of times to faithfully care for Detroiters.

We got right to work. Vision deficits were a clear low-hanging fruit. Our department already performed state-mandated vision screenings in every school in Detroit. We knew that for every three kids we identified as having trouble seeing, one of them wouldn't get the corrective eyewear they needed. Perhaps we could go the rest of the way and get a pair of glasses delivered to all three kids free of charge.

As a kid who'd gotten into my fair share of trouble growing up, I know what boredom can do to an otherwise promising kid—and that's as a kid *who could see the blackboard*. I shudder to imagine what might have been if I couldn't. I would have found one way or another to entertain myself, probably at my teachers' expense. Once you're labeled a troublemaker, particularly as a child of color, the label becomes a self-fulfilling prophecy.

We had to act. We set out to build a program to provide every child with a free pair of glasses. The project became an exercise in wrangling bureaucracy. First, just as we were about to execute our plan, the state notified me that they wanted to cut the limited funding we had for basic vision screenings. Their justification was that the city's population had shrunk with time, so health departments in suburban counties, which had grown, should get that funding. I put together a basic analysis showing why funding shouldn't follow people— it should follow *need*—and that the money would be far better spent in Detroit. I sent the state administrators my analysis. A few days later I got a call: they were sorry, but nothing could be done. The decision had been made already.

"I understand," I said. But I had something I wanted to send over, just in case. I prepared an email including my analysis to a *Detroit Free Press* reporter who had been covering the Flint water crisis. It made the case plainly that the Michigan Department of Health and Human Services was going to cut vision screening funding to kids in Detroit and send that money out to the suburbs despite the fact that kids in Detroit had more need—and the money would be more efficiently spent in Detroit. In my email to the administrator I included one extra line: "I'm sending this in a week."

Just before my deadline, I got another call. They had found the money to make our program whole for the next two years after all.

With the vision program funding secure, it was time for the hard part: getting the schools on board. It wasn't just the Detroit public schools but also the plethora of charter schools that had taken over much of Detroit's educational system. Every principal, school administrator, and teacher needed to know why we were building this program. Most importantly, we needed to earn the trust of parents, who were now being asked by their kids' schools to fill out yet another permission slip.

We also had to help secure $500,000 in funding to support Vision to Learn, the nonprofit we were working with to build a mobile optometric unit—literally a van with an optometrist in it. The van would follow our screeners. That way kids who were identified as having impaired vision could receive a full optometric exam right on the premises and get fitted for free glasses. Thankfully, the nonprofit's leadership had many strong connections in philanthropy, and one of our U.S. senators' spouses was instrumental in the effort.

The program would be reimbursable through Medicaid, so we needed to expand our ability to bill for every pair of glasses we delivered to keep it sustainable. For a department that had been crammed into the back of the parking building a few months earlier, this would be a big lift.

Six months after we started, I got to offer a boy one of the first pairs of glasses the program would deliver. As he held his glasses in his hands, I watched him look them over, slowly unfolding them. When he put them on, he looked up at me, then back down at his hands and back up again. "My hands have wrinkles in them," he said. Thinking that this might be a problem, as he'd never seen them before, he looked back up at me inquisitively and asked, "Do yours?"

"Yep, mine do, too," I reassured him. "I think all of ours do, but you'll have to check with your new glasses."

* * *

One of our key goals was to reduce asthma hospitalizations, largely a consequence of industrial air pollution in one of the most polluted cities in the country. Southwest Detroit is particularly hard hit, its airshed poisoned by several factories and idling trucks crossing the Ambassador Bridge to Canada. One of the worst polluters was the Marathon Petroleum refinery, the biggest emitter of sulfur dioxide in an area that the Environmental Protection Agency had determined had too much of that chemical in its air in the first place.

Early in 2016 we noticed that the refinery had applied for a permit that would have allowed it to increase its emissions of sulfur dioxide. The mayor and I discussed the matter, realizing that the community had had enough and we needed to act. I also saw an opportunity to show the department what we could do if we were willing to be bold—a critical step in its resuscitation.

The Michigan Department of Environmental Quality was holding a hearing in the community, and I prepared a list of ten facts to register as testimony; when I read them out in an auditorium packed with several hundred in attendance, I could tell they were resonating with the community members when the "Mm-hmms" and "You tell 'ems" got louder with each fact.

I followed up with an op-ed in the *Detroit Free Press*. By the next hearing our advocacy efforts had forced Marathon Petroleum to the table—particularly after Mayor Duggan threatened a lawsuit in federal court if they persisted. They came back with a plan that would invest $10 million to reduce their emissions overall, where they had previously wanted to increase them. They also offered to spruce up and invest in several local parks and pay for a street sweeping program to reduce dust.

We had won. It was the first time that anyone could remember when the city had stood up for its residents against pollution. The *Free Press* editorial board put it best: "Residents objected, as they've done before, to little avail. But this time, something changed."[1]

This first win for environmental justice propelled the department onward, providing us with a sense that we could really accomplish something—that we could take on big fights and win. I knew that kind of confidence would mean everything to a department that hadn't even *existed* just a few years before.

We kept up our efforts. We blocked a local corporation from trucking radioactive fracking waste into the middle of the city and stood up against another petroleum company storing metallurgical cokes—by-products of the petroleum refining process that release dust into the air—in uncovered piles by the Detroit River.

The water crisis unfolding in Flint brought the full scope of environmental poisoning back into view. Beyond the air and groundwater, we had to examine the places that our children learned and played. Alongside the mayor and other city leaders, I personally inspected a number of city schools after the teachers' union in the district conducted a massive sickout to draw attention to the poorly kept facilities. Walking into a first-grade classroom at 11:00 a.m., I saw six-year-olds huddled together in coats because the boilers in their building didn't work. I found a dead mouse in the corner near an entryway. And when we walked into the gym—the place that those kids were supposed to be able to go play on frigid mornings like this one—you could see the mold growing underneath the floorboards. You could smell it wafting in the air.

Given the state of our schools, it was clear that our kids might be exposed to the same lead we were reading about in Flint in the places where we systematically concentrated them most of the day, most the year. We needed to have schools, day cares, and Head Starts test their water for lead. Yet, because the schools were technically independent of city government, we knew we didn't have the jurisdiction to mandate this. Many schools—particularly charter schools—would balk. So instead we created a screening protocol that was optional, along with a website where families could track the results from their children's schools. By promoting the website in the media, we knew we could turn up the pressure on schools, angry parents flooding the phone lines, asking why their kids' school hadn't complied.

In the first round of tests, nineteen of sixty-two schools tested positive for lead. In the end, we were able to get every single school to comply with our protocol, which was named a Model Practice by the National Association of City and County Health Officials.[2] We forced every school that tested positive into a mitigation procedure to protect kids from lead-tainted water. Yet most of these mitigation efforts were temporary. In 2018 another round of testing found that many schools had tested positive once again—a reminder that the work always continues.

We knew there was much more work to be done to address the most common cause of lead poisoning in Detroit: homes. The rate of lead poisoning in Detroit was higher at baseline than it was in Flint at the height of the water crisis—not because of water but because of the lead paint that is ubiquitous in homes built before 1978, when lead-based paint was outlawed. A full 93 percent of homes in Detroit were built before then. In many of these homes, particularly in lower-income communities, this lead can chip off. Tragically, leaded paint is sweet to the taste, and children crawling around will seek it out, putting it on their tongues—and into their brains.

While there were many organizations working on the challenge, there was no coordination—one of the central responsibilities of a health department that was only now coming back to life. To get everyone on the same page, we created a program called Lead Safe Detroit, an effort to provide every available service to every affected family.

Every two weeks we'd pack representatives from organizations including the Housing and Revitalization Department, the Buildings, Safety Engineering and Environmental Department, the Water and Sewerage Department, and the Green & Healthy Homes Initiative, an organization that conducts home investigations for lead dust, into a conference room in our new department headquarters. Case by case, we would track every child who had had a positive lead test and, department by department, would offer a status report: Did that child get a visit from Green & Healthy Homes? Had siblings of an affected child been tested? Had the water department offered an in-home lead screening kit?

We used the meetings to identify holes in what we could offer affected children and families. For example, we learned that parents were being threatened with eviction by their landlords—which was illegal—if their kids tested positive for lead. This led many families to avoid testing altogether. We needed to make sure that we could provide legal support for families if this occurred. Some families needed hotel vouchers during lead abatement procedures. Still others required that grandparents' homes be tested if children spent most of their days there.

This knowledge would be helpful grist for anti-lead policy. If we could give landlords the right incentives to fully remove lead from their rental units, for example, we could free them of costly annual inspections. Working with the Buildings, Safety Engineering and Environmental Department, which certified rental units in the city, we were able to advocate for a smarter, healthier ordinance governing lead policy for landlords.

Every Friday afternoon I would leave the department to do my own fieldwork, dropping by some neighborhood or another in the city. I would find a random door. I'd tell residents that I was with the Detroit Health Department and show them my nifty badge that came with the gig. It conveyed just enough authority to prove that I was with the department but not enough to reveal my role there.

I'd ask them what they thought the Health Department should be doing. How were the kids? What would they like to see us working on? I'd use this gumshoe public health reconnaissance to inform our approaches at the highest levels. It was applied epidemiology à la Snow.

I'd been in countless homes over the course of my time in Detroit, but none hit me harder than the first ride-along visit I made with one of our infant health nurses. Hers was probably the hardest job in the department: visiting mothers who had lost their babies way too early.

We were visiting a mother who had lost her baby boy a few months earlier; he had been born premature, the most common predictor of infant mortality.

As she cuddled her two-year-old to sleep, she recounted her experience at the hospital: her concerns waved off, her complaints of pain ignored, hospital staff blaming her for her child's condition.

I had seen it all before as a medical student, on the other side of that divide. There is a not-so-subtle bigotry in the condescension and inattention, the snide complaints about patients "thinking they know it all." The truth is that poor patients face a double jeopardy: although they often lack the means to do so, they are blamed for failing to "take control of their lives."

She struggled, caught between pangs of guilt and profound grief. There was nothing we could do for her but bear witness to her sorrow and reassure her that we cared and wouldn't judge her. And we could learn from her loss to make sure that we were building a city where mothers didn't have to grieve for their babies so often.

As we got up to leave, I asked if I could use her restroom. She directed me to a room off the foyer in the small bungalow in which she lived with her mother, her child, and the haunting memory of her son.

I pressed the handle to flush as I turned around to wash my hands. My subconscious caught the absence of the noise it so reflexively expected to hear. I looked back and realized that there was no water in the bowl. Then I noticed all the water bottles next to the sink: this family was one of twenty thousand that had had their water shut off in the past year alone.

* * *

In 2013 and 2014, Detroit made headlines because the city, then under emergency management, began to crack down on residents in arrears on their water bills. The debt obligations associated with the Water and Sewerage Department were valued at $5.7 billion[3]—nearly a third of the value of the city's full debt burden. Willfully ignorant of the havoc that losing water access would wreak upon households struggling under poverty, the emergency manager began simply shutting off people's water—in a state surrounded by more than one-fifth of the world's fresh water. The crisis became so dire that the United Nations Human Rights Commission called it "an affront to human rights."[4]

Under Mayor Duggan's administration, the city established a few stopgap measures, offering warnings and payment plans, trying to stave off some of the loudest public pressure. But the shutoffs continued, leaving too many Detroiters without the most basic human necessity.

I had met several times with the very same activists who had brought attention to the crisis at the UN in my office at the Health Department. Here were activists who had their focus on people; they wanted my help to end the shutoffs, and I promised that I would do my best.

My best was not enough. I brought the issue up in every meeting I could—with the mayor, his staffers, and in meetings with other department heads. Every time, people who knew that the city's policy was completely and utterly wrong would balk at the mention of it. Bringing up the shutoffs would usually trigger one of three responses: some would ignore that I had even brought it up; others would rationalize the policy; and still others would explode defensively, "That's not your issue; it's above your pay grade."

City leadership was often more interested in massaging the media narrative on a problem than actually solving it. As my advocacy came to a head, I was called a "bleeding heart" in a meeting, implying that I didn't understand how the real world worked. In truth, I hope to always be a "bleeding heart"; I'd rather have my heart bleed over people's suffering than be callous about it. After that, I realized that I was being excluded from meetings having anything to do with water. When I inquired about it, I was told that I shouldn't be concerned: "Water shutoffs have nothing to do with public health."

Meanwhile, I was being pressed—rightly—by the water activists. They wanted me to declare a public health state of emergency on the matter. But if I did, I knew I'd be replaced with some yes-man, and the rebirth of our department would be aborted.

To this day I think a lot about whether or not I made the right choice—or if there was something more I could have or should have done. Leadership always comes with tradeoffs that feel nearly impossible at the time. I was caught between throwing a Hail Mary pass to try to end the shutoffs or continuing forward with the rest of the critical work we were doing.

The battle over the shutoffs showed me how politics dictated so much of what was considered "feasible" in Detroit. Feasibility was not just a measure of how much political capital elected officials wanted to use to accomplish something; it was also a measure of how much they could manage the narrative. When we presented the best available statistics about lead poisoning in Detroit in the mayor's cabinet meeting, he shut down the presentation, unwilling to believe the numbers (which turned out to be underestimates). Lead poisoning was impolitic in the era of Flint.

There was no program more politically sensitive in Detroit than the city's demolition program. Detroit demolishes more abandoned structures than any other locality in the country: nearly nineteen thousand to date in 2019.[5] For comparison, in 2016, when Detroit demolished its ten-thousandth home,[6] the next biggest program—run by the state of Ohio—had demolished less than a quarter as many.[7]

The demolition program was the capstone of Duggan's election platform during his 2013 campaign for mayor, when he argued that demolishing abandoned homes would eliminate blight and raise the property values of nearby residences. A recent report by outside organizations suggests that there may be some merit to this: the report found that the value of a home within five hundred feet of a demolition increased 4.2 percent.[8]

But the funding scheme and operations have been questionable at best. To fund the majority of the demolitions, the city relied on the U.S. Treasury's Hardest Hit Fund, which was intended to support homeowners struggling to stay afloat, not to demolish abandoned homes.[9] Almost immediately, Detroit's demolition program was dogged by allegations of corruption and mismanagement: it was far more expensive than comparable programs in other cities,[10] and there were questions about how contractors were chosen and how (or if) they followed protocol.[11] Investigations centering on allegations of bid rigging, antitrust violations, and wire fraud rained down.[12]

The Health Department also began to investigate the program when a nurse suggested that one of the children with lead poisoning we had discussed at a Lead Safe Detroit meeting might have been exposed because of a demolition near her home.

While anecdotes aren't enough to confirm that a demolition caused lead poisoning, the relationship is more than plausible. After all, lead paint permeates the walls of almost all of these structures. In fact, the program's administrators at the Detroit Land Bank were well aware of the risk and had done their due diligence before kicking it off. They carefully studied best practices established by other cities to tailor an approach for Detroit that would avoid potential hazards. They had innovated a process that involved soaking a home slated for demolition in two different ways and then flattening it to reduce fugitive dust release. This preventive measure contributed to the skyrocketing expense of the program.

But no one had ever demolished houses on this scale. And even a little bit of lead dust per house—multiplied over seventeen thousand houses—can lead to a lot of lead dust. Worse, demolitions cluster in the poorest communities, where abandoned homes are more common.

We began to collect data to ask a simple question: Were demolitions increasing the likelihood of lead poisoning among children who lived close to demolished homes? For all the reasons that identifying causation in epidemiology is hard, this question was particularly knotty. Kids who live in neighborhoods where there are more demolitions are more likely to be exposed to lead in the first place because these neighborhoods are poorer and the homes are more likely to be in disrepair. Also, how long does lead dust stay in the air? And how far does it spread? Is there a seasonal difference? Perhaps it's worse in the summer months, when people are more likely to open their windows . . .

We consulted some of the top spatial epidemiologists in the country— experts in understanding how the environment can shape health. And when we finally finished our analysis, the outcomes were startling. We found that if a demolition occurred in the summer months within four hundred feet of a child's home and within forty-five days of the day the child got tested for lead, the child had 20 percent higher odds of testing positive for elevated blood lead. That jumped to 38 percent higher if there was more than one demolition. It was also higher if a child lived closer to a demolition.[13] The trend of risk increasing with proximity or an increased number of demolitions is called a "dose-response" effect in epidemiology—meaning the more of a bad thing there is, the higher the probability of the outcome. It's a good indicator that the exposure you're considering—in this case a demolition—actually causes the effect: lead exposure.

Something had to be done. I immediately notified the mayor's office of our findings. Predictably, some members of his staff began to stonewall, denying the study's validity, second-guessing our intentions, and downplaying the results. The mayor himself was far more receptive, although he demanded our findings be independently replicated before giving them full merit.

Given how robust the findings were and the lengths to which we had gone to verify our methods with other experts, I immediately kicked off a task force to audit the demolition process relative to best practices. We devised eighteen recommendations that could eliminate lead exposure before, during, and after a demolition. The recommendations included things like early notification of a forthcoming demolition, training contractors on lead safety, real-time demolition monitoring, and covering neighboring homes. As of 2019, the full list has yet to be implemented.

* * *

In February 2017, eighteen months after I walked into that office in the back of the municipal parking building, I resigned. My tenure at the Health Department was shorter than I had expected, but it was certainly eventful. The Health Department had grown from five employees and eighty-five contractors to a team of 220 across four campuses. We had multiplied city investment in public health tenfold and attracted hundreds of thousands of dollars in competitive philanthropic support to provide children with eyeglasses, stand up to polluters, protect city schools, empower new moms through mentorship support, clean up lead, and reduce asthma. We even reduced dog bites and saved thousands of pups.

Our work was epidemiology applied—posing questions as problems and then building their solutions into our institution. Kids need glasses; how do we provide them? Kids are getting poisoned with lead; what are the causes and how do we systematically end them? Kids can't breathe; how do we reduce the pollution that is choking them?

This was the work, I hoped, that would justify my privilege—the kind my Teta would be proud of. I had given up a lucrative career as a physician and the academic prestige of a tenure-track job at an Ivy League school to come home to Detroit and serve. I walked into my role as a fresh-faced, overeducated thirty-year-old with no experience in an applied public health role, let alone as a city's top public health official. Walking out, I hoped that our results would continue to serve children like Marcus and empower and protect the community for years to come.

And although we made headway, it's impossible not to feel like we were still failing. After all, we were working against a set of problems that went far beyond what one health department in one city could solve. Marcus is a poor Black child in an America that has forgotten about poor Black children—and poor white children don't fare much better. Growing inequality has left people like Marcus's mother working multiple jobs to try to make the ends of an unraveling rope meet. His father is a Black man in jail in a society with racist public policies that have criminalized Black men. His grandmother's heart failure has been exacerbated by the difficulty of getting her medications without a car, in a city that destroyed its own public transit system at the behest of car manufacturers who have since failed it.

In Marcus's America, we've decided that corporations are people and that they deserve government support—although we are questioning whether schools do. And because we've allowed our culture to blame the victims of poverty for their suffering, many would look at Marcus's family and say they're failing. Rather, *we* are failing *them*.

And that's because our politics, which I got to see up close for the first time, are failing all of us. The administration I worked for seemed more concerned about power and sound bites than leadership and substance. I refused to play that game any longer; I wasn't going to be a health director who sat idly by while people went thirsty in their own homes. I wasn't going to justify serving under leadership that did not leap at the opportunity to protect our kids because of "optics." Perhaps there is no room for bleeding hearts in politics. And yet, there is no choice but to try.

* * *

Before I left, that long "arch of the moral universe" so often referenced by Dr. Martin Luther King and President Obama—which, in their telling, bends toward justice—had been mangled in a new direction. After a long, confusing, and at times dystopian campaign, Donald Trump—reality TV star and shameless political manipulator—won the 2016 presidential election.

President Donald Trump? I remember thinking as I clicked off CNN, which had just declared him the victor that early November night. Sarah had already gone to bed; she had an early morning the next day. Trump had defied the odds to everyone's shock—and to the dismay of anyone who knows what it's like to look into the icy stare of dehumanizing hatred. Red "Make America Great Again" hats had replaced Shepard Fairey "HOPE" posters—the worst of our history claiming revenge on the best of our future.

Dressed in all black the next day, I ambled, dazed and dejected, into our Wednesday morning cabinet meeting. Nearly everyone else who worked on the eleventh floor of the Coleman A. Young Municipal Center, which houses City Hall, registered the same melancholy. Trying to mollify us, the mayor addressed the previous night's political earthquake: "We'll do our best to find shared wins."

While I know he meant well, it was neither the time nor the place. No one was thinking about "wins." The majority of people in that room were from communities the president-elect had spent the last two years marginalizing or scapegoating: some combination of female, Black, Latinx, queer, or Muslim. To the mayor, a middle-aged white man born and raised in a suburb that voted overwhelmingly for Trump, this new president was simply not his cup of political tea, rather than the existential threat he posed to so many of us.

I began to think about what Trump's policies would mean for our work at the Health Department. So many of the programs that we had instituted were funded, directly or indirectly, by federal grant programs. Those programs would likely face cuts or consolidations that would likely hurt the poor Black communities like Detroit that Trump would characterize as "American carnage" in his inauguration speech.

I couldn't shake the fact that people in my own family had voted for Trump—people I know and love and who I know love me and the rest of their Egyptian- and Muslim-American family. Then I thought about the endless lies Trump had told, how he had played on the fear and anxiety—on the insecurity—of so many people in our country. He spoke to the worst in our public discussion, exploiting division and inflaming anger. Rather than come together to build, as Obama had so masterfully inspired us to, he wanted us to separate and destroy.

I have always believed that people are fundamentally good, although they may do bad things. Trump's election left me with some doubts. *If people are so good*, I thought, *how could we elect someone so bad as our leader?* This was the irreducible kernel of my deepest frustrations with the election and the politics that had decided it.

Taken together, I kept asking myself if this was the best place to keep doing my work. Or did the 2016 election signal something? Did the fight for the kind of justice, equity, and sustainability we were waging on the streets and in the neighborhoods of Detroit need to be taken up elsewhere to be effective?

On January 3, 2017, I was buttoning up my crisp white shirt for another day at the office—the first day back after the winter holidays. I'm normally excited to go back to work after a long holiday. But not this time: it all felt futile. *This isn't what I'm supposed to be doing right now*, I thought. I had my answer. A month later I would submit my resignation letter.

* * *

I had decided to run for governor. It was a crazy idea, to be sure. But to my surprise no one really tried to talk me out of it. Everything we had thought we knew about politics had been dashed by Donald Trump's rise to the presidency. And the idea of a thirty-two-year-old Muslim doctor named Abdul being elected to the state's highest office, though not the likeliest outcome, was not as far-fetched as it had seemed just a few months earlier.

It was the work that called to me. I knew my public health expertise could be critical in reforming a state government that had created the Flint water crisis. Having served on two state commissions in the aftermath of the crisis, I began to realize that the previous administration was more interested in putting paper over the problem in the form of report after report rather than actually solving it. Furthermore, I knew my experience working in the bowels of one of the most challenging municipal governments—post-bankruptcy Detroit—to resurrect a health department would serve me well in the role of governor. Others vying for the Democratic nomination lacked any experience in government operations whatsoever, and although my time at the Health Department had been short, I believed that voters would judge the record of my work, rather than the time I took doing it. After all, they might want someone who had accomplished something tangible and lasting in government in a little time, rather than someone who had accomplished little in a lot of time.

Finally, I was—and remain—leery of politicians who take contributions from corporations that have been the engines of inequality in our society while talking about how much they worry about the victims of that inequality. And having worked on the front lines of healthcare and environmental justice, I believe that achieving universal healthcare and tackling climate change are the defining public policy challenges of our time. I would be the only candidate who pledged to raise campaign funds without touching corporate money from health insurers or the oil and gas industry—and who was articulating a real, comprehensive approach to universal government-sponsored healthcare and fossil fuel reduction in Michigan.

So it was off to the races . . .

CHAPTER 11

Running for our lives.

On June 6, 2018, I was scrolling through Twitter on a long ride home in Michigan, and I happened upon a retweet from a progressive group that had just endorsed me for governor. It was yet another viral video of a young woman from the Bronx named Alexandria Ocasio-Cortez before she became universally known as "AOC," her very own three-letter moniker marking her ascent to the pinnacle of political stardom. She was fierce, honest, and bold. And whatever the "it" is—that rare amalgam of fearlessness, authenticity, and raw charisma that people look for in leaders—she had it.

I clicked the blue "follow" button on her profile, and it turned out that she had been following me, too. I sent her a direct message to let her know how much I appreciated her and her campaign. The next morning she messaged back: "Thank you, and likewise!" followed by a brown fist emoji. "So proud of what you're doing in MI. We're doing the dang thing!" Purple heart emoji. "Wishing you all the strength and grace in the world."

Two weeks later my grandpa Jan, who lives in Hamburg, Michigan, texted me: "Just watched an interview of Alexandria Ocasio-Cortez, running in NY 14th district primary. She is amazing! Have you met her?"

"Yeah—she's great. Not formally, but a big fan of hers!" I responded.

"She sounds a lot like you?"

"Very similar positions"

"It's good to see young capable people getting into politics."

That was the first inkling I had that this out-of-nowhere young Latina woman from the Bronx who'd been bartending just a year earlier was going to upset the political establishment and realign the stars of the political universe. As her race heated up in the last few weeks leading up to the primary, I messaged her in support: "You are BLOWING UP. My grandpa—Jan Johnson from Hamburg, Michigan—just texted me about you. Keep going."

On June 28, I was on my way out of the office after a day spent fundraising on the phone when I ran into a few of my campaign staffers. After we caught up on some of the day's happenings, the conversation turned to the Ocasio-Cortez primary. One of my staffers was a grizzled veteran of tough congressional primaries—having upset the political establishment before. But this one was too much.

"Crowley's got that district on lock," he said knowingly. "He's the king of Queens!"

"No way can she win," another staffer agreed, shaking his head.

"I don't know, guys. She's got that *spark*," I said.

Had I been a betting man, I would have made some sweet cash that night. We had just finished dinner, and I was holding Emmalee in my lap as Sarah's family and I sat around the family room watching CNN. The coverage was focused on the Supreme Court's disastrous decision to uphold "Muslim Ban 3.0," the Trump administration's third effort to make good on a campaign promise for a "total and complete shutdown of all Muslims entering the United States." The monotone blare of the talking head explaining the court's rationale dimmed as my thoughts wandered to what this country might look like when the little girl in my arms—Brown and Muslim—grew up to be my age. *How much time and effort will her generation have to spend cleaning up after our failures? Or will they be so overwhelmed by them as to stop trying?* I wondered.

The host wrapping up his interview with the monotonous legal expert brought my focus back onto the television screen. After all, I hadn't been watching for the legal analysis tonight but for the election ticker underneath. And just then I saw it flash to New York's Fourteenth District.

With 60-something percent of all precincts reporting, they had called it for Alexandria. I erupted, waking up my half-sleeping daughter and startling everyone else in the room.

"She won! I can't even believe it! SHE WON!"

The ticker had changed again, so it took a few moments for me to show the family what I was celebrating—that I hadn't just gone mad. Meanwhile, I rocked my baby girl back to sleep as I paced nervously—giddily—back and forth. *Maybe it won't be so bad*, I thought.

Exactly a month later I'd get to tell AOC in person what it meant to watch her shock the world with my little girl on my lap, something I will never forget. She had graciously flown in for a rollicking day of rallies across Michigan in the lead-up to my primary, just a few short days away.

* * *

As we barreled toward Election Day, our campaign picked up real momentum. From the inside, my day-to-day campaign experience didn't really change. But as the crowds got bigger, the requests for interviews more frequent—and from more prominent national publications—and the donations came rolling in, I began to appreciate that I was in the eye of a growing storm.

To be honest, though, it all happened too fast to remember. It was like living several weeks' worth of experiences in a day—every day for a year and a half. Experiences that would have been momentous at any other point in my life, a meeting or an event I might have circled on a calendar, became one of three important things I did on Tuesday. What's left are indelible memories of people and moments that capture what it meant to me.

* * *

About ten days before Election Day, I was supposed to meet with a group of neighborhood block club captains at one of our campaign offices in Detroit. I was running late, a perpetual consequence of having too many draws on my attention and not enough time to give any of them. As I dashed through the door into the office, I realized that the office was too quiet for a place where I was supposed to be meeting with twenty to thirty local leaders. In fact, the office was almost empty; there were only three people. I had come to the wrong office . . .

Or maybe I hadn't. It had been a particularly hard week, as several of the endorsements we were hoping for—from a few labor unions and newspapers—had gone the other way. I felt defeated. If I wasn't winning, what was the point of this campaign? All that time, effort, and money that people had invested would be simply wasted on another also-ran.

When I walked in, I immediately recognized Amal, one of my campaign organizers, but I had never seen the other two, a younger man and an older gentleman, before that. The young man was on the phone. When he saw me, his eyes lit up.

I could tell that he was disabled. He quickly explained. "My name is— is Anthony," he said in halting language between giddy chuckles. "I have cerebral—palsy, a lot of people think that means my mind—doesn't work. But it—does."

By that point I had realized that the other individual in the room was Anthony's support aide, helping him make calls to voters on my behalf.

I had positioned myself near Anthony, crouching down so that he and I could look each other in the eye.

"I love—politics. But I've never—been able to work—on a campaign before. It's so—cool that you let me—work on your campaign!"

"Anthony did twenty hours already!" Amal told me.

His support aide, Peter, looked up from the dialer they were using. "I've never seen him so excited about *anything*. He's watched, like, every one of your videos—twice."

Those tears that Sarah had taught me to cry came streaming down my face as Anthony, still giddy, started telling me about how I was his candidate because of my stances on Medicare for All and universal Wi-Fi.

"I'm so—lucky to—meet you," Anthony said as we gripped each other's hands.

"No, Anthony, *I'm* so lucky to meet *you*. Thank you for working so hard on my campaign."

Jordan, my bodyguard and all-around support man, reminded me that we had to go. And I realized that I was already a good twenty minutes late for my meeting with the block club captains. With traffic, I'd be lucky to get there before half past the hour. My tardiness would be interpreted as a sign of disrespect.

As I walked out into the stifling midday heat, I was overcome with an overwhelming feeling of gratitude, and I broke down sobbing. Anthony reminded me what I was doing this for. I had never set out to run to earn some newspaper's endorsement. I had run to earn the endorsements of people like Anthony, folks who had felt excluded—not just by our politics but by society—for too long. That he had found purpose in this movement we were building—that he had been empowered through it—that was enough.

* * *

I was so proud of the team that had formed around me. On many campaigns, a paid staffer spending her time helping one person on the phones might have been chided, even fired. But that was exactly what *I* would have done. And that our campaign ethos reflected that suggested that we were living out our ideals, not just talking about them.

Indeed, my team was built on ideals, not experience. I did that on purpose. Most of our senior staffers hadn't even worked a campaign before. But I knew that if I hired a bunch of veterans who had only worked run-of-the-mill campaigns, I'd get a run-of-the-mill campaign as well.

And I was no run-of-the-mill candidate. That much became obvious when I started interviewing polling consultants. As I began to meet prospects, each had a different approach. "Let me give it to you straight," said one. "You're young, a doctor, and a Rhodes scholar. I know how those things will poll," he said reassuringly. "But you're also an Arab Muslim named Abdul who's got a beard, and I can tell you how that will poll." Less reassuring. "To be honest, I have no damn clue what voters will think about you." At least that was honest. Some suggested that I should change my name, some that I should shave my beard. Some thought that images of me with my wife—who chooses to wear a hijab, the traditional Muslim headscarf—shouldn't be shown *anywhere*.

Here I was being parsed into my "ingredients" as if I could be reduced to some weird politician version of Chipotle. But—and I only learned because I ate so much of it—Chipotle *always* tastes the same. It doesn't matter if you go with chicken or barbacoa, load with queso or sour cream. It's the same with politicians: they overemphasize the same things in their appearance, message, and approach—and end up looking, talking, acting just like every other politician. As a hyphenated kid growing up between two worlds, I had worked hard to figure out exactly who I was. I wasn't going to change my name, shave my beard, or hide the person I love most in this world because she wears a hijab.

Nearly all the experts were pretty much in agreement on one thing: I should "stick to my base." My base was young people, people of color, and progressives who agreed with me on things like Medicare for All, and that we shouldn't be allowing corporations to corrupt our politics. In short, I shouldn't be wasting my time in low-income white suburbs. I'd never win those votes, they told me. I should stick to my tribe.

But that's the problem entirely, right? That kind of defensive politics cannot solve the problem at our core. The divisions that Trump has exacerbated and the tribalism that he has unleashed will only heal if and when we have the courage to address them directly. That means we need the empathy and humility, as real people, to show up and listen.

I needed a team who believed in the expansive brand of politics I wanted to embody, could grow and adapt, and had the grit to work harder than anyone else. And that's the team I got. We built it around a culture of mutual respect, hard work, and joy in the privilege of devoting ourselves to this cause.

They were led by Max Glass, the only member of the team who had worked in his current position for more than one candidate. In campaign circles he's known as a "primary whisperer" with a penchant for outside-the-box candidates with something to prove. Max might be the only person I know who hates losing more than I do. His brilliant deputy, Claire Sandberg, was an "organizing engineer": she helped build Senator Bernie Sanders's distributed organizing apparatus in 2016—and is leading his organizing team in 2020. She helped pioneer an approach to organizing that empowers volunteers to take on leadership roles, vastly increasing the power of the campaign. Aside from a few others with bona fide campaign experience—like Tara Terpstra, my trusty executive assistant at the Health Department, who'd worked in a congressional office and was now managing the whole campaign operation; and Connor Farrell, my human Swiss Army knife of a finance director, who had worked a few congressional races before—most of the team was new to this. They were people like Adam Joseph, who ran my communications team, his only previous political experience was writing speeches for a member of the Indian parliament, Shashi Tharoor, while in India on a Fulbright scholarship. Lama Alzuhd, who oversaw community outreach, had put law school—and her full-time job as a chemist—on hold to join the campaign.

But perhaps nobody captures the spirit of our campaign quite like my policy director, Rhiana Gunn-Wright. I met Rhiana, a Rhodes scholar with a master's degree in public policy from Oxford and an undergraduate degree from Yale, at a leadership retreat for Rhodes scholars when she was still in grad school. I was immediately struck by her razor-sharp intellect coupled with her "I don't give a damn" approach to power, honed on the South Side of Chicago, where she grew up. She has the rare ability to break complex topics down to their elements quickly and then apply a moral force of will to identifying what ought to be done and by whom. When our funding came through at the Health Department, I immediately reached out to see if she'd be willing to come on as a policy analyst for the department. And when I decided to run, I asked if she'd join the campaign as our policy director.

When I told Max that I had already found a policy director, he balked. "What do we need a policy director for?" Most campaigns, after all, prefer not to talk about policy. And what about the added expense? But our campaign wasn't going to sell empty promises: we were going to tell people exactly what we wanted to do and how we wanted to do it.

Rhiana was reticent at the beginning; she'd never taken on a role this big. But, together, Rhiana and I developed policies that would, in stark detail, shape a vision for the kind of Michigan we could become. In total, Rhiana and her team crafted more than three hundred pages of policy, ranging from a detailed state-level single-payer healthcare program called "MichCare," to a comprehensive "urban agenda," to a public option for Wi-Fi we dubbed "Mi-Fi," to a plan to reduce Michigan's disastrously high auto insurance rates. At one point a journalist called our campaign "one of the most high-powered progressive think tanks in the country."[1] More rewarding was watching Rhiana grow into the role, take on bigger, more ambitious policy projects—and finish them to rave reviews from supporters and the press.

Since the campaign, Rhiana has exploded onto the progressive policy scene—and was chosen to architect AOC's marquee policy proposal, the Green New Deal. Since then, Rhiana's appeared in the pages of *Time*, the *Atlantic*, and *Current Affairs*; she even had a feature story in *Essence*. And one Sunday evening I was randomly channel surfing and came upon Rhiana's face on the *New York Times* news show *The Weekly*. Other alumni are leading key departments for 2020 presidential, senatorial, and congressional campaigns and starting businesses. Although we did not win our race, I'm proud of the incredible people my campaign has helped showcase—and the careers it has helped accelerate.

* * *

Ady Barkan is one of the most inspiring souls I have ever met. I got to know him as we both campaigned for the kind of country we want for our children. But Ady was campaigning under very different circumstances. As I campaigned for an office I was hoping to hold, he was campaigning for the

America he wanted to leave behind. Ady was diagnosed with ALS in 2016, just after his son Carl was born. Carl's not much older than Emmalee. In 2018, despite being wheelchair-bound, Ady toured the country stumping for progressive candidates.

I was lucky to earn his endorsement, but even more, I was honored to earn his friendship. He was gracious enough to come to Michigan and do a town hall with me and an incredible labor rights organizer, Cynthia Thornton, who leads Pride at Work Michigan, an LGBTQIA+ labor rights organization. As I watched Ady struggle to speak that day, I couldn't help but reflect on the incredible courage and selflessness of this person. He was losing his ability to talk: his diaphragm and the muscles of his mouth and throat—muscles whose function most of us get to take for granted every time we so much as utter a word—were wasting away. Yet, rather than spend his last moments with his wife, Rachael, or their young son, he was fighting for them—and the rest of us.

After the event, a receiving line formed. Amid the usual group of folks waiting for post-event handshakes, to take selfies, or to ask questions, I noticed a group that looked out of place. There were four middle-aged men, each cradling something in their hands. They looked like they were trying *too* hard to fit in, awkwardly wearing "Abdul" shirts over whatever else they had walked in wearing that evening. With them was a youngish woman who was clearly the ringleader. I paid them little heed, focused rather on my conversations with the folks ahead of them in line.

Then they got to the front—and pounced. The woman reached out to shake my hand, and then asked her question. Immediately, the four skeevy guys, two on each side of her, pulled out their cameras. "I just wanted to know how you reconcile your own personal practice of Islamic law with your Marxist Socialist political platform that directly contradicts tenets within Islamic law?" The woman, a notorious far-right provocateur, had ambushed many prominent progressives in the past, and she'd chosen this moment of vulnerability to do it to me.

I knew what she wanted: tape of either her yelling at me or me yelling at her. I'd give her neither. Instead, I politely rebuffed the premise of her line of questioning, which became more hostile and angrier as she came up empty-handed. As she started yelling, my staffers caught on to what was happening and pulled me out of the situation. Supporters in line swooped in to confront her.

Although the woman would later get booted from Twitter and Facebook for her hate speech against Muslims, her edited video is still making the rounds. The last time I saw it, it was linked in a message from a concerned friend who had found it on a Facebook page called "The United West," on which it is hosted and had been shared 2,700 times.

The emotional whiplash of the whole experience shook me. In minutes I had gone from a moment of profound vulnerability as I listened to my friend— a man fighting for our lives as he fights for his own—to having to confront an embodiment of the evil we were fighting against. I could feel myself drawing the wrong lesson from the experience: *Don't ever let yourself be vulnerable like that again!*

I went to the bathroom to wash my face. I stared at myself in the mirror. The will to be vulnerable, to listen and empathize with people in pain—that's the substrate of leadership. Without it, you're just another one of those talking-point politicians, too numb or closed off to the world to even look like you believe what you're saying. And I never want to be that. The cost? Sometimes the world smacks you where it hurts. I thought about my friend, Ady, about his courage and his persistence. *It's worth it*, I told myself.

* * *

Exactly two weeks before Election Day, we got word that Senator Bernie Sanders would officially endorse our campaign—and that he had agreed to come and campaign with me in the week leading up to the election. I had spoken with him a few weeks earlier. He asked what I was fighting for. But perhaps more importantly he asked *why* I was fighting for it. I told him about my grandmother and my work as a health official in Detroit. "Good, good," he responded. "Let me see what we can do."

My team had gotten pretty good at putting together rallies by this point, having pulled off four impressive rallies for AOC in one day, each attended by upwards of a thousand or more people. But we knew that bringing Bernie to Michigan was going to be a whole new ball game. He'd upset Hillary Clinton in Michigan during the 2016 primaries, and he commanded a strong and serious following of Michiganders who were supporting me as well. He only had a half day to spend with us, so we planned two rallies, one in Detroit and one in Ypsilanti, where we'd been with AOC just a few weeks earlier. We expected more than a thousand people for each one.

I met Bernie face-to-face for the first time in the bowels of the TCF Center, Detroit's main convention space downtown. It was odd meeting this individual to whom I had looked up for so long—whose take-no-prisoners brand of politics had so marked the political moment in which I was running.

He was taller than I had expected—a good five inches taller than me. Watching the familiar countenance display the usual range of emotions one goes through in a regular conversation was odd. He asked about my family. I introduced him to Sarah. His face snapped a broad, toothy smile, something I had realized I'd never seen Bernie Sanders do. I'd only ever really seen him portrayed one way. It's odd meeting celebrities: almost instantly you're forced to reckon with them in three dimensions, a stark contrast to the single dimension that you're usually shown.

I reflected on the many people I had come to meet throughout the campaign. In the beginning, nobody knew who I was or really cared. "You're running for what? Well, you look awfully young," they'd say. But after our commercials started to air on TV, I began to get recognized in public. "Are you that guy . . . Abdul, I think it is . . . who's running for something?"

"Yes, that's me. I'm Abdul, running for governor. Hope you'll come out and support me on August seventh!"

Sometimes, usually in rural parts of the state, I'd see people look at me inquisitively—then watch their brows furl as they registered who I was, turned on their heels, and marched away in disgust. *They must have seen that chain post on Facebook*, I figured.

But sometimes people would look intently at my face—and then smile, rushing over as they pulled their phones out for a selfie. These moments were always the most interesting, as people would have the same reaction to me that I was now having with Bernie, squaring the somewhat less on-brand version of me in real life with the one they'd come to know on TV and social media. "You're a lot . . . shorter than I thought you'd be" was a common remark.

As we conversed in a holding room and the early speakers warmed up the crowd, we could hear the nearly 2,500 people who had come. Periodically one of my staffers would give me an update: "It's raucous up there."

Ohio state senator Nina Turner, then chair of Our Revolution, a progressive advocacy organization built out of the 2016 Sanders campaign, introduced me as I waited in the wings, just beyond where I could see the crowd. I could feel their energy, though. I've always loved big crowds, especially big crowds with a purpose.

As Senator Turner introduced me, I walked out to the roar of the attendees, emotionally crowd-surfing the audience of 2,500 people. My inner voice kept asking me, *WTF are you doing here? Those people can't actually be here for you.* They weren't: they were there for Bernie, I reassured myself.

But this was still, at least in name, an "Abdul" rally. And I was going to give them the best I had. As I climbed onto the rostrum, the crowd chanted my name. My inner voice was flabbergasted. *They're chanting "Abdul!" Like, this is a crowd of people at a political rally chanting your foreign-ass name. Are you serious?* That, I had to admit, was something that thirteen-year-old kid boarding that airplane to Egypt in 1998 could *never* have seen coming.

Among the sea of humanity, I was close enough to make out particular faces as I spoke. *There's Baba and Mom, and Osama and Samia, and Grandma and Grandpa!* They were all sitting together in the first row. *I wonder what Baba's thinking?* my mind's narrator asked as I recounted his story as I had a thousand times before in my stump speech. I could see the corners of his eyes glistening.

The ammus *came!* Many of the leaders in the Muslim community who had told me that I was on a fool's errand—that the campaign would embarrass the community—were sitting together in the front, too. Two of them were even wearing Abdul shirts, albeit over collared shirts and pleated khakis, the classic *ammu* uniform. The Sunrise Movement—the young people whom America would come to know through their protest at House Speaker Nancy Pelosi's office and their advocacy for the Green New Deal that had just kicked off—were one of the most organized forces behind our ground effort to knock doors. They were sitting pretty close to the *ammus*—two groups of people who might as well have lived on different sides of the globe. *I wonder if the Sunrise kids and the* ammus *are going out for lunch after this? Hah!*

Indeed, this was a mass of people who, under no other circumstance, would have ever come together. Young and old; Black, Brown, and white; gay, lesbian, queer, trans, and straight; women and men; girls and boys; poor and rich—all of them in one big well of support.

As I hit the crescendo of my speech, I could see the crowd starting to stand up and clap. With each line, more and more people got to their feet—and they weren't sitting back down. When I finished, the roar was unlike anything I had ever experienced. *Not bad. Not bad at all*, my inner voice said.

And then I introduced Bernie. It was bedlam.

Not only did they stand, people just left their chairs and started walking to the rostrum. He and I shared a moment on the stage together, his hand holding mine triumphantly toward the sky.

After I left the stage, I found a small space just behind it where I could watch Bernie and the crowd he was speaking to. *This is a pretty cool seat for this Bernie rally*, my inner voice observed. By that point it had definitely become a Bernie rally.

* * *

Once Election Day rolls around, the candidate's job is basically done. There's nothing you're really going to do that's going to swing the election anyway. Sarah and I spent the day visiting polling places all over Michigan, particularly precincts that we knew would vote heavily in my favor. We wanted to thank our supporters for their energy, their enthusiasm, their well wishes—and their votes.

We began our morning in South Dearborn, in the city's Yemeni enclave. It was a relatively slow morning, but some of our poll watchers told me that it was more traffic than they'd seen in years. That was a good sign.

We were getting ready to leave, climbing into the SUV we'd rented for the day, when a brick-red minivan pulled in. It was full beyond capacity, and as it stopped, the doors opened and the family inside came tumbling out. The driver had launched out of his seat, hailing me. Just before we pulled out, I asked Jordan to stop the car and got out to meet him.

The driver, probably five years younger than I was, called back to his family in Arabic as he approached me: "It's him! It's him!" He gave me a big handshake and a hug and then pulled his phone out for a selfie. Meanwhile, my eye still on the van, I saw an elderly gentleman finally emerge from the passenger seat. He was dressed in traditional Yemeni garb, complete with his *janbiya*, a traditional ceremonial dagger worn in a scabbard on a belt. The younger man took me by the hand to meet his elder.

"This is Dr. Abdulrahman," he told the elder man in a thick Yemeni dialect. The elder man was his grandfather—a U.S. citizen for ten years now who had never once voted in an election. He didn't believe in them. But when he learned about me a few months earlier, he not only pledged to vote but called all of his friends to make sure that they and their families were planning to vote, too. He was there to make good on that pledge.

As I extended it to shake his and thank him for his support, he took my hand—but not to shake it. Instead, he raised it to his mouth and kissed it. In Arab culture, to kiss a hand is a tremendous gesture. It bestows honor and respect: it's a gesture reserved for one's grandparent, or one's teacher. To kiss the hand of someone forty years your junior is unheard-of. Immediately embarrassed, I tried to repay the honor, but he pulled his hand away. I settled for the traditional hug and kiss on the cheeks. Afterward he looked me in the eyes. "Today I am a real American," he said in Arabic. "Thank you. You've raised our heads. We are proud of you—no matter what happens."

* * *

We had gained so much momentum in the last month of the race that even late polls that had us losing were in doubt. But from the jump on Election Night, the returns looked awful. Within an hour after the polls closed, I knew that I'd been beaten. Although I earned 340,560 votes—enough to win any of the last several Democratic primaries—I lost by 22 points, finishing second of three.

I had prepared myself for the possibility of losing, and yet it still stings. I knew we had put it all on the line: we ran the best race we could have, inspiring hundreds of thousands to get behind a political newcomer named Abdul with no previous political experience. What's more, we had shaped the debate, driven the public conversation about the deep injustices in our system and solutions to address them. I was so proud of my team, who had given their all for a year and a half. They had learned, grown, and innovated in the process.

Truth be told, our campaign would have an impact on state and national politics for a long time to come.

And every cloud has its silver lining. As I prepared to give my concession speech, I asked one of my staffers how it was looking for Rashida. Rashida Tlaib was running for Congress in Michigan's Thirteenth District, encompassing most of Detroit and a few other suburbs, including Dearborn Heights, another town with a large Arab-American community. "Too close to call."

It would be that way late into the night. But when it was finally called, Rashida had won—by a mere 887 votes. Make no mistake: Rashida won because she was an excellent candidate who ran an excellent campaign. She was articulating a vision for her district that had a legacy of leadership on issues like universal healthcare, reparations, and labor rights. She knocked on every door in her district several times over and out-fundraised her opponents by hundreds of thousands of dollars.

It was comforting to know that even though I didn't win my race, she did—and our campaign might have helped. So much of our approach was focused on mobilizing communities of color across the state, with a particular focus on Arab- and Muslim-American voters in Dearborn, Dearborn Heights, and Hamtramck, a heavily Yemeni- and Bangladeshi-American enclave in the middle of Detroit. And in communities where we overlapped, if they were coming out for me, they were coming out for Rashida too. And vice versa.

I wouldn't be going to Lansing, but Rashida would be going to D.C.—one of two people to make history as the first Muslim women in U.S. congressional history.

* * *

I had spent eighteen months traveling Michigan—the state in which I was born and raised, a state I thought I really knew—learning it afresh. Bouncing between urban neighborhoods in Detroit and Flint and rural communities like Kalkaska and West Branch, I got to look people in the eyes as they shared stories and reflected on worries they'd kept buried, things they wouldn't dare tell a neighbor or even a loved one. I loved that parallel between medicine and politics: that people unburden themselves to you in hopes that you might help.

I thought that the conventional wisdom would be true—that the stories I would hear across these diverse communities would differ radically. After all, there's just no way that people dotting Michigan's farmland and populating its cities see their lives the same way. Yet in watering holes, VFW halls, and cozy living rooms in town after town, I'd hear the same stories, followed by the same questions. People would ask why, in a state literally defined by its fresh water, people still couldn't get potable water while corporations like Nestlé were bottling unlimited amounts of it for a few hundred bucks a year. Why did their kids' school look exactly the same as it did thirty years ago, while people like Betsy DeVos, a Michigan native, were cutting budgets and privatizing public education? Why do people still have to go bankrupt when they get sick—even if they have health insurance?

As an epidemiologist, I was trained to identify the patterns that converge from arrays of data. Here, those patterns were converging in real time, from interactions with thousands of people across our state. And rather than the differences that I had expected, I found that one glaring experience united the folks I met: they were suffering from the epidemic of insecurity. In the next two parts of this book I'll define America's insecurity epidemic. I'll describe its causes and its consequences. And then I'll discuss what it means for our politics—and how we can heal it.

PART II

AMERICA'S INSECURITY EPIDEMIC

CHAPTER 12

The syndrome.

When we finally reached the back entrance to the Detroit High School where he works, Darren apologized. "I know it's a really long trip—sorry to take you so far out of your way."

It *was* a long trip. I was shadowing Darren, a custodian and Service Employees International Union (SEIU) member, that morning. The journey— comprising about a mile's walk and two legs on city buses—had taken us about two hours. Darren makes this commute every day. In fact, both he and his wife do. They form the two-person custodial crew who make sure the school is neat and tidy every evening after a hectic school day. Each of them earns eleven dollars an hour. They haven't had a real vacation since they started—four years ago.

The drive from their home to the school would take about ten minutes in a car. And they have one, but they couldn't afford the car insurance. Few people in Detroit could: it was five times the national average. In Michigan all car insurance must, by law, include personal injury protection, covering medical costs for accident victims. This made it a form of health insurance, too, vastly inflating the overall cost. Worse, auto insurers can adjust rates based on where people live and credit information. Drivers in Detroit have routinely paid thousands of dollars more than their counterparts across city lines. Auto insurance has become a shadow form of redlining in Michigan. Facing higher premiums, too many are priced out of the insurance market, forcing the burden of insurance costs on the few who can pay, which raises their rates even further. Economists call this unraveling of an insurance market "adverse selection," and it has left about 50 percent of Detroiters "driving dirty"—without auto insurance coverage. New reform measures in mid-2019 have sought to address this, though advocacy groups fear that they won't go far enough.

The consequences can be dire. When I was in court for a hearing connected to an arrest I took at a union protest, I watched an elderly gentleman get fined and sentenced to one hundred hours of community service for driving dirty. If he couldn't afford the insurance, it's only logical that he probably couldn't afford the fine. Worse, the community service requires that he have transportation—the lack of which wound him up here in the first place. Poverty had set its trap, potentially leaving him mired in the legal system for years.

So, instead of all that, Darren takes two buses and walks a mile every day, both to and from work. His gig doesn't come with healthcare. No 401(k), either. The couple's daughter suffers from cognitive disabilities, and she's hit her maximum number of treatment visits covered under Michigan's MIChild program. They try to do the treatments with her, but they haven't been able to keep up between their work hours and the fact that, between them, they spend four hours commuting every day.

A defining feature of their life is insecurity. They lack the means—and the support—they need to live a dignified life. Without a good job or dependable public services, they always have to agonize over which needs in their lives to put first: car insurance or rent, treatment for a disabled child or the food she'll eat for dinner.

* * *

One evening after a five-stop campaign tour on the west side of the state, I got another perspective on insecurity. We were driving down east on I-94, a freeway that runs along the palm of Michigan's mitten, on the way back to our headquarters in Detroit. The sun was setting over the horizon behind us. As usual on any downtime between the hours of 9:00 a.m. and midnight, I was on the phone, dialing for dollars—those last hours reserved for California. This process, called "call time," is one of the worst things about running for office. Call after call after call, having the same conversation over and over again—only to be rejected. Call time is like baseball: if you're batting .300, you're killing it.

Because of the role that corporations and mega-donors have been allowed to play by our lax campaign finance laws, modern political campaigns have become a money game. Who can raise the most money fastest? Early money is a powerful indicator of your general appeal: the kind of coverage the media will give you, and the mind-space that the chattering class will afford you. More importantly, early money lets you stockpile funds for those all-important last eight weeks, when campaigns blow millions on television ads.

That evening I was on the phone with an old friend, Mike, with whom I'd grown up. After opening a successful medical practice, he made some smart investments, earning him quite a sum. He had the money to give, to be sure.

I was trying to convince him that he should make a five-hundred-dollar investment in my campaign. Chances are that if someone donates to your campaign once, they'll donate again. I knew that if he decided to get on board, he'd stay on board—and come through in the clutch as we rounded the bend toward Election Day.

But that first donation is always the hardest to earn. My friend was the kind of person who'd never given to a political campaign. Beyond voting, his engagement with politics amounted to what he watched on CNN or the conversations he shared with his friends on WhatsApp. After all, for most folks in our country, active engagement with politics is rare: unfortunately, to most, politics is something to be observed, but not participated in, save the first Tuesday after the first Monday in November every fourth year.

"It's an investment in the future of our state—a future that is more just and equitable," I told Mike in my most chipper, hopeful tone.

"Look, Abdul, I love you," he said, and having grown up together, I knew he meant it. "But why do you have to go after people like me?"

"What do you mean?" I asked. While I didn't know *for sure*, I had a pretty good idea. A few days earlier I had tweeted about how the 1 percent had dominated our politics—and that everyday folks needed to take our politics back.

"Dude, I'm part of the 1 percent you like to go after so much," he admonished. "I know you're a good guy and you want to do some great things for people, but why do you have to go after me to do it? It's already hard enough. Between the house, the kids' schools, and everything else, I'm struggling." And then a pregnant pause—to carefully consider what he wanted to say next: "It's like I'm poor—just in a different way."

In the same breath my friend had identified himself as part of the richest 1 percent of Americans and then called himself poor. An objective assessment of my friend's finances clearly supports only one of those claims. And the two are mutually exclusive: there is no such thing as a "poor" 1 percenter. Yet, although Mike is by no objective measure poor, he still thinks of himself as poor "in a different way." He feels anxiety about his future, and his kids' future, that robs him of the security his wealth would otherwise afford him.

* * *

Epidemiologists have to be specific when defining a disorder. That makes the "case definition" one of the most important early decisions: What does it mean to actually *have* the disorder and how do we measure it? After all, only after you've defined *exactly* what you're talking about can you then start to ask coherent questions about its causes—and that's the whole point of epidemiology. But defining disease is deceptively hard to do.

Consider this: What does it mean to have a "common cold"? Well, most of the time we think about it as some constellation of a set of symptoms—a runny nose, a sore throat, and a cough, perhaps—lasting somewhere between one and three days. But do you have to have all three to have a cold? And doesn't the flu cause similar symptoms? What if it lasts five days? Or two weeks?

It turns out that even a disease with the word "common" in its name is really hard to define, because there are more than two hundred different viruses that cause the same constellation of symptoms that we believe constitute the common cold. And symptoms can differ with each virus—and with each host. Some people get bad backaches when they have a cold. Others get teary eyes. Some get mild sniffles. Others feel like they've been hit by a truck.

You may be thinking, *Look, I just know when I have a cold.* That may be true for you, but epidemiologists think about populations, so it would have to be true for everyone. And perhaps you *can* self-diagnose a cold. Are you as confident about appendicitis? Misdiagnose a cold, and you'll probably be fine. Appendicitis? That's another story. It's why we have doctors.

When doctors talk about disease, they can't just talk about symptoms, because lots of diseases can have the same symptoms. A really bad headache can mean you're suffering a potentially life-threatening aneurysm. But it can also just mean you have a really bad headache. So doctors also talk about "signs." Whereas symptoms are subjective experiences that a patient reports to a physician, signs are objective observations that a clinician can make that aren't necessarily distinguishable to the patient.

Consider high blood pressure: high blood pressure doesn't cause symptoms unless it's dangerously high. No one shows up to their doctor's office complaining, "Doc, my arteries just feel terrible." Yet the sign of blood pressure can be measured quite precisely, easily, and cheaply; all you need is a blood pressure cuff, a stethoscope, and a trained eye. But despite the fact that we can measure blood pressure so readily, the precise definition of "hypertension," the medical name for high blood pressure, has been hard to pin down: what exactly constitutes high blood pressure has been an endless debate among medical researchers and physicians. In fact, in 2017 the American Heart Association and the American College of Cardiology moved the definition from 140/90 to 130/80 millimeters of mercury.[1] To appreciate how much that definition matters, particularly for a condition as common as hypertension, consider this: it resulted in a 44 percent increase in hypertension in America, overnight. Now 46 percent of all Americans—nearly half of them—are diagnosable as hypertensive.

But there's a bigger question here: If blood pressure doesn't actually cause any symptoms, why do we care about it in the first place? Well, even though hypertension may not cause symptoms, hypertension causes heart attacks (and strokes), and *heart attacks cause symptoms*: they kill more people than any other disease.

Importantly, just as there's not one common cold—a syndrome caused by hundreds of viruses—there isn't just one kind of hypertension, either. Hypertension also has a number of causes. In some people it can be caused by kidney problems; in others a tumor on the gland that secretes the hormones that regulate blood pressure; in yet others it can be a side effect of medication, or age, or a lack of exercise, or excess body fat, or some combination of intersecting causes. There can be many pathways to the same disease.

* * *

Compare Mike's life with Darren's: although the physical distance separating Mike and Darren is a mere twenty minutes down I-75, their lives could not differ more starkly. One lives in a mansion in one the richest counties in the country; the other lives in a small bungalow in one of its poorest cities. One drives a Mercedes; the other rides two public buses to get to work. One has a medical degree; the other never went to college. One owns real estate that augments his substantial earnings as a physician; the other earns eleven dollars an hour. Yet both suffer an anticipation of future helplessness—a sense of anxiety about what the future holds for them and their families. In fact, both Mike and Darren suffer insecurity. One's insecurity is motivated by a fear of loss, and the other's is motivated by the fact that he never had.

The same can be said of insecurity—what I believe is the defining economic and social disorder of today. What *is* insecurity? Psychologists talk about the more colloquial, internal "insecurity"—a subjective feeling of inadequacy or lack of confidence—as a consequence of repeated experiences of vulnerability to painful external stimuli like childhood trauma, rejection, or failure. The politically virulent strain of insecurity to which I refer here is, in short, fear for our and our loved ones' futures.

Like any disorder, insecurity has its symptoms. It can present as anxiety when contemplating one's finances. It can present as a sense that things are getting worse, not better. Or it can present as a feeling that our children will be worse off than our parents. Other symptoms of insecurity include longing for an idealized past, blame or hatred for a particular group, cynicism, and resistance to investing in the collective good for fear that others will benefit more.

And just as with the common cold or hypertension, there are several paths to insecurity.

* * *

American life expectancy has fallen for the third straight year—the longest-lasting downturn since World War I, when war casualties and pandemic flu combined to take hundreds of thousands of lives. Today, American war casualties are limited (although the casualties we inflict on the world are numerous), and, thanks to the flu vaccine, flu deaths are far less common than they used to be. Rather, Americans are losing their lives prematurely to a more ethereal but equally deadly set of diseases. In their analysis of the 2015 mortality data that first showed the beginning of the decline, economists Anne Case and Angus Deaton coined these "diseases of despair." Alcohol use, drug overdoses, and suicide have taken hundreds of thousands of American lives way too soon. They found that deaths attributed to these causes were much more common in a particular demographic: "Ultimately, we see our story as about the collapse of the white working class after its heyday in the early 1970s, and the pathologies that accompany that decline."[2]

The pathologies cluster. Substance use and mental illness co-occur often, as those struggling with mental illness often self-medicate with drugs and alcohol. These in turn exacerbate mental illness by introducing stressors that arise from chronic substance use.[3] Although Case and Deaton chalked these deaths up to what they call "despair," they may just as well have attributed them to insecurity.

This is the insecurity of the marginalized—of people like Darren. It afflicts poor and working-class Americans of all backgrounds. And though it is spiking among white working-class Americans, it has chronically affected Black- and Brown-Americans, Americans with disabilities, Americans of minority faith, and LGBTQIA+ Americans, especially—and those who fall into more than one of these groups even more.

And then there's paradoxical insecurity. It's the syndrome that Mike suffers from. It's the insecurity of the affluent in an unequal society, driven to acquire to protect their affluence, to guard their position lest they drop in class and join the marginalized. This syndrome of insecurity is rarer, given that affluence is less common. Nonetheless, it has outsized implications in our increasingly unequal society, which I'll discuss later.

* * *

A 2017 representative poll asked Americans about their levels of anxiety—a key symptom of insecurity.[4] It found that nearly two in three Americans reported that they were "extremely or somewhat" anxious. More than one in three were more anxious overall than the previous year. Young people were more anxious than previous generations.

In 2018, just one year later, another poll found an increase among all ages and demographic groups. When asked about their anxiety across five major areas—safety, relationships, health, finances, and politics—finances were a particularly important driver of overall anxiety. Nearly three in four women and the same proportion of young adults aged eighteen to twenty-four reported they were "extremely anxious" about paying bills.[5]

That may be because 78 percent of Americans report living from paycheck to paycheck.[6] That leaves Americans at risk of financial disaster if they suddenly lose a job or have to endure a payless payday—like the federal employees held hostage during the government shutdown over Trump's border wall during the 2018–19 holiday season. Complicating things further, three-quarters of workers reported being in debt, meaning lost jobs or paydays would mean even more debt to make ends meet, loan defaults, and destroyed credit scores, with long-term consequences.[7]

The situation is particularly dire for those earning minimum wage. Four in five U.S. workers report having worked a minimum wage job in the past, and 71 percent of them reported not being able to make ends meet. More than half had to take another job to make ends meet while working for minimum wage.[8]

Even among those earning $100,000 or more per year—which would translate into earning approximately $50 an hour over fifty weeks, or nearly seven times the federal minimum wage—nearly one in ten reported living from paycheck to paycheck. Six out of ten are in debt.

Indeed, even among millionaires worth between $1 million and $5 million, nearly half live with the anxiety of losing it all.[9] That number jumps to 63 percent for millionaire parents working full-time jobs. In fact, "most millionaires are worried their grandchildren will not have the same opportunities as their children."[10]

This insecurity is driven largely by the declining economic outlook of the middle class. Importantly, a 2015 report by researchers at the Federal Reserve analyzed economic realities among this broad swath of Americans—the 25th percentile to the 75th percentile of earners, earning from just over the poverty line to nearly six figures. The report concludes that the changing structure of our economy has meant that these families may "be under downward economic and financial pressure."[11] In fact, they found that today's middle-class children had to reach higher educational levels than their parents a generation ago to achieve similar real incomes, adjusted for inflation with time. The real incomes of those with similar educational levels declined over a generation. But these financial statistics offer only a glimpse of the quagmire of insecurity in which many Americans are struggling. Like quicksand, economic insecurity is both devastating and hard to escape.

* * *

Diagnosing an epidemic is one thing; healing it is another. And if we aim to heal it, we have to understand its causes and the mechanisms by which they cause disease. As discussed earlier, the concept of causation in epidemiology is by no means simple; rather, we discuss causal chains that intersect to weave webs of causation. This is particularly true for complex disorders, where feedback loops and social interaction influence the probability of disease.

Insecurity is a complex social disorder that is rife with feedback loops and interactions. To appreciate the complex causal mechanism of insecurity, it's worth revisiting the story of John Snow. Snow was a contagionist, meaning he believed that cholera was spread through some "poison" that later science would demonstrate to be microscopic bacteria. His main opponents in that debate were the miasmatists, who argued that there was something about the environment of poverty that was transmitting disease.

They had a point. In reality cholera, like insecurity, is a complex epidemic. Although exposure to the *V. cholerae* bacterium is sufficient to cause the disease, exposure is not a chance event. Rather, it is the function of various social, political, and economic dynamics. In Snow's time it was a matter of where different companies procured their water. In our time it's about the collapse of social and governmental order in places like Yemen, themselves the function of intricate geopolitics whereby more powerful countries like the United States and Iran compete for regional dominance through client states that both cause and sustain long, drawn-out civil wars. What the miasmatists were getting at is that our environment can shape our health in profound ways.

The thing about the environment, though, is that its impact can be hard to ascertain, because we're usually *all* experiencing it at the same time and so we can't readily identify how its variation may affect us.

To appreciate how subtly impactful the environment can be, ask people what they need to survive. High on every list are food and water. We appreciate how important these things are to our livelihood because we consume them several times a day. But rarely do people list air or oxygen. If all of the food on earth were to suddenly disappear, most of us would survive between three and four weeks; if all the water disappeared, perhaps three to four days. But if all the oxygen were to suddenly disappear, we would all suffocate in a matter of three to four *minutes*. It is because oxygen is so ubiquitous, such an intimate a part of our existence, that we don't pay it as much attention. It's almost *too* important.

And not only is our environment such an essential part of our experience that we forget about it, but that proximity makes it hard to appreciate small changes to it. Philosophers call this the "sorites paradox." It goes like this: If you had a heap of sand, and little by little you began to remove small amounts, when is it no longer a heap?

There's also the parable of the boiled frog. If you throw a frog into a pot of boiling water, the frog will reflexively jump out. But if you put that same frog into a pot of water at room temperature and slowly heat it, the increase in temperature would be imperceptible to the frog, and it will boil. (Who would want to boil a frog, anyway?)

Going back to our oxygen example: if, rather than removing all of the oxygen at once, it were to be removed slowly over the course of a month, it would be extremely challenging to perceive the changes over time. Nonetheless, the loss of oxygen would be just as lethal, suffocating us just the same.

To this end, it's extremely challenging to appreciate the consequences of changes in something to which everyone is exposed over a long period. This is a particular challenge for epidemiology. If everyone experiences the exact same thing, it's almost impossible to understand the consequences of that thing because there is no counterfactual—no all-important hypothetical contrast. Not only does the problem of the ubiquitous environment hobble our ability to answer certain questions, but, perhaps worse, it distracts us from even asking them.

Consider obesity. In 2011, scientists announced that, globally, the number of people who are obese had doubled since 1980.[12] Obesity is a worldwide epidemic and its consequences are profound, increasing the risk for heart disease, stroke, diabetes, myriad different types of cancer, and nearly every other bad thing that can happen to a body. Today, about 40 percent of American adults are obese. And so, in an effort to understand obesity, we ask whether there are any systematic differences between obese and non-obese people, as if that will tell us why obesity is increasing so rapidly. Reams and reams of epidemiologic research—including my own doctoral dissertation—have tried to understand this. Researchers point to genetic differences, psychological differences, community differences, and so on. But they're probably missing the biggest point of all: people, who have been around for millennia, really haven't changed that much in thirty years; what has changed is the global food environment.

However, appreciating the consequences of gradual changes that affect all of us is really hard to do. What happened thirty years ago? Let's start with the present and work backward: American farmers produce more than a third of the world's corn exports today.[13] They didn't always produce that much corn, though. During the Great Depression, grain farmers—who at that point constituted a much greater share of the overall population—suffered tremendously from the boom-or-bust cycles in agricultural markets. New Deal policies sought to remedy these. First, they instituted production limits to reduce the volatility resulting from production surpluses. In exchange, they instituted limited subsidies to support farmers to stay within the limits they had set.[14] And for the most part it worked.

Under Richard Nixon, though, that all changed. His overeager USDA secretary, Earl Butz, who served on the boards of several agribusiness firms, abolished production limits in favor of driving down the cost of commodity crops—and driving commodity food production.[15] He argued that, rather than limit production to keep prices high, global trade could off-load any excess American production.

That worked—for a while. Then President Jimmy Carter issued a grain embargo against the Soviet Union. That, coupled with a recession, devastated American agriculture. In response, the Carter administration vastly inflated farm subsidies to prop up America's suffering farmers.[16] And the subsidies only grew. Between 1995 and 2010, the American taxpayer spent $170 billion in subsidies for seven commodity crops[17]—much of that money going to corn.

The excess corn being subsidized by the American taxpayer flooded our food environment. It was packaged into new, innovative products, like the now infamous high-fructose corn syrup, as well as corn oil. Corn became ubiquitous in the American food supply, including in meat: rather than grass, livestock farmers began to feed their animals corn on the cheap.

The tragic irony here is that increasingly obese American taxpayers are subsidizing the means of their own obesity. Indeed, nearly half of the earnings of the average Iowa corn farmer comes in the form of federal subsidies.[18] And a study by researchers at Emory University found that higher consumption of these subsidized grains was associated with a higher probability of being overweight.[19] Yet, throughout the 1990s, the real price of fruits or vegetables—which are not subsidized—increased by 40 percent. The real price of a can of Coke dropped by 80 percent.[20]

But because these changes have been both ubiquitous—affecting the global price of food for everyone—and gradual over decades, their effects are extremely difficult to appreciate. What's more, it's nearly impossible to test them scientifically. To run a hypothetical experiment to see whether or not the changing food environment changed the probability of obesity, we would have had to compare the global obesity rates according to two situations: the present reality and an alternative, counterfactual one where we could go back in time and hypnotize Nixon into naming a different USDA chief who would keep the New Deal production limits where they were.

* * *

Like our food environment, our sociopolitical environment has changed drastically over the past several decades. Yet, like frogs, because it has happened gradually, we can't fully appreciate just how hot it's gotten. Drastic increases in inequality, the changing structure of the economy, persistent structural racism, racial and socioeconomic physical segregation, ideological segregation resulting from structural changes in the nature and consumption of media—all of these have, over time, created the circumstances for insecurity. They have created a miasma, if you will. Alone, each of these factors would be dangerous enough—but their consequences in concert have created the circumstances in which we find ourselves today.

In the next several chapters, I explore this miasma in parts. I draw larger and larger concentric circles around our lives. I start with our health—the most intimate and individual cause of insecurity—and then move outward to our households, our communities, our economy, and our politics.

CHAPTER 13

Insecure health.

American life expectancy lags behind other high-income countries. American maternal and infant mortality outcomes are woeful. But perhaps worse than the averages are the deep inequalities that characterize American health. Epidemiologist Christopher Murray and his team set about articulating demographic clusters of health patterns in our society and suggest that, rather than one, coherent American experience, there are actually *eight* different Americas.[1] Across them, the team identified a twenty-one-year life expectancy gap between the longest-lived group, Asian-American women, and the shortest-lived group, urban Black-American men. These inequalities are stunning, considering that twenty-one years is a quarter of a life span—even among the longest-lived Americans.

Those at the bottom end of American life expectancy are those for whom insecurity is a clear fact of life—their lives cut short because of it. Today the diseases of despair mentioned above are disproportionately affecting low-income non–college-educated white Americans. However, one should not forget that they've been devastating low-income communities of color for decades, creating inequalities in health by race and socioeconomic position that have long been traceable if one chose to look for them.

American healthcare is ineffective. It is inefficient. And it is inequitable—and that is principally because the healthcare system has been constructed around the goal of profiteering on sick bodies rather than healing them. American healthcare is simultaneously among the most advanced and impressive in the world—and dollar for dollar the worst performing. That said, if you're insured, the United States is statistically one of the best places in the world to get cancer: your likelihood of surviving it is higher than almost anywhere else.[2]

But that's only if you're insured. Nearly 10 percent of Americans are not—an oddity among high-income countries, of which we are the only one that doesn't guarantee basic health services to its people. Millions more are underinsured. They have insurance, yet they lack reliable access to health-care because they can't get to a doctor who takes their insurance or they can't afford the high out-of-pocket costs. So mortality because of more preventable diseases, like heart attack or stroke, is substantially higher in the United States than in other high-income countries.[3]

For the under- or uninsured, illness lands a one-two punch. If illness itself doesn't ruin their lives, the financial calamity that follows is sure to. Insecurity takes root when people are more concerned about the financial hardship of illness than the illness itself. Nearly 2 million Americans a year are forced into bankruptcy by healthcare debt.[4] In fact, it is the leading cause of personal bankruptcy, outpacing credit card and mortgage debt.[5]

In fact, even those cancer statistics I quoted above—the fact that the United States is one of the best places to be diagnosed with cancer if you're insured—come with a cost. Nearly 62 percent of cancer patients report going in debt to pay for their cancer care.[6] And 42 percent of cancer patients reported depleting their life savings within two years of their diagnosis.[7]

How do we explain this? American healthcare has been dominated by powerful industries that have put their bottom lines ahead of our collective wellbeing. They include the insurance industry, the hospital industry, and the pharmaceutical industry. They work together to sustain the system and their primacy in it, all the while maintaining the illusion that they're protecting choice and preserving the "free market" in healthcare. In truth, they have done more to decimate any semblance of choice. They offer the greatest healthcare money can buy, but because they have built the system around their financial gain, they have all but left out those without the means to pay.

To explain: Imagine I were to start clutching the left side of my chest, a sign that I might be having a heart attack. I should hope that the good people around me would call 911. An ambulance would appear and rush me to the nearest hospital. And that's where my false choices would begin.

There are far fewer hospitals in the United States than there were even twenty years ago. In fact, there have been 1,600 hospital mergers during that period, leaving many communities covered by a single major health system. But this alone already means that any semblance of choice I had regarding where I might get my care is gone. Once I'm at the hospital, being seen by an emergency room doctor, I await the results of a series of tests that the doctor will interpret to decide how I'll get treated. Do I have a choice regarding my doctor? No. Do I have a choice about my treatment? Not really. I'm at the mercy of the doctor, hoping he or she has diagnosed me correctly. I can't really shop around, because every second counts.

This is what economists call an "information asymmetry" between the doctor and me. Doctors both diagnose and treat us when we're ill, meaning they both tell us what to buy and then sell it to us. And because most of us don't know enough to disagree with our doctors, we are at their mercy and can only hope they will be honest with us. It's a classic conflict of interest, a situation analogous to going to the mechanic. If your car were to start making an odd sound when you hit the gas, and your mechanic tells you that you need a new cranking fly, which will cost you $1,500, you don't know enough to object that a cranking fly is not actually a thing. That's called "upselling." Of course, you might choose to get a second opinion, but that's hard to do when you're having a heart attack.

One would think that doctors, who've taken an oath to "first, do no harm," would never try to sell you healthcare you don't need. But the evidence suggests otherwise: like mechanics, doctors who make more money offering more services routinely offer more services.[8] In fact, if you're a doctor looking to learn how to upsell, you can find a handy article on Practice Builders (PracticeBuilders.com), a website that will teach you how to do it; it's titled "Increase Your Practice Revenue by Up-Selling and Cross-Selling."[9]

So we've established that I have almost no choice about where I get care, which doctor I see, or what care I get. There's another oddity. If you were to walk into any other establishment to buy something, they'd show you a price list. But no one ever showed me a list of the costs I would incur for my care. And when it's time to settle up with the hospital for the care that I received, I get a bill for the services, with prices I'm only seeing now for the first time. But then, I don't actually pay that bill. I'm insured, thankfully, so my bill actually goes to my insurance company. Instead, I'm left to pay some proportion of the cost based on my co-pay and deductible, depending on what kind of insurance I have.

Unfortunately for many Americans, high-deductible plans, which don't kick in until you've paid several thousands of dollars, are increasingly common today because health insurance has gotten so expensive. They're a big reason why so many people facing catastrophic or chronic illness are pitched headlong into debt even though they have health insurance. The average deductible for a family health plan is around $2,500 dollars, and nearly a quarter are $5,000 or more.[10] That's nearly 10 percent of what the median American family of four earns every year.

And that's if my insurer agrees to pay. One tactic insurers use to protect their all-important bottom lines is to flat out reject certain claims. If my insurer rejects my claim, I'll be forced to spend hours on the phone haggling for the coverage.

But how did they come up with those prices? Well, my insurer negotiated the prices they'd pay for various services in a supersecret process that only the insurance company and the hospital are privy to.

This is why hospital consolidation is closing down so many rural hospitals. Hospitals and insurance companies use their negotiations with each other to reward size and scale. Both use these negotiations to try to price out smaller competitors and then buy them. In the end, each region is usually left with just a few dominant hospital chains and a few dominant insurers, basically local micro-oligopolies. And then they jack up prices. One study found that after hospital mergers, even though operating costs for hospitals decline, the average cost of hospital care increases by 6 to 18 percent on average.[11] With higher hospital prices come higher insurance prices. Fewer people can afford insurance, and more people go without it. But the bottom line for hospitals and insurers always stays strong.

Americans also pay more for prescription drugs than any other country in the world. That's because we're one of the few high-income countries that has no public system that negotiates with drug manufacturers to reduce the prices of prescription drugs or to buy them in bulk. For example, if I were to receive a medication prescription in New Zealand, the country's Pharmaceutical Management Agency, or Pharmac, would have negotiated the price for me—which is why New Zealand's prescription drug costs have stayed relatively stable. In the United States, there is no such negotiation. While insurance companies have an incentive to negotiate prescription drug prices down, they're usually not big enough to have the bargaining power they need to do this. Medicare— the public insurance provider for Americans over sixty-five and with certain disabilities—covers nearly sixty million Americans. In theory, Medicare would have the size and power to negotiate on behalf of this huge group of people. But Medicare is barred from negotiating the price of prescription drugs on behalf of its beneficiaries *by federal law.*

All told, the costs of prescription drugs in America—already the highest in the world—are skyrocketing. The average American spent twice as much on prescription drugs in 2017 as she did in 2001.[12] And in a 2019 public opinion poll, nearly one in four Americans reported that they found it difficult to afford their prescription drugs. And for that reason, three in ten reported not taking their prescribed medications at some point in the past year.[13]

Big Pharma likes to tell us that our prescription drugs are so expensive because of all the innovation that they're doing. But these costs aren't driven by innovation, just corporate price hikes. That was the finding of a report published in *Health Affairs*, which found that, though the medications themselves hadn't changed much, prices for brand-name oral prescription drugs increased by more than 9 percent a year, while prices for injectible medications increased by more than 15 percent a year between 2008 and 2016.[14]

The case of insulin—a life-sustaining medication for people with certain forms of diabetes—is instructive. Insulin has not changed substantially since it was discovered nearly a century ago at the University of Toronto. In fact, its discoverers sold the patent rights for a dollar because they knew how critical it was. Nevertheless, the price of insulin doubled between 2012 and 2016.[15] Despite a few new bells and whistles, insulin is still pretty much insulin.

And even when there is innovation, these costs keep it from getting into the hands of people who need it. My grandfather in Egypt—the one who sold vegetables in the fish market—died in the early 2000s of hepatitis C, a viral liver disease that slowly destroys that vital organ over time. He got hep C from a blood transfusion during a knee surgery he had in the U.S. while he was visiting us in the early '90s, before blood banks screened for hep C. Although far more common in Egypt, hep C is the leading infectious disease killer in the United States.[16]

In 2011, Gilead, a major pharmaceutical company, announced that they had purchased the company Pharmasset, a small company that had spun out of an academic laboratory, for $11 billion. Pharmasset had one compound of particular promise in its pipeline: a drug called sofosbuvir, which would come to be sold under such brand names as Sovaldi and Harvoni, depending on the formulation. The initial research behind sofosbuvir was conducted by Professor Ray Schinazi, a professor at Emory University, funded by grants from the federal government, through the National Institutes of Health and the Veterans Affairs Administration.

Sofosbuvir was, at the time, the only known cure for hep C. In its Sovaldi formulation, Gilead priced it at $84,000 a course (more than $1,000 per pill)—this for a course that cost Gilead $136 to make.[17] This pricing kept the potentially life-saving medication out of the hands of people who needed it. But don't worry, Gilead's bottom line is safe: in its first five years, Gilead raked in $25.8 billion on sofosbuvir, multiplying its initial investment money many times over.

That includes $4.5 billion from Medicare—in 2014 alone. It was one of the most expensive drugs on the Medicare formulary for several years running. That means that huge amounts of federal money are being spent on a medication that originated as a federal research project, leaving the American taxpayer paying twice. And because Medicare is barred from negotiating drug prices, they're left to the whims of the drug manufacturer.

Which brings us back to Egypt. Given the high prevalence of hepatitis C in Egypt, the Egyptian government realized that the existence of a cure meant that it could set up a plan to try to eradicate the disease. But for a country with one-twenty-fourth the GDP per capita of the United States, the $84,000 price tag was steep,[18] so the Egyptian government rolled up its sleeves and negotiated with Gilead, denying them a patent in Egypt and allowing manufacturers to sell generics in the Egyptian market. Gilead responded by licensing the drug at a 99 percent discount, selling a twelve-week course for $900.[19]

* * *

Whereas other aspects of American healthcare have been hijacked for private gain, America's mental health infrastructure is just woefully inadequate. But mental illness is on the rise nationally, increasing substantially over the past several years.[20] Among young people ages twelve to twenty, the prevalence of mental illness jumped from 8.7 percent in 2005 to 11.5 percent in 2014.[21] One in five American adults will experience a mental illness in a given year.[22] And mental illness and substance abuse go hand in glove.

But the burden of mental illness and substance abuse in America vastly outstrips our ability to treat it. The federal Health Resources and Services Administration estimates that by 2025 our country will be short of behavioral health professionals by 250,000 workers.[23] In fact, in 2016, more than half of all counties in the United States had zero psychiatrists.[24] And more than half of practicing psychiatrists are over fifty-five.[25]

Worse still, community mental health clinics and hospitals are woefully under-resourced. Even as we face growing need for mental health services, states have passed $5 billion in cuts to mental health services in the past decade. Between 2005 and 2010, the number of state psychiatric beds decreased by 14 percent. Thirteen states eliminated at least 25 percent of their state psychiatric hospital beds.[26]

Amid chronic underfunding of state mental health systems, corporate healthcare is chomping at the bit to take this over, too. In Michigan, for example, state mental health services are organized through a system of ten regional authorities that manage services. The system is by no means perfect, although most of the issues that arise are in some way connected to chronic underfunding. A report by the Community Mental Health Association of Michigan outlined five key improvements, every single one of which was designed to improve funding to the system.[27]

And yet, when the system ran a $92.8 million overage in 2018, state officials were receptive to a move by the Michigan Association of Health Plans, a trade organization for the state's private health insurance corporations, to privatize mental healthcare in Michigan. Indeed, as early as 2016, Governor Snyder had proposed privatization of the system. However, part of the reason regional mental health authorities had been running overages was because of a massive influx of patients, as outlined in the Community Mental Health Association of Michigan report.[28]

Substance abuse—in particular opioid use—has become a national emergency. Over the past decade, what started as a rural epidemic has invaded suburban and urban communities alike, decimating lives and livelihoods. Between 1999 and 2017, drug overdose deaths in the U.S. nearly quadrupled.[29] Opioid use has also led to a resurgence in heroin use, and the increased sharing of syringes has caused massive spikes in blood-borne diseases such as hepatitis C and HIV.

The opioid epidemic is a corporation-created crisis. Manufacturers of prescription opioids knowingly and calculatingly peddled their medications in low-income rural communities, which were particularly susceptible to drug dependence. Purdue Pharma, makers of OxyContin, the wildly addictive opioid medication widely blamed for setting off the epidemic, waged a full-frontal lobbying campaign to drive prescriptions for its drug.

In fact, when I was in medical school, I was taught that pain was the "fifth vital sign": that if a patient's pain was not properly medicated, I had failed my duty as a clinician. I was never taught how addictive opioid medications could be or warned about the risk of overdose. Purdue purposely misrepresented the academic literature and manipulated medical boards to perpetuate the myth that opioid painkillers were safe and effective, with risk of addiction lower than 1 percent.[30]

The rural communities that opioid manufacturers targeted were particularly susceptible to this disease of despair.[31] Insecurity had long since taken hold in these economically depressed areas, which had been ravaged by mass migration and the loss of jobs due to automation. In that respect, these diseases are both a cause and a consequence of insecurity: a consequence because those most susceptible to substance use and addiction often turn to substances to numb the anxieties of financial, social, and psychological vulnerability; a cause because they exacerbate those circumstances, forcing opioid users to dig themselves deeper and deeper into debt to escape the dope sickness that trails ever closer that last high.

Without the resources to treat rising and overlapping epidemics of mental illness and substance abuse, we will inevitably shunt these problems onto the criminal justice system. But consider that one in six men and one in three women in jail have a serious mental illness.[32] Choosing not to invest in treatment and resources for people with mental problems means that, in many cases, we will have to pay for their incarceration instead.

* * *

Health is *the* fundamental resource; without it, little else matters. In that respect, our failure to ensure equitable access to affordable healthcare has become a deep source of insecurity in America. The risk of losing your healthcare or the consequences of having to give up your life's savings to regain it are a critical source of insecurity for too many Americans.[33] A representative survey found that 15.5 percent of Americans in 2016 were "healthcare insecure," meaning they reported "not having enough money in the past 12 months to pay for necessary healthcare or medicines for themselves or their families."[34] Nearly one in six Americans reported being unable to afford their medications in the past year.[35] And even among those who can afford healthcare today, the anxiety of losing health insurance is profound: The majority (57 percent) of Americans lack confidence that they or their loved ones will have access to affordable health insurance sometime in the future.[36] By allowing our healthcare system to be dominated by massive corporations, we have ceded power over our bodies and minds to the financial greed of very few, leaving most of us with the precariousness of having to pay for increasingly unaffordable healthcare in the moments when we can least afford it—when we and our loved ones are ill.

CHAPTER 14

Insecure households.

Unlike many children of divorce, I grew up in a home with two parents, my father and stepmother. I also maintain a loving relationship with my mother. And yet, the emotional challenges of my childhood—the divorce itself, the distance from my mother throughout my grade-school years, and the work of reengaging with a parent and siblings with whom I did not grow up—challenged me in profound ways. They still do.

I think often about my parents' choices—both to marry and to divorce. My parents married because they shared the same values. While they were together, each was committed to the other and the concept of marriage itself. They had barely met each other when they got married, but my mother put her blossoming career as a physician on the back burner to join her husband halfway across the world, where they were immigrants, struggling to build a life for themselves without the help of their families. And within a short time they had a new son.

Conservatives often decry the loss of "family values." Yet, conveniently, these family values are left undefined. It's an "if you know, then you know" kind of thing. But it seems that by "family values" they mean the ideals and mores of a mythical white, suburban, upper-middle-class Anglo-Saxon Protestant nuclear family with a male breadwinner, a female homemaker, and their biological children. But families that have to deal with the adverse circumstances that the real-world poses—even those that match the (extremely limited) demographic I just described—are rarely able to live up to the standard of that mythical family. But that hardly matters to the folks who believe in this ideal, because it really only serves as a foil for shaming all the other real families—families like mine with real people, real problems, and real adversity to face. Worse, this image has been used to actively discriminate against families that don't look like it—like LGBTQIA+ families—with respect to marriage, adoption and child-rearing, and inheritance rights.

In his book *The Conservative Sensibility*, columnist George F. Will argues that "the nation's most destructive social problem" is "family disintegration." Not rising inequality, not devastating poverty, not stagnating earnings, not unaffordable healthcare or metastasizing war or the rising cost and diminishing quality of our education system, but "family disintegration."

The problem with "family values" as a concept is that it ignores the circumstances that shape the dynamics of a family. It assumes that every family has agency over their own lives. Speaking with thousands of voters across the state, it became clear that the fate of most households—like mine—is less a function of values and more a consequence of external circumstances.

The household remains the principal unit of human organization in most of our lives, whether we live in something that looks like *Leave It to Beaver* or a loft with five of our friends. The household is the most important lens through which we come to understand ourselves and our place in the world. And the circumstances facing households has never been more dire.

In the 1980s, when my parents got married, divorce was at its peak: fully 50 percent of marriages broke off in divorce. Furthermore, because couples married younger and had children earlier, the probability that these divorces affected children was higher, too.

I was born in 1984, and my parents divorced soon after having me. I am not alone in my generation. Many of my childhood friends and classmates were also children of divorce. We lived the reality, at best awkward and at worst deeply and profoundly painful, of watching our parents struggle through it. We lived through the complications of multiple households, sometimes pawns in the conflict between parents, with the double jeopardy of somehow feeling to blame for it all. The costs of our parents' divorces are written in the long-term outcomes of our lives. Indeed, a twenty-five-year follow-up study of children of divorce found that 25 percent experienced serious long-term psychological or emotional challenges. These issues were 2.5 times more likely to occur in children of divorced parents than in children whose parents had not divorced.[1]

Today the probability of divorce is down to around 40 percent. It would be tempting to assume that this is because couples are simply choosing to stay together. However, the available evidence suggests it's because they are being far more selective about whom they marry in the first place. This, I believe, is in part a function of my generation's intimate understanding of the human costs of divorce.

There's something else, too. A 2019 study that considered the causes of the decline in divorce showed that millennial couples are marrying later than previous generations.[2] The average age at marriage was thirty for men and twenty-eight for women in 2018, compared with twenty-seven and twenty-five, respectively, fifteen years ago.

Although marriage is happening later, cohabitation has become far more common. In 2018 the proportion of Americans aged twenty-five to thirty-four who were living with a cohabiting partner was 15 percent; it was 8 percent in 2000. By contrast, the proportion living with a spouse in 2018 was 40 percent, compared with 54 percent in 2000. As attitudes toward partnering and cohabitation have changed, marriage is becoming a destination in a relationship rather than an early step.

This certainly *feels* true. Sarah and I are an anomaly for our generation: we got married at nineteen and twenty-one, respectively, and have stayed together for thirteen years (and counting!). But only over the past several years have we been inundated by wedding invitations, followed a few years later by birth announcements, from our classmates from college and graduate school.

These couples who "reach" marriage have often tested their relationships for longevity and, perhaps more importantly, addressed in advance the structural issues that often lead to divorce. In her book *Marriageology: The Art and Science of Staying Together*, journalist Belinda Luscombe argues that these structural and often financial issues are a critical hurdle to a stable marriage. She writes: "Young couples are delaying marriage not because they're waiting to find The One, but so that they can feel financially secure. And as jobs for those who stopped their education at high school have become more tenuous, and as income inequality has pushed the have-lots and have-somes further apart, that security recedes further into the distance for a lot of young couples."[3]

In that respect, material insecurity may be robbing young couples of the potential to marry. It may also be driving them to cohabit in the first place: less-educated Americans tend to cohabit sooner, and those who cohabit sooner are less likely to get married in the long run.[4] The secondary effect for children is devastating. Nearly 50 percent of children born to cohabiting parents are unplanned.[5] The children of unmarried couples are nearly 2.5 times more likely to endure a parental breakup by age nine than the children of married couples,[6] and nearly one in three solo parents is living in poverty.

Among the 40 percent of marriages that dissolve, 21 percent cite money problems as a key a reason. To complicate matters, nearly 60 percent report being driven into debt by the divorce itself.[7]

* * *

Debt is a major source of insecurity for American households. The average American household carries more than $137,000 in debt, including credit card, student loan, auto loan, and mortgage debt. That's more than twice the median household income.

Two forms of debt are particularly toxic. The first, because of its incredibly high interest rates, is credit card debt. The average American with credit card debt owes just under $7,000—although they have to make more than $1,000 a year in interest payments alone. In fact, one in ten Americans say they don't see a path out of their credit card debt.[8]

The other form of toxic debt, and one of the fastest-growing, is student loan debt. The average family owed $5,400 in student debt in 1989; that's ballooned more than sixfold to $34,200 today.[9] This has largely been driven by the explosion in the cost of higher education.

Young people recognize that the prospect of student debt hamstrings them at the very moment they are most vulnerable: when they first enter the job market. Meanwhile, we keep hearing statistics about how young people aren't buying houses, when in fact they are too bogged down with student debt to even dream of homeownership.

At a town hall I attended in an affluent suburb while on the campaign trail, a seventy-two-year-old gentleman made the best argument for addressing the student debt crisis that I have heard yet. A middle-aged woman asked a question about my position on student loan debt. When I began my answer about the exploding cost of higher education and the need to address this, I heard an audible harrumph from the corner of the room. My answer always seemed to get the boomers angry.

But today, this older gentleman stood up and bailed me out. "I went to the U of M in 1968. I had to pay seven hundred fifty bucks for my tuition—and another fifteen hundred for my room and board. I could make about three thousand bucks working odd jobs over the summers, so I'd have a little extra for beer money."

I could see the more silvered heads nodding in agreement. "Now my grandkid's a freshman at the U of M. Her tuition is fifteen thousand bucks, and her room and board are another fifteen thousand bucks. Now, I don't know many folks who can make thirty thousand bucks in a summer, especially not as a freshman in college."

Student debt hits us multiple times. Servicing their own student debt is one of the key costs young people face just as they're starting their careers, while saving enough to send their own children to college bedevils them thereafter. Furthermore, only about 32 percent of Americans have a college degree, although an additional 18 percent have some college education but never completed a degree.[10] The prospect of student debt remains an important reason for both dropping out of college and for never attempting to go to college at all.

Consider Keisha, the young Flint woman I mentioned in the Prologue. She was one of the top graduates of her high school class—receiving a partial academic scholarship to the University of Michigan–Flint. However, she was forced to drop out, caught between unpredictable hours at her part-time job at McDonald's and the need for income to help offset the costs of her uncle's medical care. Keisha told me she wants to be a nurse—I have no doubt that she'd be great one, and we need more nurses. But material insecurity may rob her of that opportunity.

* * *

It's not just how little money people have that causes insecurity; it's how they bank it. In a 2017 survey, the Federal Deposit Insurance Corporation (FDIC) reported that 8.4 million households—nearly one in fifteen—were unbanked, meaning that nobody in the household had a checking or savings account. An additional 24.2 million were underbanked, meaning those households had to rely on an alternative financial services provider, something like a money order, check cashing service, or payday loan.[11]

The primary cause of being un- or underbanked is poverty. More than half of respondents to the FDIC survey of unbanked households said they simply didn't have enough money to keep an account open. Nearly a third reported they simply didn't trust banks. A third also suggested that banking fees were prohibitive. Indeed, many banks require high minimum balances or high start-up fees that serve as obstacles to lower-income consumers.

Being unbanked introduces households to huge financial risk. First, being unbanked is extremely expensive.[12] Alternative financial services carry serious fees. Walmart charges six dollars just to cash a check greater than a thousand dollars. Payday loans, for example, can charge annual percentage rates as high as 500 percent. But the poor lack the resources to maintain an account, so instead they end up paying substantially more for these alternatives, adding another source of insecurity to their lives.

* * *

When Sarah and I realized that she was pregnant, Sarah was a medical resident and I was in the middle of a statewide campaign for governor. We knew that one of the most immediate challenges we'd face was providing care for our daughter, given the challenges of our careers—and the fact that neither of us was making much money. Running for governor pays nothing, and we were living on Sarah's residency salary.

Maternal leave is not a consistent benefit for many Americans, including medical residents. Sarah's hospital—one of the few hospitals in the country where residents have unionized—had granted her the union-negotiated six weeks of paid maternity leave. But Sarah had complications from labor and was instructed by her providers (at that same hospital) that she would need another four weeks. When she notified her department, they tried to deny her disability and any further paid leave. The union had to step in to enforce their contract. After ten weeks, she was back at work.

Thankfully, both Sarah's parents and mine live in Michigan, and my heroic mother-in-law agreed to care for Emmalee during those crucial first eighteen months. So we bid adieu to our apartment in downtown Detroit and moved in with my in-laws. We were lucky to have a loving, capable family member who could care for our baby, but here's the rub: my in-laws live in Macomb County, Michigan, a full sixty miles from Sarah's residency in Ann Arbor—meaning she had to make a ninety-minute commute each way.

Providing childcare shouldn't require women (or men, but almost always women) in our society to make such sacrifices. And yet, for so many families in America, it does. On average, childcare costs nearly $10,000 a year, and it is more expensive on average than college in twenty states.[13] That is nearly one-fifth the median family income. It's no wonder that half of U.S. families report difficulty finding childcare.[14]

Worse, of thirty-five countries in the Organisation for Economic Co-operation and Development (OECD), the United States is the *only one* that doesn't guarantee some form of paid maternity leave or family leave. The Family and Medical Leave Act of 1993 only requires employers to give twelve weeks of *unpaid* leave, meaning you can't be fired but you probably won't be paid; only 17 percent of employers in the private sector provide any paid maternity leave at all for their employees. The rest of American mothers are either expected to go without any income or immediately return to work after having gone through childbirth—assuming, of course, that the new mothers are healthy enough to work after labor.

The consequence of the overwhelming cost and logistical challenges of child-rearing is that working parents are forced to work less or take pay cuts—and sometimes are forced out of the workforce altogether—to care for a child. Because of the structural inequity in our society, this burden disproportionally falls on women. A survey by the Center for American Progress, a public advocacy group, found that women were 40 percent more likely to report that they had sustained a negative impact on their careers due to childcare.[15] Furthermore, women who had challenges finding adequate childcare were significantly less likely to be employed.[16] Beyond the injustice borne by women, this has substantial implications for families, too. The lost earnings can delay or stop a family from buying a house and also reduce how much they can invest in college funds or retirement savings.

This also has important implications for society at large. The nonpartisan Council for a Strong America estimates that our childcare crisis is costing our economy nearly $57 billion a year in lost earnings, revenue, and productivity.[17] Since more of the burden for childcare falls on mothers, the childcare crisis only perpetuates the gender pay gap and the shortage of women in key positions of leadership in business and government. Being forced out of the workforce often sidelines promising women just as they are ascending in their careers, damaging their long-term prospects. In 2018 a paltry 5 percent of Fortune 500 companies had female CEOs.[18] Meanwhile, women account for a mere 28 percent of state legislators and less than a quarter of the United States Congress. Here, too, our broken parental support policies may play a role. When Liuba Grechen Shirley ran for Congress in 2018 in New York, she had to petition the Federal Elections Commission—which oversees election spending—for permission to use campaign funds for childcare while she campaigned.

* * *

Finally, one of the key targets of "family values" arguments is a person's right to comprehensive family planning. Antiabortion arguments are flawed for many reasons. Antiabortion activists and politicians completely undercut the rights of women to have autonomy over their own bodies—and that's simply unjust.

Their arguments are also illogical. First, they tend to completely misunderstand the complexity of obstetric medical care, abstracting away the fact that abortions late in a term are often medically indicated, resulting from life-threatening risk. Second, and perhaps most illogically, though the best way to prevent an abortion is to prevent an unwanted pregnancy in the first place, opponents of abortion, by and large, are unwilling to embrace universal contraception access, defaulting to ineffective "abstinence-only education."

Furthermore, the same conservatives advocating "pro-life" policies out of one side of their mouths tend to oppose support for children and families out of the other—whether in the form of paid family leave, or universal childcare, or even investments in the foster system. Although they claim to value the lives of children, they consistently undercut our society's means of doing so.

* * *

Our daughter was born into a family of privilege: the financial security of her parents' socioeconomic positions, and a two-parent household with the love and care of grandparents on both sides. Too many children are not so fortunate. One in five children lives below the federal poverty line. An additional one in five is considered low-income.[19] Furthermore, nearly five hundred thousand children are circulating through the foster system on any given day—and that number is increasing.[20] Additionally, 39 percent of children live in a home with only one parent or neither parent (but with another relative).[21]

This is often the consequence of household instability, which can expose children to trauma with deep, long-lasting consequences. In 1998, Dr. Nadine Burke Harris and her research team began to explore the results of adverse childhood experiences (ACEs) on long-term wellbeing. ACEs are all-too-common experiences that can range from neglect and abuse to markers of household dysfunction, like substance use, divorce, physical abuse by a parent, and parental incarceration. The team's research estimates that at least 64 percent of adults have experienced at least one ACE during childhood,[22] Using a ten-question battery, they created an ACE score—a simple tally of yes answers[23]—and found that higher ACE scores predicted everything from alcohol use and divorce rates to cholesterol and autoimmune disease.[24]

Most profoundly, they found that adverse experiences in childhood can even rewire young brains. Studies have shown that institutionalized children had less gray matter[25] and that children who had been exposed to adverse childhood experiences had weaker connections between parts of the prefrontal cortex and the amygdala—leading to a higher probability of anxiety and depression.[26] There's also evidence that ACEs change the way our bodies behave at their most elemental level: that they lead to changes in the way our genes are switched on and off—particularly across genes that may help control stress and the wiring of the brain[27]—with possible implications for disease risk later in life.[28]

* * *

Americans are, thankfully, living longer lives than ever before. The Census Bureau projects that in 2030, nearly one in five Americans will be over sixty-five, and seniors will outnumber children.[29] That's because diseases that would have been a death sentence in the past—like a heart attack or a stroke—are regularly survived today. However, they often leave considerable disease and disability in their wake, and the burden of providing care and support to survivors too often falls on the generation below them.

However, too many seniors lack support. And more need it. When President Franklin D. Roosevelt signed the Social Security Act in 1935, he said, "The civilization of the past hundred years, with its startling industrial changes, has tended more and more to make life insecure . . . [W]e have tried to frame a law which will give some measure of protection to the average citizen and to his family against the loss of a job and against poverty-ridden old age."[30] But in 1935, living through one's eighties was far less common. Today, seniors must ration their savings over a much longer time, putting too many in financial strain.

What's more, the cost of living longer has increased dramatically. As noted earlier, prescription drug costs have skyrocketed, and more than three-quarters of adults over sixty-five take at least one prescription medication a day, and more than half take at least four.[31] Nearly a quarter of seniors chose not to fill a prescription they were given, most of them because they could not afford it.

Today, nearly 10 percent of seniors live below the poverty line. Poverty in old age is particularly common for seniors of color, women, and people living alone.[32] Poverty and disability often leave seniors dependent on people whom they cannot trust, which has increased the incidence of elder abuse. One in ten elder adults in our society is the victim of abuse, which includes neglect, physical, emotional, or sexual abuse, and financial exploitation.[33] And yet, because seniors are often dependent on those who abuse them, cases are rarely reported.[34]

The advent of material insecurity in old age has secondary consequences for younger Americans as well. In fact, sixty-five million Americans—nearly one in three—are providing care for a member of their family, and spending an average of twenty hours per week doing so. The Caregiver Action Network estimates the value of the services they provide for free at \$375 billion, twice as much as is actually spent on nursing services and home care.[35] And nearly 78 percent of adults in need of long-term care depend on a friend or family member as their only source of support.[36] As with childcare, the burden of care falls disproportionately on women, who account for two-thirds of family caregivers, and nearly half report that the care burden caused them to use up most or all of their savings.[37]

Many of these caregivers have children, compounding the challenges. One survey found that a third of parents with children ages eight to fourteen were also caring for an aging family member.[38] This "sandwich generation," caught between the challenges of providing for both children and aged adults, feels the strain most acutely.

* * *

Housing is another serious driver of insecurity in our society. Sociologist Matthew Desmond, author of the landmark book *Evicted: Poverty and Profit in the American City*, estimates that in 2016 there were 2.3 million evictions; that's one every four minutes. For families who are evicted, it shakes the literal bedrock of their lives. Along with their homes, they lose the place to situate themselves, their belongings, and their relationships. They are forced to move and sometimes to scatter, disrupting the lives of family members and straining the bonds that hold the family together. Eviction is particularly devastating for children.[39]

When I was working in Detroit, I saw how the threat of eviction on trumped-up grounds intimidated renters into not testing their children for lead. We realized that getting families access to tenant defense lawyers had to be a critical part of our lead program.

Eviction is on the rise in large part because the cost of housing has skyrocketed even as median household income has stagnated. Between 1995 and 2018, the median asking rent increased nearly 70 percent. Although there are federal and local housing assistance programs available, they are limited in availability: only one in four families who qualify receives aid. That leaves many families paying upwards of 80 percent of their income on rent.

Because rental applications ask about previous rentals, an eviction can mark a family for years to come, reducing their access to available housing or putting onerous restrictions on their rental, increasing the probability of the next eviction.

We cannot ignore the role that race has played in the skyrocketing of rents in major U.S. cities, which has been largely driven by upper-middle-class white Americans leaving the suburbs their parents and grandparents built a generation earlier and returning to cities. In doing so, they have driven up rents and largely displaced low-income Black and Brown residents. For example, between 2000 and 2007, New York City lost nearly 570,000 units of affordable housing.[40] Homelessness soared.[41] When a Whole Foods Market opened in the middle of Harlem in 2017, I knew the neighborhood was long past the gentrification tipping point.

Evictions have important implications for neighborhoods, too. Beginning in the 1990s, social scientists began describing factors like "social cohesion" and "collective efficacy," markers of trust and goodwill in local communities. They used these factors to explain why different neighborhoods with similar socioeconomic characteristics experienced different levels of crime and social disruption. Evictions devastate a neighborhood's social cohesion, breaking the neighborly bonds, which take time to form.[42] This has long-term consequences for the social welfare of those living in these neighborhoods—even if they never experience an eviction themselves—as property values decrease and social disruption and crime increase.

* * *

Insecurity strikes American households not just through broken relationships, debt, education, childcare, senior care, and housing but also through the food we eat. Food insecurity remains an epidemic in America, affecting one in eight Americans, twelve million of whom are children. The USDA defines "food insecurity" as the "household-level economic and social condition of limited or uncertain access to adequate food."[43] Food insecurity results because a family lacks the resources to buy food—but also because they may not have affordable food readily accessible.

This was often the case in Detroit, a massive city where the low population density makes it hard to support much commerce, including quality grocery stores. Furthermore, because few Detroiters can afford to drive in the city, and public transit is notoriously spotty, families are often limited with respect to their ability to travel to buy food, so they spend too much money on a limited supply of unhealthy foods available nearby. People are left eating foods that are high in the *macro*nutrients that grow a belly (fats and carbohydrates) but low in *micro*nutrients that nourish a brain.

* * *

For too many American households, particularly Black households, many of these forms of insecurity result from having fathers, brothers, or sons stolen away by mass incarceration. To get a sense of the scope of this, consider that for every one hundred Black women who are not in jail, there are only eighty-three men.[44] The equivalent number among whites would be ninety-nine. In New York City alone, that adds up to a deficit of 118,000 men.

That's because we've allowed the erection of a prison state in the United States. Under the guise of "law and order," we've constructed a system of policing, sentencing, and incarceration that systematically targets men of color. In the thirty-five years between 1980 and 2015, the prison population quadrupled from nearly 500,000 to 2.2 million.[45] Black-Americans bear the brunt.[46] Nearly 70 percent of incarcerated people in America are people of color.[47]

How did this happen? Under President Nixon and then President Reagan, "tough on crime" attitudes were leveraged to deconstruct the "war on poverty"—era policies of the Kennedy and Johnson administrations. Rather than invest in housing, education, and jobs, tax dollars were spent on police forces, war matériel, and prisons. In the late 1990s, criminologist Jim DiIulio advanced the theory of the "super-predator," which gave a veneer of intellectual rigor to age-old racist tropes and conspiracies that young Black men were lazy, hateful, and prone to acts of violence.

Writing in the *Weekly Standard* in 1995, DiIulio described these super-predators: "We're talking about elementary school youngsters who pack guns instead of lunches. We're talking about kids who have absolutely no respect for human life and no sense of the future . . . And make no mistake. While the trouble will be greatest in black inner-city neighborhoods, other places are also certain to have burgeoning youth-crime problems that will spill over into upscale central-city districts, inner-ring suburbs, and even the rural heartland."[48] DiIulio was invited to brief then president Bill Clinton in late 1995, and in 1996 in New Hampshire, then first lady Hillary Clinton said, "They are not just gangs of kids anymore. They are often the kinds of kids that are called 'super-predators'—no conscience, no empathy."

Words have consequences. When I had my run-in with the two cops in the early 2000s in a swanky Detroit suburb, I wonder how much this stereotype played—directly or indirectly—in the police officers' minds. For too many young men and women, boys and girls, these kinds of encounters have ended in lost lives. These lives are disproportionately likely to belong to Black-Americans.[49] That's what happened to Terence Crutcher, Philando Castile, Alton Sterling, Shereese Francis, Aiyana Jones, Walter Scott, Darnesha Harris, Alesia Thomas, Eric Harris, Tony Robinson, Miriam Carey, Sharmel Edwards, Rumain Brisbon, Tamir Rice, Laquan McDonald, Michael Brown Jr., Eric Garner, Tanisha Anderson, Aura Rosser, Freddie Gray, Sam DuBose, Jamar Clark, Malissa Williams, Natasha McKenna, Jeremy McDole, William Chapman II, Akai Gurley, Stephon Clark, Paul O'Neal, Christian Taylor, Keith Scott, Sean Bell, Shelly Frey, Shantel Davis, Oscar Grant, Amadou Diallo, India Kager, Yvette Smith, Rekia Boyd, and, unfortunately, many others. We must remember their names because statistics without names and stories only serve to obscure the humanity behind the statistics.

These words have also driven the election of "tough on crime" prosecutors and judges—leading to harsh sentencing and putting many more lives behind bars. Statistically, the National Research Council found that arrests per crime haven't increased over the past thirty years: we're not catching a higher percentage of "bad guys."[50] Instead, even as crime rates have fallen, incarceration rates have skyrocketed, driven by punitive sentencing by prosecutors and judges. "Three strikes" laws, mandatory minimums, and truth-in-sentencing laws have landed more people in prison for longer. Again, the burden has fallen disproportionately on Black-Americans. For example, although illicit drug use is no more common among Black-Americans than it is among the rest of the population, they account for 29 percent of those arrested for drug-related offenses and a third of those incarcerated in state facilities for drug-related offenses.[51]

Beyond the staggering human cost of incarceration, the financial cost is immense. In a 2015 study of forty-five states, the average overall cost of incarceration was just under $1 billion annually per state—up to $8 billion in California. That represents an average cost per inmate of $33,274 a year.[52] In Michigan it's about $47,000 per prisoner.[53] For context, the University of Michigan estimates that it costs about $31,358 to attend the university as an in-state student for a year—inclusive of tuition and fees, books, supplies, housing, meals, and other costs.[54]

Even after release, the consequences of incarceration are clear. Like Ammu Othman, a criminal record reduces the chance that a prospective employer calls you back by 50 percent.[55] Unable to find jobs in an economy actively allowed to discriminate against them, the probability of recidivism among formerly incarcerated people remains high, perpetuating a vicious cycle.

* * *

Perhaps one of the most peculiar aspects of household insecurity in America is how many of us feel *alone*. A survey of about twenty thousand Americans found that nearly half of Americans report sometimes or always feeling lonely or left out, and about half report that they share meaningful, daily face-to-face social interactions with others. One in five report that they rarely or never feel close to people. Worse, younger people report the highest likelihood of loneliness.[56]

Loneliness hurts. Not only is it emotionally painful on its own terms, but it's also bad for our physical health, increasing the probability of chronic illness and shortening our lives. It also has profound implications for our culture.

The cultural advent of "incels," short for "involuntary celibates," a misogynistic online community of men who blame women for denying them sexual relationships, speaks to the ways that extreme loneliness can be dangerous. Incels have become synonymous with a spate of mass murders: one shot up a yoga studio, killing two, in November of 2018; another went on a rampage near the University of California, Santa Barbara, in 2014, killing six.

* * *

If insecurity emerges from anticipating future helplessness, then nowhere is it more apparent than in the decisions we have to make about our future. But these are the decisions that make a life. The decision to get an education, to marry, to have a child, to buy a home—each of these has become a source of insecurity for too many Americans.

Insecurity creates feedback loops, being both symptom and cause. The choice to pursue higher education is blocked off from too many promising young people because they can't afford to take on the debt. Lack of higher education traps people in poorly paying jobs with limited benefits. Those limited benefits make the decision to have children an economic calculation: Can you afford a safe home for that child? Can you take leave to care for her? What if you get sick? What if you're living in fear of eviction or struggling with a father, brother, or son (or mother, sister, or daughter) in prison?

We are afflicted by an epidemic of insecurity because the circumstances within which we live no longer support us in the ways they used to. In the next two chapters we will explore how the very places in which we live, learn, work, and play have become sources and compounders of our insecurity. I will first consider the role of our social environment and then the role of our physical environment in driving the insecurity epidemic.

CHAPTER 15

Insecure communities.

Metro Detroit is one of the most segregated metropolitan areas in the country: the city is 80 percent Black, while neighboring counties are nearly 80 percent white. And although the economic challenges of the region extend across the city border, there is a difference. In Detroit, structural and institutional racism—economic discrimination, residential exclusion, and systematic disinvestment—compound those challenges, resulting in more poverty, more pollution, worse schools, and fewer opportunities. Not only do suburban residents largely avoid this structural racism, but suburban policies vis-à-vis Detroit have also helped to amplify them.

There's a rare birth defect called twin-twin transfusion syndrome, in which two fetuses share one placenta, which shunts a disproportionate amount of the mother's nourishment to one of the infants, all but starving the other. But the condition is potentially fatal to *both* twins. Between 1992 and 2019, when he passed while in office, L. Brooks Patterson, the longtime Oakland County executive helped architect Detroit's demise through a municipal version of twin-twin transfusion syndrome. By attempting to deprive Detroit of business development opportunities, control of its own water and sewerage, or its main convention hall, and consistently opposing regional collaboration, like public transit, Patterson set the stage for the entire region's current challenges. Young people are leaving the region in droves for places like Chicago, New York, Los Angeles, and Washington, D.C., thriving urban communities that seamlessly connect to their residential suburbs. Meanwhile, starved for young talent, our region in metro Detroit has struggled to attract new industries, contributing to its economic stagnation.

But instead of pointing at the folly of failed leadership like Patterson's to explain regional economic stagnation, suburban residents often point to government programs that focus on Detroit (and often fail to deliver). *Why them and not me?* creeps into the subconscious and turns their political attention toward undoing these programs (which is why they often fail), rather than building desperately needed regional infrastructure that might support metro Detroit as a whole.

This is how segregation drives our epidemic of insecurity. And Americans are extremely segregated—by race, socioeconomic position, and even political preferences. Even decades after the *Brown v. Board of Education* decision, the abolition of the Jim Crow laws, and the passing of the Fair Housing Act, segregation is the truth of American geography. The average white-American lives in a community that is 75 percent white, while the average Black-American lives in a community that is 65 percent people of color.[1] Although the redlining and racial covenants that were once used to enforce this segregation may have been outlawed, many of the policies, norms, and pressures that maintain segregation still exist.[2] For example, zoning that requires large lots and high square footage per unit is often designed to keep lower-income, often Black and Brown people out of high-income, usually predominantly white communities.[3] And housing discrimination by landlords and real estate agents persists.[4]

As discussed, as wholesale gentrification continues to relocate white Americans into historically Black and Brown neighborhoods, increasing rents have forced those very same people of color out of them.[5] Segregation by socioeconomic position is vastly increasing.[6] And school segregation is patterning the next generation in the same mold. Today, 75 percent of Black students attend "majority-minority" schools, as do 80 percent of Latinx students.[7] Both are more likely to attend schools where 60 percent or more of the students live in poverty.[8] In the South, school segregation has been increasing since the early 1990s, approaching levels similar to when *Brown v. Board of Education* forcibly integrated them.

Segregation changes the character of a neighborhood. As wealth leaves, poverty concentrates in a community, reshaping its businesses, lowering the quality of its schools, and devaluing its homes—the most critical wealth assets of low-income homeowners. Worse schools, worse options for healthy food, increasing crime—these all shape life opportunities in poor neighborhoods. Several studies have even documented the influence of living in segregated communities on reducing the life expectancy of Black-Americans.[9]

* * *

Segregation by income and race has led to segregation by political preference. "Red" states are becoming redder, "Blue" states bluer: In 1976, only about 25 percent of Americans lived in a county where one of the candidates for president won by 20 percent or more; in 2016 that was up to 80 percent.[10] The Pew Research Center considered why and found that lifestyle preferences may differ with political leanings: liberals preferred smaller homes in more walkable communities, whereas conservatives tended toward larger homes that are farther apart.[11] Ultimately, urban communities increasingly vote Democrat, while rural communities run to the GOP. Coastal states—more cosmopolitan and diverse—vote for Democrats, while the South is deep Republican territory.

The implications of segregation for our polarizing politics are clear. In 2008, journalist Bill Bishop wrote *The Big Sort: Why the Clustering of Like-Minded America Is Tearing Us Apart.* In an interview with *Governing* magazine after the 2016 elections, he said, "The result is that you have increasing populations where people talk to those who agree with them politically. They hear stories and facts and figures that support their beliefs.

"Over time, social psychology research will tell you that these like-minded groups become more extreme in the way that they're like-minded. Put a group of conservatives in a room and they'll become more conservative. It's just the same with liberals."[12]

Our media environment has also segregated, tailored to reinforce our preconceived beliefs. It serves as an echo chamber and magnifier of these trends. But it wasn't always that way. There *was* a time when the media brought Americans together. In a 2013 paper, a pair of economists at Harvard considered the impact of the introduction of broadcast radio and television in the 1920s and 1950s, respectively, on political polarization.[13] They hypothesized that broadcast media would draw Americans closer together politically with similar, unifying messages. In analyzing historical data from that time, that is in fact what they found. It follows that the modern era of hyper-tailored media would have the exact opposite effect.

In fact, in a recent report by Reuters and Oxford University on seven hundred thousand surveys from thirty-six different countries, American media was found to be the most polarized: only 51 percent of left-leaning Americans reported trusting the news, and a mere 20 percent of right-leaning Americans reported the same. About the same number (19 percent) of conservatives visit Breitbart.com, while a whopping two out of three watch Fox News.[14]

Nearly all media, but especially the conservative media, are notorious in their portrayals of people of color to play up racist stereotypes.[15] Considering that such stereotypes are disproportionately consumed by people who, as a consequence of demographic physical segregation, rarely interact with people of color in real life, it is no wonder that our tax dollars flow to prisons largely filled by Black men and we fight wars abroad to protect ourselves from people who look like me. Never mind that, between 9/11 and the end of 2016, more acts of terror were committed on U.S. soil by white supremacists than by people acting in the name of radical interpretations of Islam.[16]

But traditional media is quickly becoming an anachronism. More than two-thirds of Americans get their news on social media today. And this is where it gets weird—because so much of it just isn't real. One analysis of engagement on Facebook during the 2016 presidential election found that the top twenty fake news stories about the election earned more engagement than the top twenty real news stories from nineteen major news outlets.[17] These can be traced to fake news farms like RealTrueNews.org originating in places like Veles, Macedonia, where young people looking for a few extra bucks of ad revenue have figured out how to dupe us all.[18]

But they're not alone: Facebook is a platform that purposefully built out and implemented algorithms designed to serve us only what they think we will click, not what is accurate. In 2016 the *Wall Street Journal* launched an interactive project called "Blue Feed, Red Feed"—a side-by-side view of two Facebook feeds, one that a "very liberal" Facebook user might see, the other what a "very conservative" user might see. The feeds can be toggled across issues, like healthcare, Trump, and immigration. The results display our national polarization in a shocking side-by-side comparison.

When I clicked on "Immigration," the first post in the liberal feed was from the ACLU: "Officials are not doing enough to detect and respond to incidents of sexual abuse in immigration detention," with a link to the article. In the conservative feed, the first post was from Breitbart (though I reject the premise that the ACLU is at all comparable to Breitbart!): "Presenters and winners at Sunday's Academy Award's [*sic*] ceremony once again took the opportunity to preach their political opinions, with Hollywood stars lecturing viewers at home on everything from Holocaust-level racism in America today to the importance of immigration."[19] Facebook has sorted us into our own echo chambers, where every piece of "news" is tailored to our preexisting beliefs. Couple that with a tailored broadcast television environment—and racial, economic, and political residential segregation—and you can see why our national conversation is so polarized. What's in it for Facebook? The all-important ad revenue. And that's not changing anytime soon. Facebook spent $12.6 million in lobbying and $2.2 million in candidate contributions in 2018 to make sure it doesn't.

The polarization of our traditional and social media, coupled with the advent of fake news (*actually fake* news), has muddled truth and falsehood. When you have a hard time knowing what is real, how do you construct a perspective on the world? These two trends have played right into the frankly fascist narrative that actual journalism by actual journalists at actual news organizations is "fake news." When your president tells you that the news media are the "enemies of the people," who do you believe?

Oh, and that "friend" who shared that article from RealTrueNews.org probably wasn't real, either. Whole armies of sock puppets (I bet you've never imagined an army of sock puppets; I told you it was going to get weird)—people who are paid to pose as someone else on social media—and bots—fake online accounts used to propel a message on social media—were created by Russian intelligence's "Internet Research Agency" to expressly interfere with the 2016 election. Their goal was to sow discord and misinformation in our electorate—and ultimately to undermine faith in our democratic institutions.

In their book *LikeWar: The Weaponization of Social Media*, P. W. Singer and Emerson T. Brooking detail how this new online reality came to pass—how the confluence of tech trends that put a smartphone in every hand, put the Internet on every smartphone, and targeted content on every platform made social media a weapon of war. In an interview with the Verge, Singer noted that social media has enabled "simultaneous personal connection as never before, but also the ability to reach out to the entire world. The challenge is that this connection has been both liberating and disruptive. It has freed communication, but it has also been co-opted to aid the vile parts of it as well. The speed and scale have allowed these vile parts to escape many of the firebreaks that society had built up to protect itself. Indeed, I often think about a quote in a book by a retired US Army officer, who described how "every village once had an idiot. And now, the internet has brought them all together and made them more powerful than ever before."[20] We can only expect these trends to get worse, as new machine learning technologies are allowing people to create "deep fake" videos portraying real people saying things that they in fact have never said.

* * *

There is no issue that better captures the insecurity inspired by segregation than immigration. We have a unique national dissonance about immigration: on the one hand, we hear the familiar popular mythology celebrating America as a "nation of immigrants" (implicitly ignoring the experiences of Black- and Native-Americans), and on the other we hear the fascist cries of "Go back to your country!" Often these views are held by the same people.

Although the United States hasn't always been kind to immigrants, immigration has been kind to the United States. A recent study by the Brookings Institution found that every percentage-point increase of immigrants with a college education raises the average number of patents per person by 12.3 percent, while each percentage-point increase in immigrants with an advanced degree raises the average patents per person by 27 percent.[21] Immigrants grow the American economy and pay their taxes. In fact, more than half of America's billion-dollar start-ups were founded by immigrants. Collectively, those companies are worth about $248 billion and employ about sixty thousand people. And anyone who's ever watched the Scripps National Spelling Bee can tell you that the children of immigrants perform relatively well in school.

But immigration is an easy target for insecurity. There is no greater manifestation of the "other" you don't know than people who were born and raised in another country. By definition, they are foreign, and the notion of having to compete with them over scarce jobs exacerbates the material insecurity of an unequal, unjust economy.

Donald Trump understood how to play this issue up in the national psyche throughout his 2016 presidential campaign. He had one clear message—so clear, in fact, that his supporters would chant it at rallies: "Build that wall!" In three words, he excavated his base's latent insecurity and made it tangible.

To his supporters, the wall was meant to protect "us" from "them" after all, implicitly pegging all of "our" economic woes on immigrants who are coming to take our jobs. Indeed, Professor James Gimpel of the Center for Immigration Studies in Washington, D.C., argues that immigration "was one topic of consistent message discipline in an organization that many called untidy and haphazard."[22]

Since his election, Trump has used his platform as president and his control of the country's immigration infrastructure to create more discord around immigration—by means of the Muslim ban, family separations, shutting down the government over border wall funding, and concentration camps at the border. All of this serves to unify his base. All of this seeks to exploit their insecurity.

* * *

Gun violence is another serious contributor to insecurity in our communities. I was in the eighth grade in April 1999 when one of the first major mass shootings, at Columbine High School, left thirteen dead and twenty-four wounded. I remember talking about the incident with my class—the shock and horror of armed students coming into school to kill their classmates.

Few of us could imagine that it would become the new American reality. Since Columbine, the epidemic of mass shootings has only grown. In December 2012, a gunman entered Sandy Hook Elementary School in Newtown, Connecticut, and killed twenty children, only six or seven years old, and six adults. And in February 2018 an expelled former student walked into Marjory Stoneman Douglas High School in Parkland, Florida, and killed seventeen people with a semiautomatic rifle.

And these are just major mass shootings at schools. Between Sandy Hook and the twenty-year anniversary of Columbine, in April 2019, there were more than two thousand mass shootings in which four or more people were shot. They took nearly 2,300 lives and wounded almost 8,400.[23]

But the most common homicides by gun don't happen en masse. While these mass shootings are horrific, gripping the national attention for days on end, gun homicide usually only takes one or two people at a time— usually people who knew the gunman. There are nearly thirteen thousand

gun homicides per year.[24] The victims of these homicides are disproportionately likely to be Black. Black-Americans make up 54 percent of all victims of homicides by gun but only 13 percent of the population. Indeed, gun
homicide is the leading cause of death among Black-Americans ages one to
forty-four.[25]

But the most likely person to die by gun is the person who pulls the trigger. Nearly 60 percent of all deaths by firearm in the United States are deaths
by suicide.[26] That's an average of fifty-nine deaths a day—and that number is
on the rise.[27] The increase is sharpest among children, increasing 61 percent
over the past ten years. Half of all deaths by suicide are by gun,[28] and guns are,
by far, more fatal than any other means of attempted suicide.[29]

American gun violence—and gun access—are a complete outlier relative
to similar countries. In 2017, America's rate of deaths by gun violence was
nine times higher than in Canada.[30] Meanwhile, there are nearly ninety guns
per one hundred Americans—almost three times as many guns per capita as
in Canada. In fact, Americans own nearly half of all civilian-owned guns in
the world.

The reason is simple: America has some of the laxest gun access laws in
the world. Military-style assault weapons, banned in many other high-income
countries, remain perfectly legal. And we lack laws that allow for the removal
of guns from owners if they are reasonably suspected of using them for violence against themselves or others.

In other countries, major gun reform has followed mass shootings. For
example, after a student killed fourteen of his classmates at a Montreal engineering school in 1989, Canada passed major reforms, including a twenty-
eight-day waiting period before purchased guns are delivered; detailed
background checks; bans on high-capacity magazines and military-style guns
and ammunition; and mandatory safety courses.[31] After gunmen killed wor-
shippers at two Christchurch mosques in New Zealand, their parliament voted
119 to 1 to ban military-style semiautomatic weapons.

Our lax gun laws are due to major political opposition by gun advocacy
groups like the National Rifle Association (NRA), who lean on an extremist
interpretation of the Second Amendment to mean that anyone should be able
to have any gun at anytime, anywhere. And they have spent millions of dollars to make this extremist view an inviolable plank of the Republican Party.

Meanwhile, because of this advocacy, Americans continue to die at gunpoint. These deaths are preventable. Gun advocates argue that the problem is not the weapon but the person who pulls the trigger. They point to stabbings and other forms of violence in countries with strong gun laws. But knives are far less deadly than guns. They require close-range contact, can't be used in rapid-fire succession, and are more difficult to conceal. There's a reason we don't send troops into combat armed only with knives. The weapons of war that the NRA and others are defending are designed to kill many people quickly. And that's exactly what their users choose them for.

Watching the parents of children sob on television because of completely preventable violence drives our insecurity. After all, what's to stop our children from being next? Meanwhile, gun advocates tell the vast majority of gun owners who use guns responsibly that it's a slippery slope to ban the kinds of weapons that are used to kill people rather than hunt deer—that their weapons will be banned next. Meanwhile, Americans are dying around us.

* * *

Our segregation—physical and intellectual—tends to leave us interacting with people who look like us: same race, same income, same education, same political preferences. This narrows our thinking by secluding us from people whose lives are different from ours. Rather than engaging with people from different walks of life through interactions at a VFW hall or bingo night, we're surrounded by those who reaffirm our worldviews. More commonly, we're alone, scrolling social media feeds designed to serve us material that certifies our worldviews. This drives our insecurity by convincing us that we're constantly under threat by some "them" just beyond the edge of our own community—and that we have to protect ourselves.

It also has serious implications for a diverse, pluralistic, multiracial, multiethnic, multifaith country like ours and makes it difficult to forge a path of collective action, as our democracy was intended to. In the next chapter we'll consider what it has meant for maintaining our shared public infrastructure.

CHAPTER 16

Insecure places.

In Michigan in August 2016, days of heavy, humid heat alternated with days of torrential rain—as if the atmosphere were wringing itself out like a giant wet sponge. Over time, these cycles have gotten more severe—not just in Detroit but across the country. For residents of Detroit's East Side, these cycles usually mean one thing: flooding—and 2016 was a particularly bad year. Although I usually had to pay more attention to the heat side of the equation rather than the rain side, this year was different.

That month I learned that two men had been diagnosed with hepatitis A, the least serious of the forms of hepatitis, though still deadly. Hepatitis literally means inflammation of the liver, and that's exactly what it does, causing abdominal pain, vomiting, stomach upset, and the characteristic dark urine and yellowing of the eyeballs that indicate liver disease. Rather than being transmitted by blood or sexual intercourse, the hepatitis A virus moves from victim to victim via what scientists call "fecal-oral" transmission, cloaking it in scientific terms to spare listeners the gut-churning (both literally and figuratively) implications. A bout of hep A usually only lasts for a few weeks, and most healthy people recover without any lasting complications—but it can be far more serious in seniors or people with underlying liver diseases.

Hepatitis A is a reportable disease, meaning that providers who diagnose it are required to contact their local health department. And given the route of transmission, the first thing I wanted to know was if they had come in previous contact with anyone who had had the disease. Neither man had any known contacts. In fact, the only potentially relevant history—one they shared in common—was that they had both been cleaning basements that had been flooded with sewage because of the rains.

According to the CDC, contact with sewage is not a risk factor for hepatitis A, meaning that the incidence of the disease does not increase among those who have been in contact with it. While that may be true at the population level, it certainly remains plausible that contact with raw sewage *could* transmit the disease; it's just that hep A is so uncommon in the United States, the chances of someone introducing the virus into the sewage system are exceedingly low.

Considering that contact with raw sewage was the only plausible exposure for two different people, I was concerned. The implications were daunting. Hundreds of homes had flooded. That meant that potentially thousands of people might have come in contact with hepatitis A–infested waste.

Hepatitis A has a long incubation period, meaning the symptoms don't appear right away. Instead, the virus has to make its home in your liver before it starts to cause its characteristic problems. That can take up to fifty days but averages about twenty-eight. And critically, if the hep A vaccine is administered during that period, it can avert the onset of symptoms. If we assumed that the two men were in fact exposed while cleaning sewage out of their basements, and the sewage was the cause of their disease, then there was still time to provide city residents with the vaccine and prevent countless cases of hepatitis A.

We had to act. My team and I decided that we needed to immediately set up a makeshift vaccination clinic in multiple locations across the city, then get the word out to residents about the potential hepatitis A risk and urge anyone who might have come in contact with sewage to come to the clinic for a vaccination.

When I called the state's health department, I asked for their advice. They cited the CDC guidelines in an effort to avoid having to get involved. I shot back that the CDC guidelines don't tell you what to do when you have two cases of hep A whose only plausible source of exposure was sewage.

"Sorry, we're just following protocol," they said. It was a classic bureaucratic dodge, the kind of bureaucratic obstinacy that leaves so many people so frustrated with government. Worse, some in the mayor's office were worried it "wouldn't be good optics." If bureaucratic intransigence is one reason for people's frustration, brazenly putting political interest over government responsibility is its flip side.

Optics be damned: hepatitis A is a potentially deadly disease. I demanded to see the mayor. Although he was understandably annoyed at the situation, he assented to my request both to set up our makeshift clinics and to hold a press conference to educate people about what had happened and what our response would be.

Within a few days we had erected two vaccination clinics in the city. To procure the vaccines that the state's health department had denied us, we sidestepped them entirely, instead going directly to the manufacturers.

Beyond the immediate need to avoid a possible outbreak of hepatitis A, there was another reason for offering the vaccine. Put simply, Detroiters had little reason to trust their health department, which didn't even exist a few years earlier. In the context of rebuilding the Detroit Health Department, it was critical that we be proactive. Had we failed to act, it might have confirmed their low expectations and distrust.

The old adage that "it's better to be safe than sorry" is basically the operating credo of public health, and I'm glad we were proactive, although there's no telling how many cases of hepatitis A our intervention prevented.

* * *

We don't often have to think about infrastructure—whether its infrastructure we can see, like roads or bridges or streetlights, or infrastructure we can't, like water and sewer pipes. That is, until it fails us. And the fact that we pay it little heed before it fails makes its failure all the more alarming. It's jarring to realize that something to which you paid so little attention can impact your life so critically. It's more jarring to realize that it's failure can literally kill you.

And when it fails often—as American infrastructure has begun to—it becomes another source of insecurity. Our transit, electrical, and water infrastructure have all shown their vulnerability in recent years. The American Society of Civil Engineers (ASCE) issues infrastructure report cards across the United States. Their last federal report card, in 2017, gave the United States a D-plus overall.[1]

What's worse, in the grandest sense, is the fact that the earth offers (for now) the absolute limits of our infrastructure. Climate change has clear implications for our infrastructure—just as our infrastructure has clear implications for climate change.

* * *

"Social infrastructure"—a term coined by sociologist Eric Klinenberg, who wrote a book on the subject titled *Palaces for the People: How Social Infrastructure Can Help Fight Inequality, Polarization, and the Decline of Civic Life*—was defined by him in an interview with CityLab as the "set of physical places and organizations that shape our interactions."[2] It refers to libraries and community gardens, parks and public athletic fields—places that foster social engagement between people in a community. Klinenberg argues that, just as investing in social infrastructure can facilitate public interactions between friends, loved ones, and strangers, when we neglect our social infrastructure, it can promote loneliness and isolation.

American social infrastructure is decaying. Although the ASCE doesn't grade social infrastructure just yet, Klinenberg argues that if it did, our grades would be "shameful."[3] That's because of cuts to important social infrastructure institutions like libraries and parks. For example, the Massachusetts Department of Conservation and Recreation has seen its budget cut by $30 million between 2001 and 2015.[4] Similarly, the Trump administration's fiscal year 2019 budget proposed a $481 million cut to the National Park Service—one of the most beloved social infrastructure agencies in the country.[5]

* * *

That's not the only infrastructure we're underfunding. Whether it's an obnoxious pothole we have to veer around every morning on the way to work, absurd lines on the subway in cities like New York, or our crumbling airports, we have to navigate our transportation infrastructure every day.

We travel 3.2 trillion miles a year on our roads and make more than 188 million trips a year over our bridges. Yet America's roads and bridges are in bad shape,[6] largely because we're nearly a trillion dollars behind in funding their repairs. One-fifth of our highways are in such bad condition that they cost us an estimated $160 billion annually in wasted time and fuel.

Fixing our transportation infrastructure would offer an almost immediate return on investment: the Federal Highway Administration estimates that every dollar spent on repairs would result in about $5.20 in savings—on everything from reduced delays and fuel consumption to auto repairs.

Our bridges aren't faring much better.[7] Forty percent of our 614,387 bridges are over fifty years old and nearly 10 percent are structurally deficient. The ASCE estimates that fixing them would cost the government about $123 billion.

Michigan has the country's worst roads.[8] Less than a third of our major roads were in "good" condition per the Federal Highway Administration; 42 percent were rated either "fair" or "poor." The average Michigan driver spends nearly $650 a year on additional auto repairs.[9] In fact, my opponent ran on a simple message: "Fix the Damn Roads." She won.

We have equally neglected public transit.[10] Americans take about 10.5 billion public transit trips a year, and it's increasing. However, nearly 20 percent of public transit systems are in a state of disrepair. That includes 35 percent of tracks and 37 percent of stations.

New York City's subway system, the country's largest, is a testament to this. Anyone who has taken the subway more than a few times in recent years has a story to share about rats (on the tracks, on the platforms, even on the trains), about being stuck in a tunnel, or having to endure a long wait on a hot or dangerously crowded platform. Indeed, an analysis by New York City's Independent Budget Office found that the number of delays in a month increased from twenty thousand in 2012 to more than sixty-seven thousand in 2017.[11] That translates into a 45 percent increase in passenger hours wasted. For some, a delay is merely an inconvenience. But if you work part-time, showing up late could cost you your job.

Too many communities have no reliable public transit at all. Detroit has become synonymous with the automobile. But for most of the twentieth century, Detroit had one of the country's best public transit systems: streetcars that could efficiently move people from one part of the city to the other. At one point it was the largest municipally owned transit system in the country. In 1929 alone it moved five hundred million passengers in more than 1,700 streetcars over five hundred miles of track.[12] But lobbying by GM eventually destroyed it. Today, Detroit is serviced by an underfunded bus system that services many stops just a few times a day.

Ultimately, Detroit's streetcar system fell victim to a network of hulking freeways, which were built atop some of the city's most vibrant Black neighborhoods. Similar construction took place all over the country following the passage of the 1956 Interstate Highway Act, promising federal support for 90 percent of highways.[13] They facilitated exurban sprawl all over the country—the death knell of public transit systems nationwide—leading to a decades-long cycle of traffic jams, construction to add lanes, more sprawl, more traffic, and more construction. This "induced demand" has started to abate, because millennials are choosing to move back to the cities, and those who aren't are demanding more public transit. Experts argue that the positive feedback loop that led to huge highway systems could work to expand public transit, too: more investment leading to more demand leading to more use.[14] Not only would these investments improve transit overall, but public transit is far more energy efficient and may help reduce the numbers of gas-guzzling cars on the road, which are contributing to climate change.

* * *

Air travel is becoming increasingly common despite how bad it is for our environment. In 2015, 55 percent of Americans never boarded a flight. However, that's changing quickly. In 1997, nearly half of all flights were for business purposes. However, by 2015, that had fallen to less than one in three.[15] This increase in leisure travel has led to a growth in air travel more generally. Airports service more than 2 million daily passengers, and the number is growing. And as you probably guessed, our airports aren't up to it. The ASCE suggests that, sometime soon, twenty-four of the top thirty American airports will experience "Thanksgiving-peak traffic volume" at least one day a week.

While the airline industry is extremely safe, there are nearly seven thousand planes in the air at a given time, which requires a lot of logistics. Thankfully, our nation's air traffic control system is about to get an upgrade, which is estimated to save 1.46 billion gallons of gasoline and reduce air delays by 41 percent. That should save about $38 billion a year—which is a good thing, because our airport infrastructure is about $42 billion short on funding.[16]

All of us have spent hours in traffic or waiting for a train or at the airport because of a flight delay. Those delays wreak havoc on your best laid plans, forcing you to miss important meetings or, worse, time with loved ones. Every hour is not created equal: a good friend of mine missed out on spending the last few hours of his father's life with him because of a flight delay. Instead, he spent them with angry fellow passengers at the Detroit Metropolitan Airport. I nearly missed my interview for the Rhodes scholarship because of a flight delay; if I had, it would have altered the trajectory of my life. The fact that these delays are often unpredictable and so costly makes them a tremendous source of insecurity in our lives.

Worse than lost time, however, is lost life. In 2007 the I-35W bridge in Minneapolis collapsed, sending dozens of cars and even a school bus careening into the Mississippi River, killing thirteen people and injuring 145. In 2017 alone, more than forty thousand people lost their lives on the roadways,[17] and that's been increasing over time. And it's not just that people are driving more; it's attributable to our failing infrastructure—potholes and road debris causing accidents that rob drivers of life and limb. The AAA foundation estimates that $146 billion in investments in highway infrastructure over twenty years could prevent 63,700 deaths and 353,560 injuries during that period.[18]

* * *

Five years after the cameras left, after the world turned its attention elsewhere, the people of Flint are still reeling from one of the worst water crises in modern history. Ask Flint residents if they trust their water—water their government tells them is now okay to drink; water that it told them was okay to drink even as the crisis was unfolding—and, to a person, they will tell you no. That's because trust, once lost, is hard to ever get back. It's a matter of insecurity.

"Out of sight, out of mind," as they say. That is true both for Flint and for our water infrastructure in general, buried under the ground. But as I discussed above, that infrastructure—which allows us to obtain clean, fresh, pure water to drink, cook with, bathe in, and clean with at a turn of a tap—is the cornerstone of public health. It protects us daily from communicable diseases like typhoid and cholera, diseases that ravaged our families just a few generations back. And when it fails, it kills.

There are more than a million underground pipes in this country. Together they deliver that fresh water we have come to rely upon so intimately. Most of that piping was laid in the middle of the last century.[19] It wasn't intended to last forever, and it's reaching the end of its lifespan. As it breaks down, we lose to waste nearly 6 billion gallons of clean water every day—up to 18 percent of all the clean water consumed.

Public investment in water systems has declined. Between 2009 and 2014, state and local government investment in water systems declined by 22 percent.[20] More of those costs have been pushed onto rate payers, many of whom cannot afford them. That's the case in Detroit, where thousands of households a year have their water shut off. After all, the exorbitant cost of city water in Detroit—surrounded by the Great Lakes, the world's largest repository of fresh water—isn't about the water; it's about the infrastructure to purify the water.

Although we pay little attention to the water coming into our homes, we pay strikingly less attention to the water leaving our homes—until it backs up into our homes. The country's nearly fifteen thousand wastewater treatment plants service nearly 80 percent of our population through eight hundred thousand miles of sewer lines. The Environmental Protection Agency estimates that sewers back up and overflow as many as seventy-five thousand times a year.[21] In the spring of 2019, unusually warm weather created a major string of floods in Illinois, Iowa, Missouri, and Nebraska. Three people lost their lives in the flooding, and states of emergency were called across those states. Damages were estimated at around $3 billion. The flooding is a reminder of the catastrophic consequences of inadequate stormwater drainage systems (as was the flooding in Detroit that sticky August in 2016).

To fix our water system, the American Water Works Association estimates it will cost a trillion dollars.[22] But not fixing the system would surely be more expensive.

To appreciate the way that failing water infrastructure shapes insecurity, imagine watching the sewage level rise in your basement. Imagine knowing that the water in which you were bathing your child—brushing her teeth— was causing that rash you were finding all over her body, that that water was leaded, and that the lead would stay in her body for months, leaching into her developing brain.

* * *

I wake up every morning because my smartphone tells me to. It then brings me the mornings news, tells me the day's weather, and reminds me of the meetings I have and to-do list I have to churn through. When I have questions during the day, I use it to answer them. If I'm feeling like a tune, I stream it. But usually, being a nerd, I stream a book or a podcast. When I need directions, I use it to get me where I'm going. And when I want to connect with friends, it offers me several platforms to do so.

Throughout the day, I take for granted that my smartphone is constantly exchanging information with the outside world to enable these activities—because its constantly connected to the Internet, whether Wi-Fi or LTE.

And that's why it was always so jarring when I lost coverage for miles on end as I traveled through broad expanses of the state of Michigan during the campaign. Indeed, although upwards of 95 percent of Americans carry a cell phone, nearly a third of rural communities in America have no wireless LTE connectivity.[23] Furthermore, one in ten Americans lack access to broadband Internet, defined by the Federal Communications Commission as download speeds of 25 megabits per second or greater.[24] Under the current system, corporate Internet service providers are left to lay the infrastructure for broadband, which they then sell to subscribers. But in communities with low population density, the number of new subscribers would be so low that the providers choose not to do it. Urban communities may have the infrastructure, but the costs are unaffordable for many.

In the twenty-first century, Internet access is like having a paved road. And not having it puts you at an ever-deepening disadvantage. That's why our failure to lay adequate broadband infrastructure in rural communities—and make it affordable in urban communities—is a source of insecurity for too many. Worse, knowing that the lack of access to basic learning tools that other children take for granted may be stunting your child's intellectual development compounds insecurities that Americans in urban and rural communities have about the future they can provide for their offspring.

* * *

But that pales in comparison to the ways that our schools fail those kids every day. Every morning, when I drop my child off at her day care, I trust that the building in which my most beloved person—the most vulnerable human in my family—will be spending the day won't be poisoning her because of mold growing underneath the floors or lead paint chipping off the windowsills. I trust that when it's cold, the building will be adequately heated, and when it's hot, it will be adequately cooled. Millions of Americans put that same trust in schools all over the country—institutions that they rely on to provide safe environments for their children to learn. When those schools break that trust by failing to care for our young ones, it strikes at the very heart of our insecurities—that our future, and our children's future, is in doubt.

Beyond this, public schools serve important roles in local communities beyond education, serving as evacuation shelters and voting places and meeting spaces—the kind of social infrastructure described above. When I walked through that school building on the inspection tour in Detroit in the winter of 2016, which I described in Chapter 10, I could not help but imagine what it meant for the future of our city, our country.

Detroit children and parents are not alone: the ASCE gave America's entire school infrastructure a grade of D-plus. The hundred thousand schools that nearly fifty million children walk into every day are lacking in some of the most basic ways. Nearly a quarter of those buildings are rated in fair or poor condition, with failing HVAC, plumbing, or windows. More than half of all buildings require repairs.[25]

A big reason for this is that many school districts, facing constraints during the Great Recession, made permanent cuts to their facilities budgets. Although enrollment has increased, these expenditures have not, leaving us with a $38 billion budget gap every year.

And that's just the school facilities. Consider what's happening inside: a recent report from the OECD found that between 2010 to 2014, U.S. spending on elementary and high school education dropped by 4 percent per student.[26] Meanwhile, education spending increased 5 percent per student on average across similar high-income countries.

This is devastating, considering current economic trends. Automation has decimated the American job market, but it should at least create the kinds of technical jobs, like software engineering, that are needed to sustain it. And it does—but our education system hasn't prepared our children adequately to do them.

Our lack of investment has resulted in middling education outcomes among American students, particularly in science and math. In 2015 an international assessment of fifteen-year-old kids showed that American students performed at the middle of the pack in these technical skills—and not much better in reading comprehension.[27] In 2015 the Trends in International Mathematics and Science Study showed that fourth graders in ten countries out of forty-eight had higher average scores than fourth graders in the United States, and those in seven countries had higher math scores.[28]

* * *

When I spent summers with Teta in Egypt, there would be regular rolling blackouts. Between the hours of two and four in the afternoon a few days every week the electricity would just go out. Sarah's family's village in India experiences the same situation. Indeed, it was a wonder that the village had electricity at all: thirty-one million homes in that country still lack access to electricity,[29] something we have taken for granted in America for the better part of a century.

And yet, because we have had electrical access for so long, our grid is starting to break down. Most American distribution lines were built in the 1950s or '60s, with a life expectancy of about fifty years—meaning that they are already past their expiration dates. And that's resulting in more blackouts. In 2009, more than 2,800 blackouts affected thirteen million people. In 2017, there were 3,500 blackouts, affecting nearly three times as many people.[30] Given that electricity is essential in an Internet-enabled world, the cost per minute of each blackout has also increased tremendously, growing 57 percent between 2010 and 2016.[31]

Energy infrastructure has obvious implications for our sense of insecurity. If you've ever had your electricity go out in the middle of your workday or as you were preparing an evening meal, you know how disruptive it can be. A power outage can cause all of the food in your fridge to spoil, a serious financial blow if you're living from paycheck to paycheck. And as electricity powers more and more technology in our daily lives—from smart cars to smart homes to the ubiquitous Wi-Fi—our reliance on constant, ready access to electricity grows. Worse, we are quickly outgrowing our energy infrastructure, leaving us more dependent on a less reliable resource.

* * *

Since 63 percent of our power is generated from the burning of fossil fuels, all of this demand for electricity comes at a cost: climate change. Climate change is *the* most important existential challenge facing our country and our world. While in the past our focus was drawn to melting ice caps and the consequences for wildlife, climate scientists have forced us to come to terms with the staggering *human* cost of climate change. We are now seeing "once-in-a-lifetime" storms, floods, and wildfires—every year. These climatic events are deadly, forcing survivors to deal with loss of loved ones, homes, communities, and livelihoods, and more and more often compelling them to migrate en masse.

In 2015, when I was a professor, I was invited to write a chapter for a textbook about the effect of climate change on mental health.[32] I and the other contributors were asked to highlight key clinical consequences of climate change—the things that social workers, psychologists, and doctors would need to focus on. Chief among them is that climate change will pitch stressor after stressor at us, challenging our capacity to accommodate. Because climate change will destroy the resources we take for granted—infrastructure, housing, food, water, jobs—it will exacerbate scarcity and all of the other causes of insecurity.

The chief driver of climate change is our addiction to fossil fuels—mostly natural gas and coal. Although the technology currently exists to harvest energy from renewable sources, like wind, the sun, and the heat of the earth's core, we lack the electrical grid necessary to store and allocate that energy. Burning fossil fuels allows humans to control the speed and pace of electrical generation. We can fire up the plants when we need more energy and then slow them down when we don't. That allows us to modulate the production of energy according to the daily and monthly patterns of use. Renewable energy sources are less controllable. The sun generates the most energy when people don't need it—during the day—and less when they do. That means that relying on solar power requires us to store and distribute vastly more of our energy, necessitating a very different type of electrical grid.

As we build the power grid of the future, we are daily making decisions that will either empower or disrupt a transition to a just, sustainable, renewable energy infrastructure. And as corporations and politicians continue to invest in the broken fossil-fuel-driven infrastructure of the past, they are wedding us to a system of energy production that will ultimately destroy us if we don't change.

* * *

Failing infrastructure is not random, although it may seem that way as a pothole develops here or flooding occurs there. As we have allowed our society to become segregated—racially, socioeconomically, and politically—we have seen the trappings of wealth and the costs of marginalization reinforce disparities in quality infrastructure across communities. The constant flooding in Detroit, a poor, predominantly Black city, is not coincidental. The fact that Detroit schools are in such a state of disrepair that first graders had to wear their coats until the afternoon is not a coincidence, either. Nor is the fact that Flint, another poor, predominantly Black city was the epicenter of the worst lead and water crisis in decades.

These infrastructure failures reflect the institutional racism and segregation that have both kept these communities poor and deprived them of the tax base needed to encourage new local investment in that very same infrastructure. For example, in 2018 the Northeast Ohio Areawide Coordinating Agency (NOACA)—the agency that governs regional planning for the region that includes Cleveland—had nine seats. Six of those seats represented the city of Cleveland and three represented neighboring Geauga County. But here's the rub: Cleveland had 385,000 residents, the majority of whom were Black. Geauga County had 94,000 residents, who were 97 percent white. That meant each Geauga County resident had more than twice the representation as each Cleveland resident. That's a problem because regional planning organizations like NOACA often control the flow of millions of dollars of federal and state infrastructure funds. Northeast Ohio isn't alone. A Brookings Institution report on metropolitan planning organization boards across fifty large metropolitan areas found that this bias toward higher-income, whiter communities is relatively common.[33]

CHAPTER 17

Insecure economy.

I met Chris when he pulled into my driveway at 6:30 one morning to take me to the airport. He was my Lyft driver. We struck up a conversation. Born and bred in Macomb County, Michigan, Chris had gone to the same high school my wife attended in Utica. He had been driving for Lyft for the last three months after being laid off by a local automotive supplier for General Motors that was forced to downsize after GM announced it was shutting down yet another factory in Detroit.

That wasn't the first time Chris had been laid off. It had happened once before, during the Great Recession, after he had been a skilled factory worker for twenty-seven years. He got the auto supply gig because a cousin's husband was the foreman. It paid two-thirds the hourly rate of his previous job—which had been a union job with generous benefits—and was technically part-time, although he'd routinely work overtime, taking him well over forty hours a week. There were no benefits. "Hell, I was just lucky to have a job," he said.

As I inquired about his job prospects this time around, he said flatly, "I ain't ever gettin' another job like that. Them times are over."

"Why?" I asked.

"They don't need people like me no more. The factories are so high-tech now, they don't need people with my skills."

Macomb County had long been home to much of the region's heavy industry. Folks in Macomb tend to be white, working-class, and reliably Democratic. But in 2016 that changed. These were the communities pundits talked about when they referred to the "Obama-Obama-Trump voters" who confounded them and the Democratic Party by supporting Obama in 2008 and 2012 but voting for Trump in 2016.

But their choices at the ballot box were written in their economic history. In the post–World War II boom, communities like these prospered. They were the substrate of a flourishing manufacturing industry. You could get a job paying in the near six figures without a college degree—and a handsome pension and benefits after you'd put in your thirty years. Unions had forged those opportunities, and places like Macomb County would deliver a reliable Democratic vote in return. But with NAFTA and other international trade deals, the corporations that relied on union labor in Macomb County began to offshore those jobs. Whole factories would crash, disintegrating in the open like corpses, a brutal reminder of the stark contrast between what had been and what is. Technology picked off many of the jobs that were left, with automation replacing skilled workers who had for so long relied on their skills being needed to operate the factories that stayed. Macomb County lost nearly half of its manufacturing jobs between 2000 and 2010.[1]

The Great Recession accelerated these trends. With the near collapse of the auto industry, a number of smaller parts suppliers and steel manufacturers vastly downsized or went under entirely. And the big three automakers— Ford, Chrysler, and GM—were forced to radically rethink their business, opting to kill once-mighty brands, like GM's Pontiac.

Although President Obama's heroics to save the auto industry helped buoy the economy in communities like Macomb County, the recovery largely failed to address the structural realities that decimated the economies of communities like these. Too many people still don't have jobs: they've been out of the economy for so long that they've stopped looking. Those who continue to search for work have found once-lucrative opportunities replaced by gigs that pay considerably lower wages.

Over time, the "recovery" from the Great Recession has left communities like Macomb County behind. Corporate profits have skyrocketed, labor participation has stagnated, and real wages have fallen. In sum, these industries have earned their profits by squeezing their labor pool, employing the same number of employees for less than they used to make. That is the reality in which folks like Chris in Macomb County are living: they feel like they've been forgotten in an economy built by elites, for elites. Small wonder, then, that Chris voted for Donald Trump, who said he'd bring back all of those manufacturing jobs.

* * *

Not all jobs are created equal. After all, what if your job doesn't afford you the basic means of a dignified life, like a wage that allows you to afford your rent, your transportation, and your meals. What if it doesn't come with healthcare or a secure retirement? Sociologists refer to these kinds of jobs as "bad jobs."[2] Chris is one of millions of Americans stuck in one of those bad jobs. Another name for a bad job is a "gig," a slightly more empowering label we've given them to relieve the embarrassment inspired by the fact that so many of us are working them.

The number of Americans working gigs, like Chris, is rising. The Center for Economic and Policy Research found that they increased by nearly a third between 1978 and 2010.[3] In fact, gigs are the new norm: short-term, temporary positions without the pay or benefits that their permanent predecessors would have offered. "The fact that so many people took temporary jobs, often as contractors, was pushed along by the downturn, in part because employers were so unsure about the future but also because workers had no choice but to take them," says Professor Peter Cappelli, director of the Wharton's Center for Human Resources. "Good employee-management practices took a big step back during this period because employees were willing to put up with anything as long as they had a job."[4]

Is Chris "employed"? Technically, yes. But through the course of his career, he's gone from a comfortable, skilled job to a classic "bad job" to a gig as a Lyft driver. He is underemployed. And Chris, in his late fifties, doesn't see any improvement on the horizon.

This is what those who point to historically low unemployment as proof that our economy is performing well are missing. Unemployment is, after all, a simple ratio: the number of people in jobs divided by the number of people who are employed or looking for a job. But just because you are technically employed doesn't mean that job allows you all the means of a dignified life—that you're working as much as you'd like, and that your work pays you a fair wage. This is the crisis of underemployment, which boomed during the Great Recession and remains high.[5]

In fact, the Great Recession cost more jobs than any economic downturn since the Great Depression. But as economic recovery began, firms took the opportunity to reorganize their businesses—automating or offshoring work that had previously employed many of these workers—making the recession's massive layoffs permanent. Without the skills to compete for new jobs, many were fundamentally frozen out of the economy. After years of looking, they've just fundamentally given up. Professor David Autor is a leading economist at MIT, and he's advanced the argument that the American economy has "polarized"—losing many of the well-paid, middle-skill jobs to automation and offshoring, helping drive income inequality.[6]

To understand how this happened, one must appreciate the politics that drove the government response to the Great Recession. Captains of industry turned politicians, like Michigan's then governor Rick Snyder, accelerated the trends that cost Chris his job.

First, Snyder decimated the unions that protected what few jobs were left. With his support, the Republican legislature passed a brutal "Right to Work" law, which in effect reneged on collective bargaining contracts by allowing workers not to have to pay union dues. They repealed the prevailing wage law that protected the trades from low-balling on government-contracted work sites by nonunion labor. Snyder and his allies in the state legislature even repealed a popular paid sick leave law and an increase in the state's minimum wage.

Snyder followed a well-worn playbook, as unions and the minimum wage have been targets of corporations and their politicians for the past century. After all, unions have been the most important protector of worker rights and wages in American history. Child labor laws, workplace safety requirements, the minimum wage, the concept of a weekend—all of these were inspired and advocated by the union movement in the nineteenth and twentieth centuries. And each of them was critical to establishing a more equal America.[7]

In the heyday of the unions in the 1950s, more than one in three workers were union members. Today it's just one in ten. The hard-won victories of the union movement have also eroded. For example, had the minimum wage kept pace with the American economy since 1968, it would be nearly twenty dollars an hour today.[8]

These losses are the consequences of direct, coordinated, and effective attacks on the union movement. Right-to-work laws, prevailing wage repeals, and minimum wage stagnation are all part of the playbook. Most damaging, however, has been the Supreme Court's ruling in the case of *Janus v. AFSCME*, which effectively made right to work the law of the land in the United States by ruling it unconstitutional to enforce the collection of union dues for those benefiting from union contracts.

While bringing union power to its knees, Snyder and Michigan Republicans set about slashing taxes for corporations. These cuts, coming off the worst years of the Great Recession, would help fuel automation, enabling investment in the very machines that had been taking jobs away from people like Chris. To pay for these tax cuts, Snyder instituted a tax on pensions, robbing seniors who had already put in their thirty years of the full benefits that they had been promised. Across Michigan, I met countless seniors who, because of these taxes, were forced to choose between their prescription medications and their property tax, their weekly groceries and their car insurance.

Automation has destroyed job prospects for people like Chris. Estimates suggest that 87 percent of the manufacturing jobs lost in Michigan were lost to automation.[9] This trend has penetrated many of America's biggest sectors. You can see its trappings everywhere if you look. Think about it: The last time you went to a grocery store, did you stand in line for a cashier or at an automated kiosk?

Amazon alone now accounts for 50 percent of all e-commerce and 5 percent of all retail in the United States.[10] With a fully electronic purchasing platform and a highly automated back-end operation, Amazon is fundamentally automating the retail industry. Ironically, Amazon has now started building what it has destroyed: brick-and-mortar bookstores and grocery stores.

Amazon's labor force of approximately 613,000 presents a microcosm of the "polarized" workforce heralded by automation that Autor describes. Their white-collar workers, mostly tech and business professionals, are well paid, earning an average of more than $110,000 a year—often to figure out new ways to automate away the blue-collar workforce. Meanwhile, those blue-collar workers are left doing increasingly mindless and menial work across their warehouses. These blue-collar employees now earn $15 an hour, their minimum wage having been raised only under extreme political pressure. Meanwhile, their CEO, Jeff Bezos, is the richest person in the world, worth more than $127 billion at one point (until he lost half of it in a divorce).

* * *

To understand the urge to automate, one has to reach further back into the financial system that drives corporations. Over the three decades between

1980 and 2010, our economy underwent what economists call "financial-ization." In a financialized world, according to Professor Greta Krippner, an economic sociologist at the University of Michigan, "financial machinations have superseded productive enterprise."[11] Here the word "financial" means "the activities relating to the provision (or transfer) of liquid capital in expecta-tions of future interest, dividends, or capital gains." In short, when it comes to valuing a company, the *potential* of their stock takes precedence over the productivity of the company underlying those stocks *right now*.

In the financialized world in which we live, in the eyes of Wall Street, the value of a corporation has less to do with its quarterly bottom line and more to do with the bets that Wall Street can make on its potential future quarterly bottom line through complex financial instruments. Ironically, this is largely because Wall Street itself has been automated: most trades are now done through complex computer algorithms. This has led to vastly more com-plex financial instruments and helped drive the overall financialization of the economy.

To illustrate the impact of financialization on our economy, consider this: In May of 2017, Ford announced that it was going to cut 10 percent of its global workforce. This news came as a shock. Ford made $7.6 billion in profits in 2017—up 65 percent over 2016![12] But real, durable profits don't matter as much in a financialized world. What matters is the all-important stock price—which at the time of the announcement had dropped 17 percent over five months. Responding to shareholders, Ford executive chairman Bill Ford said: "Look, we're as frustrated as you are by the stock price . . . Much of our—most of our net worth is tied up in the company. And the stock price matters a lot to us."[13]

The market wasn't responding to Ford's profitability, which was sky-high; they were responding to whether or not they thought Ford was making moves to anticipate a changing automotive market, focused more around electric and autonomous vehicles. Ford's competitor, GM, had, after all, cut four thousand jobs over the past seven months.[14] Ford wasn't keeping up with the Joneses, and so its stock price suffered.

Nowhere in their thought process, mind you, was there a conversation about the fact that ten thousand people who relied on Ford to earn their daily bread would suffer as a consequence of this shoot-from-the-hip decision. The only consideration was Ford's flagging stock price. Short-term reasoning was driving long-term choices—and people were suffering because of it.

A few weeks later, Ford's then CEO, Mark Fields, was sacked and replaced by James Hackett. After all, cutting ten thousand jobs is crazy, right? Hackett is on the verge of an $11 billion restructure. And Wall Street analysts are partly speculating, partly suggesting that Ford could cut twenty-five thousand jobs in total.[15] Considering that Ford headquarters is in Michigan, it's likely that a disproportionate number of these lost jobs will be American jobs. To date, Ford has received more than $4 billion in subsidies and $28 billion in local, state, and federal government loans.[16] And people like Chris, the taxpayers who paid those subsidies? They'll be driving for Lyft.

* * *

The consequence of all of this—the crippling of unions, the acceleration of automation, the emergence of the gig economy, financialization—is deep structural inequality. Howard Schultz, erstwhile Starbucks CEO turned one-time 2020 presidential aspirant, earned $13.4 million in 2018. Meanwhile, the median Starbucks employee earned $12,754—and fifty-two pounds of coffee. That's a pay differential of 1,049:1.[17] The average pay ratio between CEOs and median employees among Fortune 500 companies is about 361 to 1.[18] Beyond how straight-up huge that number is, consider it in the context of the fact that in 1950 that number was just 20 to 1.[19] The degree to which CEOs out-earn their workers has risen eighteenfold in the past seven decades.

Inequality is the new American truth, with levels surging beyond the extreme income disparities of the Gilded Age and the Great Depression. Economists analyzing inequality have shown that it's largely attributable to increasing income among the very rich while earnings among the poor have stagnated. This is particularly troubling considering what economists call the "productivity-pay gap." Over the past five decades, American productivity has increased 77 percent, yet hourly pay has only increased 20 percent.[20] Where did the difference go? To people like Schultz and Bezos. Through automation and the erosion of labor, more and more of the profits go to the very top, rather than to the people who make it possible.

What does that mean for us? Insecurity. Rising inequality puts the fundamentals of a dignified life further and further out of reach. We are left trying to pay for more of the basics with a smaller share of the productivity we create. Each of us is closer to financial insolvency: missing that rent payment, being swallowed up by credit card debt, having to ration our medications, having to skimp on simple pleasures, like birthday gifts for the kids or a trip to the movies on the weekend. To add insult to injury, the wealth of the winners in this economy reminds us of what we don't have, leaving us asking why, if there is so much wealth to be had, do we have so little of it? All of this drives our insecurity, exacerbates the tensions created by our segregation, and leaves us that much more susceptible to manipulation by those who would use our insecurity for their own ends.

In the next chapter I'll discuss how our political system—meant in a democratic society to be the great equalizer—has become a driver of the epidemic of insecurity.

CHAPTER 18

Insecure politics.

Although voting is the bedrock of our democracy, it is way too hard to do in America. I should know. My campaign for governor almost got derailed by a controversy regarding my past voting record, which brought into question my overall eligibility to serve as governor.

I finished medical school in New York. And during the 2012 election, I decided to vote there. Although perhaps I should have known better, I didn't know at the time that I could send an absentee ballot to Michigan, where in fact, because of our electoral college system, my vote would have mattered more. I still considered Michigan home at the time, and Sarah and I owned a place to which we had imagined someday coming back. As a student managing multiple research projects, I admit that my voter registration wasn't the first thing on my mind. When my Michigan driver's license expired, I applied for a New York license, and I was automatically registered to vote in New York.

That crisp morning in 2012, Sarah and I got in line to vote at a polling location in Washington Heights. We waited for four hours that day, as is far too common in low-income urban communities. Manhattan is covered by the Voting Rights Act,[1] specifically to address decades of Latinx voter suppression in communities like Washington Heights—the exact kind of efforts to subvert the will of voters we experienced that day.[2] But that four hours in line wasn't all that fateful vote would cost me.

Registering—even casting my vote—in New York did not abrogate my voter registration in Michigan. It is perfectly legal to be registered to vote in two places; it's just not legal to vote in two places, which of course I didn't do. However, five anonymous lawyers, no doubt lined up by allies of my gubernatorial opponent, told a reporter at Bridge, a Michigan news outlet, that I should have been removed from Michigan's voter rolls when I was registered in New York. Why would my opponents care about my voter registration in 2012? Because according to the state constitution "to be eligible for the office of governor or lieutenant governor a person must have attained the age of 30 years, and have been a registered elector in this state for four years next preceding his election." That means I had to have been a registered Michigan voter in good standing at least four years before the date I took office. If by voting in New York in 2012, I had somehow relinquished my voter registration in Michigan until I updated it when I registered for a Michigan driver's license in 2015, I would have been ineligible to run for governor.

Never mind the fact that I was never actually removed from the Michigan voter rolls—and had been continuously registered to vote in Michigan since the first time I registered to vote in 2003. The attack wasn't designed to be adjudicated in the court of law; it was designed to be tried in the court of public opinion. My opposition's goal wasn't just to knock me out; it was to cripple my campaign, so that even if I were to stay in the race, my fundraising would be so anemic as to keep me from really moving my message on television, the Internet, and radio in the critical final months of the campaign.

As I tried to fundraise against the cloud that the question of my eligibility cast over the campaign, call after call would end with some variation of the same question: "Are you even eligible?"

"Yes! We've had this looked at by some of the top election lawyers in the country, and they all say I'm good to go. This is a manufactured controversy designed to steer people like you off," I would implore.

"I believe you. But maybe come back to me once it's been cleared up."

Before this question of my eligibility had surfaced, between February and July 2017—the first five months of my campaign—we shocked almost everyone by raising more than $1 million. For a political newcomer who had never run before, it was an eye-popping amount, particularly considering that the front-runner had raised the same amount in roughly the same amount of time—although we had done it without taking money from corporate political action committees (PACs). We raised our second million in three months. The next million should have come even faster as our campaign started to pick up steam, with a steady stream of feature articles in national and international newspapers. But after these questions about my eligibility, I raised a paltry $500,000 over the next five months. Finally, in May—three months before the election—the Bureau of Elections ruled me eligible.

This ordeal was one of the most grueling psychological challenges I have ever endured. All of my team members, the thousands of people who had invested their hard-earned money in this campaign—the thousands more who had given of themselves by knocking on doors or making calls or telling a friend or coworker—were watching. The same questions were asked of me over, and over, and over. As I responded to them, I knew my interlocutors were looking more for the *way* I answered than for the words that came out of my mouth. They were watching for any sign that would betray something I might be hiding.

It was hardest to bear with my campaign team: people who had literally put their lives on hold to work on this campaign. I watched them withstand the constant barrage of media coverage, social media posts, and questions from friends and supporters. They were flagging. Every morning I tried my best to deliver a fresh dose of confidence and optimism.

That is, until I'd lay down to sleep every night, alone with myself, immune to my own posturing. *What if you're not actually eligible? Will you have wasted more than two million dollars of other people's money just to embarrass yourself?* And then I'd hear Sarah's voice, reassuring—but with the same doubtful premise as everyone else: "Even if you're not eligible, it's not the end of the world."

"You're right," I'd manage. I wasn't so sure. The next day I'd be right back at it, though. *I'd better get some sleep.*

Unfortunately, all of the attention paid to my voting record had brought to light questions about my previous voting record. Although I had supported Senator Bernie Sanders in his outsider bid to take the presidential nomination in 2016, I did not vote in the Democratic primary, something I deeply regret.

It wasn't for lack of trying. The primary was held on March 8, 2016. That was a particularly busy day, as all days at the Health Department were. I had gone to the polling place in a large church across the street from my apartment building. When I noticed the number of people waiting in line to vote, I asked one of the poll workers how long the line was; he told me that it would be around an hour and a half. I didn't have that kind of time. So I told myself I'd come back at lunch. During lunch I was told it would be two hours. I told myself I'd come back after work. I didn't finish up until about 9:00. The polls had closed. I hadn't voted.

It turns out that even if I had gotten to the front of the line, my Michigan registration was for a polling place in Ann Arbor, about forty minutes away, because that was where I had last been registered in Michigan. I would have been given a provisional ballot or told to go to my polling place out there.

Two weeks later I renewed my Michigan license—and therefore automatically reregistered to vote—at the polling place in Detroit.

I absolutely should have known more about the voting process and blocked out some time to stand in line and vote, knowing from experience that polling can be an exercise in patience in low-income urban communities like Washington Heights or Detroit. That's what I did in November, when after waiting a few hours in line at the church, I voted for Hillary Clinton in the general election.

I usually have my act together when it comes to juggling several balls at a time, and I have colleagues and family who help me keep those balls in the air. If *I* couldn't figure this out, I can't imagine how opaque it must have seemed to folks who have to work two or three jobs and then care for their kids—folks without nearly the level of professional or personal support that I have. Although I make no excuses for myself for not voting, I do believe that our abysmal voting numbers have a lot more to do with how difficult it is to vote than with apathy or disinterest on the part of voters. We put the pressure of voting on individuals rather than designing our voting system around empowering people to fulfill their civic duty.

Part of this is the nature of bureaucracy. When I was serving in Detroit, I realized that most bureaucracies are self-oriented: too often they ask how a new program or service would best be organized *within the bureaucracy* rather than how best to organize it *around the people we want to serve.*

But more than that, since the dawn of American democracy, politicians and their hacks have made a concerted effort to squeeze the will of the people out of it.

Voter suppression—direct efforts to introduce obstacles to voting for certain groups of people—is as old as voting itself. And although we no longer have the poll taxes or voter literacy tests that characterized Reconstruction era voter suppression efforts, make no mistake: voter suppression is alive and well.

It is no coincidence that voting in low-income communities of color like Washington Heights and Detroit is harder to do than it is in the suburbs where I grew up: when I voted in the midterm primary in Macomb County, Michigan, in 2018, the whole experience took me five minutes.

Though not as blatant, today's voter suppression efforts remain viciously effective. In July 2017, then Georgia secretary of state Brian Kemp purged five hundred thousand people from the state's voter rolls—one of the largest voter purges in American history.[3] As he campaigned for governor, his office used an "exact match" approach to matching registration applications with personal data to cast doubt on applications with even slight inconsistencies, marking them for potential removal. They closed voting precincts in communities of color. They even turned around a bus full of seniors headed to early voting. Kemp was awarded the election over his opponent, former Georgia State House minority leader Stacey Abrams, by less than 55,000 votes. She has since gone on to dedicate herself to uprooting voter suppression, founding Fair Fight, an organization committed to free and fair elections.

Voter purges, strict voter registration and voter ID laws, restrictions on early and absentee voting—all of these are tools in the arsenal of voter suppression, usually targeting lower-income citizens and voters of color. For example, explicit voter registration requirements that are not automatic, or at least same-day, that force voters to explicitly register themselves at some point before Election Day are intended to make the voting process more onerous for people with less flexible schedules—who tend to poorer. The purging of voter rolls—almost always without alerting the citizens being purged—heightens the impact.

The absence of early voting or absentee voting is similar, intended to discriminate against people for whom flexibility is difficult. Voter ID laws are intended to discriminate against people who may not habitually carry an ID. For example, a study of voters in Michigan in 2018 found that non-white voters were between 2.5 and 6 times less likely to have ID.[4] The Fourth Circuit Court of Appeals struck down a strict voter ID law in North Carolina on the grounds that it was designed to "target African-Americans with almost surgical precision." However, whether or not voter ID laws actually influence voter turnout remains unclear.[5]

Another form of voter suppression is felon disenfranchisement, which discriminates directly against people of color, who are arrested, prosecuted, and imprisoned at much higher rates than their white counterparts. In 2018, Florida voters overwhelmingly passed a state referendum to re-enfranchise most people who had been convicted of felonies but had served their sentences—welcoming 1.5 million Floridians back to the democratic process. However, in the ensuing legislative session, the Republican legislature passed a law that required them to pay outstanding fines and fees they might owe the courts before regaining their right to vote. It was a barefaced attempt to suppress their votes and overturn the will of the people.

And then there are deep inequalities in the allocation of voting resources across communities, with low-income communities routinely shortchanged. This can lead to the most convenient polling places being shut down or to the long lines I experienced in both Washington Heights and Detroit.

You might think that things are moving in the right direction. But following the 2008 elections, which saw an historic turnout in low-income and urban communities, many states passed *more* restrictive voting laws. Fifteen states passed stricter voter ID laws, ten restricted early or absentee voting, and three made it more difficult for people convicted of crimes to have their voting rights restored.

The consequences are serious. In a recent poll 9 percent of both Black and Latinx respondents indicated that they or someone in their households had been told they lacked the proper ID to vote—which happened to only a third as many whites. And nearly one in ten Black and Latinx respondents were told they were not listed on voter rolls—even though they were—compared with one in twenty whites. And 15 percent of Black and 14 percent of Latinx respondents had trouble finding a polling place, compared with just 5 percent of whites.[6] This echoes the findings of another study of voting precincts in North Carolina after it passed some of the country's most restrictive voting laws. The study showed that relocated voting places left Black voters having to travel a total of 350,000 miles farther to vote early, compared with just 21,000 extra miles for whites. In total, 68 percent of Black respondents reported that disenfranchisement was a serious problem.[7]

* * *

And even when votes are tallied, the principle of "one person, one vote" rarely holds up. That's because of gerrymandering and the electoral college. Gerrymandering is the process of drawing legislative districts to apportion voters to districts that best suit the party drawing the lines. Gerrymandering employs processes called "packing" and "cracking." Packing means concentrating many of the opposing party's voters into one district; cracking is the exact opposite: evenly distributing the opposing party's voters across districts so that they never reach a majority in any one district.

Michigan, a classic "purple" swing state, is one of the most gerrymandered in the country. In 2014 a Pew Research Center poll showed that about 47 percent of Michiganders identified as Democratic, compared to 34 percent who identified as Republican.[8] That hasn't changed much over time. In 2007, seven years earlier, those affiliations were similar, at 49 percent and 33 percent, respectively.[9] However, because of gerrymandering, the state senate has been held by Republicans for the past twenty years straight. The state house was held by Republicans in all but four years. In fact, for twelve years Republicans held unified control of the governorship, senate, and house.

That has serious implications for state policy. The infamous emergency manager laws that so devastated Flint were passed twice—the second time to override a vote of the People via a state referendum to repeal them. Yet they were passed both times by a gerrymandered state legislature. Thankfully, Michigan voters passed a referendum in 2018 to have district boundaries set by a nonpartisan commission of voters. These new nonpartisan districts will take effect in 2022.

Gerrymandering devalues the votes of members of the opposing party, whether Democratic or Republican. However, it arises from a necessary process of dividing a space into legislative districts. The other challenge to the "one person, one vote" principle is the electoral college, a completely unnecessary anachronism from a time when ruling elites didn't trust the people.

That fateful November morning in 2012 when I cast my vote in New York, a comfortably blue state, instead of Michigan, a purple state, I was sacrificing the value of my vote. Michigan's 16 electoral college votes are consistently at play in a presidential election, whereas New York's 29 electoral votes are comfortably Democratic. Michigan went for President Obama by nearly 45,000 votes—nearly 10 percentage points. New York went for him by nearly 165,000 votes—27 percentage points. Only four years later Michigan would flip, helping send Donald Trump to the White House by 10,704 votes, a mere two-tenths of a percentage point. Meanwhile, New York went for Clinton by nearly 174,000 votes, a comfortable 23 percentage points.

* * *

If our votes decide the outcomes of elections, what decides our votes? In today's politics, it's money. It may not be clear exactly how money buys votes in politics, so let me explain. Imagine you are trying to run for governor, but you've never run for office before in your life (a scenario I know well). To win the primary, you need to earn upwards of four hundred thousand votes. That means that at least four hundred thousand people need to know who you are and know enough about your politics to vote for you. How do you get people to know who you are? Well, you could crisscross the state, hit all of the counties, and invite people to hear you speak.

Let's say you use social media and send press releases to local papers, and you get an average of one hundred people at a town hall, which is pretty good. You do that in eighty-three counties. They all love you and pledge you their vote. And now you've got . . . 8,300 voters (assuming they all stick with you and show up to vote). Only 391,700 to go! Let's say you get great coverage in several local news outlets, but you can't rely on people watching, so let's say that earns you another 50,000 votes. Let's say you inspire a legion of idealistic folks from all walks of life to knock on doors for you—and they knock on 50,000 doors. If every household averages two voting aged adults, and both adults in every household decide to vote for you, you've only got 241,700 votes to go. You can see how this is an uphill battle.

How do you solve it? You buy commercials. And here's where things get expensive. I remember the first time I watched my commercial on television. It took two or three seconds to realize what it was. But when I did, I was pretty excited—knowing thousands of others in the region were seeing them, too. Within ten seconds, though, I realized that, based on the cost of our first ad buy—several hundred thousand dollars—every second that ticked by was costing our campaign $27.

We knew we'd get outraised: we weren't taking money from corporate PACs, who could donate up to $68,000 each to a campaign. There weren't any shady super-PACs supporting us, nor did I have allies who could set up even shadier accounts to allow donors to move unlimited sums of money to my campaign. And because I was a newbie, I didn't have inroads into the donor class. I had to create my own donor base: a hodgepodge mix ranging from working folks donating $5 or $10 at a time at the end of a hard-earned paycheck, to doctors and nurses who believed in my vision for healthcare, to Muslim-Americans helping to elect someone whom their children could look up to and see a reflection of themselves. I could not be more thankful to these folks for putting their money behind a political rookie, who happened to be a thirty-three-year-old Muslim guy named Abdul.

Together, we raised $5.5 million, including a state matching-funds system that kicked in an additional $990,000 because one of my opponents was financing his campaign from his own bank account. And more than half of that money was spent on TV commercials across Michigan media markets.

Yet I still got outspent nearly six to one in commercials by other Democrats in the race, one relying on millions of dollars of his own money, the other relying on a well-oiled political machine (complete with dark-money interest groups that would later be found to have violated campaign finance restrictions) to beat us. Even though our campaign had written hundreds of pages of policy; even though we had won both post-debate straw-polls by more than 70 percent—even though we were earning more coverage in the local, state, and national news media—we couldn't match our opponents on television.

Both of their campaigns underscore exactly how much money has corrupted our politics, but in different ways. One plowed $10.7 million of his own money into his campaign, allowing him to spend hundreds of thousands of dollars on a Super Bowl ad, which helped buy him name identification quickly.

The other was supported by a cadre of shell accounts that a Russian doll would be jealous of, funneling all kinds of money to support their campaign. First, there was "Build a Better Michigan" (BBM), an entity called a "527" after the section of the IRS code that governs it. These entities can accept unlimited amounts of money from any source, but they have to disclose their donors. Further, although they can spend money to influence elections, they are expressly prohibited from directly supporting candidates. All summer leading up to the primary, however, BBM was buying thirty-second commercials featuring the candidate, identified as a "candidate for governor." That was a clear violation of election law. The secretary of state ruled it as such, but only after the election was over. All told, BBM spent nearly $2 million on illegal ads.

The last time a similar violation occurred, the entity had been forced to pay a fine equal to the amount of money it had spent illegally. But BBM was given a measly $37,500 fine.[10]

But the story doesn't end there. BBM stalled on disclosing its donors, filing via paper rather than online to delay the disclosure. Among its biggest donors were two other groups, the Progressive Advocacy Trust (PAT), which donated $300,000, and the Philip A. Hart Democratic Club of Mount Clemons, which donated $250,000. Both of these groups share addresses with local Democratic clubs, and both exist as slush funds organized under the auspices of the state Democratic Party, which has special allowances that allow it to take unlimited contributions from corporations *without* disclosure requirements.

Although it remains unclear exactly where the PAT money came from (for obvious reasons), my opponent's relationship with big corporations became a serious issue in the campaign. I was running without taking *any* corporate money; my opponent had raised $144,000 at a closed-door fundraiser hosted by the Blue Cross Blue Shield of Michigan PAC. And when DTE, the region's biggest energy company, revealed its contributions, they disclosed having given $320,148 to PAT, which had funneled money through to BBM—all to run ads that were illegal in the first place.

* * *

"Corporations *are* people, my friend!" The line, spoken in response to a heckler at the Iowa State Fair in 2011 by then presidential candidate Mitt Romney, would come to symbolize an entire era of Republican thinking. He would go on to try to explain himself: "Everything that corporations earn ultimately goes to people."

When the framers of our constitution envisioned the future United States and guaranteed the right to the freedom of speech for every American, I somehow doubt that they considered that someday those rights would extend to the millions of dollars in campaign contributions made by multinational corporations worth hundreds of billions of dollars. I doubt they ever imagined a moment when a candidate for president of the United States would seek to justify those rights.

How did we get here? The Fourteenth Amendment was ratified in 1868 following the Civil War to guarantee that government could no longer "deprive any person of life, liberty, or property, without due process of law; nor deny any person within its jurisdiction the equal protection of the laws." Since then, this equal protections clause has been, along with the First Amendment, an undeniable linchpin of civil liberties litigation—cited in *Brown v. Board of Education* to desegregate schools; cited in *Loving v. Virginia* to protect the right to interracial marriage; cited in *Griswold v. Connecticut* to roll back Connecticut's contraceptives ban; cited in *Roe v. Wade* to protect a woman's right to an abortion; and cited in *Obergefell v. Hodges* to protect the right to same-sex marriage.

Ironically, as early as 1886, this provision, which was intended as a shield for the marginalized, would be co-opted by the powerful. In a headnote appended to the court's decision in *Santa Clara County v. Southern Pacific Railroad Co.*, the chief justice of the Supreme Court, Morrison Waite, was quoted as saying, "The Court does not wish to hear argument on the question whether the provision in the Fourteenth Amendment to the Constitution . . . applies to these corporations. We are all of the opinion that it does."[11] That headnote was treated as an official part of the verdict in subsequent cases. In 1978, in *First National Bank of Boston v. Bellotti*,[12] it was cited along with the First Amendment in a case granting the First National Bank the right to spend unlimited amounts in support of a ballot initiative—setting two devastating precedents, identifying corporations as "people" and campaign contributions as "speech."

Ruling in *Citizens United v. FEC*, the Court extended these precedents to political campaigns—clearing the way for essentially unlimited contributions in forthcoming elections. Corporate spending doesn't usually show up as direct candidate contributions; after all, with so many shadowy paths to choose from, why would corporations contribute in direct, traceable sums to candidates? Rather it has expanded the influx of "dark money": untraceable sums of cash that are used by outside organizations to support candidates, just as my opponent did. The elections watchdog group OpenSecrets calculates that the proportion of overall federal election spending by these shadowy outside groups has more than doubled since *Citizens United*.[13]

What are they spending the money on? Protecting their financial future. After all, the Supreme Court ruling notwithstanding, everyone knows that corporations *aren't actually people*. Corporations don't get sick; they don't fall in love; they don't care for their ailing parents or worry about how to afford college or dream of their children's futures. Rather, they exist to deliver shareholder value.

Perhaps the worst corruption of our politics comes, predictably, at the hands of these corporations. Corporations "invest" in politicians through campaign contributions, and then when their candidates win, they have direct access to them, lobbying them to vote "in the right direction" on everything from subsidies to loans to industry regulations.

The pharmaceutical industry is by far the industry with the deepest lobbying pockets. It has spent more than $4 billion in lobbying over the past twenty years.[14] Ever wonder why Medicare, one of the biggest buyers of prescription drugs in the world, can't negotiate its prices down? Pharma lobby dollars. They'll happily pay $4 billion to make tens of billions on the back end like Gilead, which made $4.5 billion from Medicare in 2014 on sofosbuvir, its hepatitis C drug.

The health insurance industry is the second biggest lobbyist by sector, spending nearly $3 billion over the past twenty years. What's it got to protect? Well, we're the only high-income country in the world that doesn't provide universal healthcare for its people. The insurance industry lobbies to make sure that will never happen. They've allied with their partners at Big Pharma, the hospital industry, and others to form the Partnership for America's Health Care Future, discussed earlier, with the explicit intent of killing Medicare for All.[15] Meanwhile, 5 to 10 percent of Americans will go without healthcare, the rest of us paying more for our healthcare than citizens of any other country on earth—for worse health outcomes.

And the mass incarceration I discussed earlier? Well, the private prison industry has something to do with that. Putting people in prison is good money—at least, that's what the private prison industry, a $5 billion industry in the United States, has found. And business is booming. Between 2000 and 2016, the private prison population grew by 47 percent.[16]

Like any corporation, protecting their bottom line is a key aim. Corrections Corporation of America (CCA), rebranded "CoreCivic" in 2016, is now one of the country's largest private prison companies. CCA's 2014 annual shareholder report muses on the potential threats to their earnings: "The demand for our facilities and services could be adversely affected by the relaxation of enforcement efforts, leniency in conviction or parole standards and sentencing practices or through decriminalization of certain activities that are currently proscribed by our criminal laws."[17] Although they state "our policy prohibits us from engaging in lobbying or advocacy efforts that would influence enforcement efforts, parole standards, criminal laws, and sentencing policies,"[18] CCA has spent tens of millions of dollars to support candidates and lobbying efforts, spending $1.23 million in 2018 alone.[19]

But here's the kicker: CCA's annual report goes on to say that "similarly, reductions in crime rates . . . could lead to reductions in arrests, convictions and sentences requiring incarceration at correction facilities."[20] Simply put, reducing crime is bad for business for CCA and its peers.

CCA has an army of lobbyists. Schoolchildren like Marcus and Aisha don't. They can't throw millions into the campaign coffers of "strong-on-schools" candidates. And their voices—and futures—are lost in these debates. So rather than invest in our kids' brains, we invest in jails that they might occupy because we didn't. The vast majority of these kids will be Black or Brown, poor and marginalized. But corporations like CoreCivic will continue to report "increases in shareholder value and profitability."[21]

* * *

These corporations have also been using their sheer size and scale to crowd out smaller entrants into the market. Rather than spark innovation or efficiency, this "late stage" of capitalism leads to a few gargantuan, market-dominant oligopolies.

Want a cell phone? Apple and Samsung control 99 percent of the smartphone market.[22] Need a carrier? You've got Sprint, T-Mobile, Verizon, or AT&T. Together, they control 98 percent of the market.[23] Perhaps you need a vacation. Booking a flight? Well, American, Southwest, Delta, and United Airlines control 67 percent of the air. Okay, maybe you'll take a car. Ten automakers account for 91 percent of the American market share. You get the picture.

With market dominance, these mega-corporations can bend the markets to their will, reducing the kinds of innovation that smaller, more agile firms might create, and buying up those that come close. Worse, as any of these companies become "too big to fail," they can leverage their size with governments to wring out more goodies: "We employ 20,000 people in your state" is a powerful negotiating tactic.

And that's the approach Amazon took when they launched their HQ2 sweepstakes. It wasn't their blue-collar jobs that Amazon was advertising. Rather, the promise of fifty thousand white-collar jobs earning an average of $150,000 a year set every major metropolitan on fire in an attempt to compete. But it was always going to be a race to the bottom. Despite earning nearly $11 billion in 2018, Amazon paid zero dollars in federal income tax, and the goal of the HQ2 contest was always to extract more and more subsidies from local communities—funds that could otherwise have been used to provide basic needs, like affordable housing for the residents now forced to compete for housing with those $150,000-a-year workers.

And when all was said and done, Amazon took a second helping from the cookie jar, opting to build two HQ2s, one in Long Island City, Queens, New York, and one in Northern Virginia. But local activists and politicians in New York were having none of it. They demonstrated against Amazon's blatant corporate capture. Amazon chose to abandon the Long Island City HQ2 project.

The argument that most corporations make for their lavish subsidies is that they create jobs. But even though Amazon employs hundreds of thousands of people, the argument that it creates net jobs is a nonstarter. It has fundamentally automated one of the economy's biggest sectors.

* * *

Early into my trip to Egypt back in 1998, I remember meeting one of my cousin's best friends, Mahmoud. The three of us were sipping fresh-squeezed mango juice from a roadside shop one blazing afternoon when an off-duty cabbie rolled by, windows down and music pounding. It was the Backstreet Boys' "Everybody (Backstreet's Back)." Had I been back home, I probably would have acted too cool to like the Backstreet Boys. But without a rep to maintain in Egypt, I just started singing along in mid-song, comforted by this small reminder of home.

Almost immediately, two other voices started singing right along with me. The car had long passed, but the three of us were holding the tune. I was taken aback: "How do you guys know this song?" I asked. Naively, I had thought that these kids, who'd never left Egypt, would have no clue who the Backstreet Boys were.

"Are you kidding? *Everybody* knows *that* song." Indeed, the impact of American culture is truly international. It turns out that my cousin's best friend was a huge hip-hop fan, and before I left, I found a shop that could burn him a copy of my "Abdul's Summer Mix" CD.

One afternoon, as we were chilling to the tunes, each sharing part of the headphones on my Sony Walkman, Mahmoud asked me what America was like. As I started to tell him about the wide-open roads where everyone follows the traffic laws, and about the boredom of having nowhere to go if you can't drive and you live in a sleepy suburb like mine, he stopped me. "But what's it like *for you*? Do the people there *hate* you?"

"Why would they hate me?" I was taken aback. "No, of course not . . . ," I told him as I searched his face, only now appreciating the gist of his question. "There are a few bad people who don't like people who aren't like them, but mostly everyone gets along," I explained.

"But I thought they hate Muslims in America." Mind you, this was 1998—before 9/11, before the Patriot Act, before the War on Terror, before the war in Iraq. It was before the media would blast images of Americans bombing Muslim cities into oblivion all over the world—before the torture in Abu Ghraib and Guantánamo.

When I asked why he thought that, this young man—who clearly *loved* everything about America and could sing every line to the whole *Billboard* top 100—answered me this way: "Because they kill Muslims."

About six years later, I was on a road trip in California with my teammates on the University of Michigan lacrosse team. I generally enjoyed my time with my lacrosse teammates, building the kind of camaraderie that spending twenty to thirty-five hours a week and long bouts of travel with a group of people united in their love of a sport can engender. Indeed, several of my teammates remain close friends today. But when it came to politics, my teammates—almost all white, mostly conservative—and I didn't always see eye to eye.

It was 2004, in the thick of the Iraq war, and I had taken to showing my opposition to the war by choosing not to face the flag during the national anthem prior to our games. This was many years before Colin Kaepernick would bravely kneel during the national anthem in solidarity with the Black Lives Matter movement, igniting a national firestorm. As any kind of demonstration involving the flag and the anthem often does, my choices offended many of my teammates: they couldn't understand how or why I felt this way. As I tried to explain, I love America—I always have. But I love it enough to demand it to be better, and to believe it can be.

One of my teammates, Johnny, a conservative-leaning, hard-charging Texan, approached me at our hotel after a team dinner one evening: "Abdul, look, I respect you and the way you live your life. And you have the right to believe what you wanna believe. But I've gotta understand something: *Why do they hate us?*" I immediately thought of the question Mahmoud had asked me that afternoon six years earlier.

As someone who's always lived on both sides of this "they" and "us" duality, I've had some version of this conversation many times since. And sometimes I wish I could just disintermediate myself, put Mahmoud and my teammate, and every other person who's ever thought that "they" hate "us" into one room—and let them see the insecurity that drives so many of their assumptions of hatred, and the fear it inspires.

American foreign policy has profound consequences—at home and abroad. The United States has been at war in 226 of 243 years of its existence.[24] In 2017–2018 alone, the United States was militarily involved in fourteen countries. U.S. troops saw combat in eight of them. Too many of these wars—both in the past and today—have been unjust, unwarranted, and inconsistent with our ideals as a country.

War is, in the simplest sense, driven by an international competition for power and resources. It is, in that way, a concentrated reflection of our national insecurity about the future. We fight nearly endless wars in other parts of the world, some of them to maintain geopolitical primacy, and some of them to maintain unfettered access to resources—many of which we don't even really need.

For example, much of our ongoing military presence in the Middle East is, in large part, about access to oil. When President George W. Bush declared war on Iraq in 2003 under the pretense of false intelligence about Saddam Hussein's possession of "Weapons of Mass Destruction"—linking Saddam

Hussein, a secular nationalist, to Osama bin Laden, a militant religious extremist—he played on our insecurities after 9/11 and Americans' general ignorance of Middle Eastern regional politics to finish what his father had started in the region. There were no WMDs in Iraq. There was no connection between Hussein and Bin Laden.

So what was there? A lot of oil—140 billion barrels' worth, the world's fifth largest proven oil reserve. And given Hussein's penchant for belligerence, having made war with Iran (158 billion barrels, fourth largest proven reserve) and Kuwait (101 billion barrels, sixth largest proven reserve), regime change would secure oil markets and American access to oil for some time to come.

This is not uncommon. In fact, a paper by Professor Jeff Colgan for the Belfer Center for Science and International Affairs at the Harvard Kennedy School, suggests that up to half of all interstate wars since 1973 were fought in part over oil.[25] But why are we still fighting wars over oil when our addiction to the stuff is accelerating the destruction of our planet? Yet again, corporate lobbying plays an important role. Oil and gas companies and their utility partners spent $2.2 billion and $2.4 billion, respectively, between 1998 and 2019 to lobby our government. Their purpose was to protect our fossil fuel–based energy system.

We are also still fighting unnecessary wars because we've built an entire industry around the American war machine. American weapons manufacturers lobbied to the tune of $1.1 billion between 1989 and 2019. There has to be a demand for weapons for these corporations—often lead by former military top brass—to continue to deliver on their bottom lines. This "military-industrial complex" needs war to survive. Peace wouldn't be good for business. So it's in their best interest that we continue to fight wars in places like Iraq and make alliances and sell arms to despotic regimes like the House of Saud in Saudi Arabia, who then use those weapons in places like Yemen, killing hundreds of thousands of people. That ballistic missile the Saudis used to kill dozens of kids on a school bus in Yemen in 2018 was a laser-guided MK 82 bomb, manufactured in the United States by Lockheed Martin[26]—a company that spent $13 million lobbying government officials in 2018.

Every time we sell short our ideals in the name of realpolitik, every time we sell arms and subsidize the militaries of despots in countries like Egypt or of countries politically held hostage by religious extremists who violate the human rights of their residents, like Saudi Arabia and Israel, we do irreparable harm to our standing abroad.

Kids like Mahmoud are watching and asking, "Why do they hate us?" They get exploited by hateful, extremist terrorist organizations like Al Qaeda or ISIS who prey on these sentiments to recruit disaffected young people into their movements of death and destruction. There is *never* justification for terrorism or extremism. But we only fan the embers that fuel it when we start unnecessary wars or back despots who drop U.S.-made bombs on innocent civilians.

All the while, the media spin machine does its part by driving the narrative of a "clash of civilizations," generating new pretenses and justifications for war—which kids like Johnny are watching. John Bolton, an architect of America's war in Iraq, became Donald Trump's national security advisor. While in the administration, until his departure in September 2019, he was the chief war hawk behind escalating tensions with Iran. Through years of careful diplomacy, the Obama administration brought the Iranian regime to the table for a historical nuclear agreement, under which the regime submitted to a regularly monitored freeze of its uranium enrichment. However, despite the fact that Iran had been in full compliance with the agreement's stipulations, the Trump administration abruptly and unilaterally pulled out of the agreement. Worse, by slapping Iran with sanctions, they pressured other signatories to the agreement to do the same or risk U.S. sanctions, themselves.

Throughout, Fox News and the conservative spin machine have been ablaze, with talking heads calling Iran the aggressor, highlighting the grievous risk it poses to American security and American interests in the region.

I am no apologist for the Iranian regime, which has blood on its hands in Syria and other countries in the region and has aided and abetted terror—and I condemn their human rights abuses against their own people. But all this warmongering is language we have heard before. If we go to war with Iran, it will be because of the aggressive posturing of a corporate-lobbied administration that is violating international norms of decency and trust to secure access to a substance that is accelerating our global demise.

The fearmongering required to justify war drives insecurity at home, exaggerating the risks we face from abroad. Worse, war is extremely expensive.

All this war requires extraordinary amounts of money. In the fiscal year (FY) 2018, the U.S. spent $649 billion on defense. That is more than the total of the next seven biggest spenders *combined*, including China, Saudi Arabia, India, France, Russia, the UK, and Germany.[27] And that spending is increasing: the FY 2019 budget included an additional $44 billion in military funding.

But the annual military budget is only a small estimate of how much our country actually spends on fighting wars. Over the ten years it was officially fought, the Vietnam War would cost $1 trillion in today's dollars.[28] But that's paltry compared to how much the Watson Institute for International and Public Affairs at Brown University estimates that we've spent on all wars since 9/11: $5.9 trillion.[29]

Imagine if we spent that money to provide Americans healthcare and health research, rebuild our crumbling infrastructure and invest in new clean technologies, and educate our children and leave them free from debt.

Perhaps the worst consequences fall on those we have asked to fight these wars. They are disproportionately likely to be young people from lower-income communities with less opportunity than their peers. Even while they serve, a startling number of our service members' families struggle on food assistance. Nearly a quarter of children attending DOD schools are eligible for free school meals—and twenty-three thousand active-duty service members rely on food assistance benefits. In 2016, service families spent $67 million in Supplemental Nutrition Assistance Program (SNAP) benefits at commissaries.[30]

Their circumstances are even worse following their tours of duty. Although the proportion returning home with traumatic brain injury (TBI) and post-traumatic stress disorder (PTSD) has skyrocketed, our response has not kept pace. Nearly one in five in a random sample of post-9/11 military veterans met the criteria for a TBI,[31] and between 11 and 20 percent of veterans of Iraq and Afghanistan had symptoms consistent with PTSD.[32] These have had important implications for homelessness, unemployment, and poverty. One study found that Iraq and Afghanistan veterans suffered food insecurity at twice the national rate.[33] Further, veteran homelessness remains an epidemic, as more than one in ten homeless people are veterans.[34] Veterans have also disproportionately suffered the consequences of the raging opioid epidemic. Between 2010 and 2016, the number of opioid overdose deaths of veterans increased 65 percent.[35] Our Veterans Affairs healthcare system, which I rotated through as a medical student, remains woefully underfunded, unable to meet the needs of our veterans as they return home. And plans to privatize the system would only open it up to the same systematic failures that the general American healthcare system suffers, as discussed earlier. We owe our veterans so much more. But perhaps most of all, we owe them the wisdom to use our military with restraint and responsibility.

* * *

If politics in a democratic society is meant to be a forum where each of us can contribute to the decisions that affect us all, the corruption of our politics stymies those ideals. Voter suppression, gerrymandering, the electoral college, the dominating role of money in politics, corporate personhood, and corporate capture of government are all meant to subvert our collective will.

As the economy accelerates inequality, our government becomes ever more critical as a tool for empowering those losing out. And yet we find that, because of the porous barrier between our economy and our politics, politics only furthers that inequality; the slow, piecemeal corruption of our politics contributes to our insecurity.

Every day as I traveled across the state, I'd hear someone say, "My vote doesn't matter." Or they'd ask me, "What can someone like me do, anyway?" Having no sense of agency in the choices made by our government, no sense of say in how our public funds are spent, leaves us worried about what might happen when those problems affect us directly—as so many of them do. Our infrastructure crumbles every day, the cost of our healthcare rises, the quality of children's schools falls. Yet we feel powerless to solve these problems.

CHAPTER 19

The spread of insecurity.

If the American dream is the notion that we can work an honest job, make a fair wage, afford the roofs over our heads and the meals on our tables, have a little something left over to enjoy—and, more importantly, believe that our children's lives might be just a little bit better than ours—our households, our communities, our economy, and our politics are slowly grinding our dream to death. They are the miasma of insecurity.

The corporations that once employed legions of Americans—offering them a living wage, meaningful benefits, and comfortable retirement because of the hard organizing and collective bargaining of unions—have sought to automate their workforces to placate financial markets. The average worker is stuck where she was in the late 1960s, while executives are rewarded to excess for the gains in "efficiency" they returned to corporate stockholders. Meanwhile, corporations lobby governments for subsidies, tax breaks, friendly regulatory schemes, and the destruction of unions in the name of the "jobs" they seek to offshore or automate. Cash-strapped governments are left without the means to fund the foundations of the public goods we rely on, like schools and public infrastructure, investing instead in prisons and wars because those, too, have corporate lobbyists. Lost in all of this are the people—real people, not corporations—whom these institutions were meant to serve.

The suffering wrought by each of these systems manipulated by narrow corporate interests, alone and together, degrades our lives, but not equally. The poor *always* suffer more. Without wealth, they are not insulated from the loss of a job or the shuttering of their local health department. Because poor and working Americans are more reliant on public services, like transit and public schools, cuts in these services are devastating for them.

Nor are these systems color-blind. Rather, structural racism shapes the ways they conspire against people of color. Ask yourself: Who is least likely to get a high-quality public education in America? Who is most likely to be arrested, sentenced, and jailed in America? Who is most likely to work a "bad job"? Who has the most debt? Who has the least wealth? Whose children are most likely to drink poisoned water or breathe dirty air? The answers to every one of these questions are the same: Black- and Brown-Americans. Likewise, they bear down on women, sexual and gender minorities, religious minorities, and disabled people.

But these systems and their unequal costs are hard to perceive. They are like the pot of water containing the frog, slowly heating up: they will destroy us, but not quickly enough for us to notice. Like the sorites paradox, the new American paradox goes like this: How many opportunities do you have to eliminate before we can no longer call America "the Land of Opportunity?"

* * *

But how did this miasma of insecurity come about? Who created it? How is it sustained and perpetuated? The answer, paradoxically, is insecurity—although not the insecurity of the poor and marginalized but the paradoxical insecurity of the wealthy. The fear of some future material insecurity compels them to put more space between themselves and the materially insecure, and in hoarding resources and creating and sustaining systems that accelerate inequality, they perpetuate the insecurity under which so many suffer. Paradoxically, insecurity forms a positive feedback loop whereby the consequences of a behavior drives that behavior even more.

But how can people who have so much feel so insecure? Because people are often more concerned with what they *don't* have relative to those with whom they compare themselves, who usually have more. One study of American millionaires concluded that "58% of millionaires say their expectations for their standard of living have increased in the last 10 years. Those whose wealth has increased significantly during this time period are even more likely to feel their standard of living expectations have gone up (64 percent). As a result, the majority of millionaires want more. Those with $1 million want $2 million; those with $10 million want $25 million."[1]

Beyond the stress of the never-ending quest for more, there is a shame that comes with wealth. As my friend Mike did, the rich defend their wealth by underselling all that it affords them. They struggle to fit their lifestyles neatly into the American narrative of "hard work" and "grit." Professor Rachel

Sherman, a sociologist at the New School for Social Research, interviewed fifty young, wealthy New York City residents undergoing home renovations for her book *Uneasy Street: The Anxieties of Affluence*.[2] Her study reveals the general unease that many of the richest Americans feel about the wealth they have—and the ways they narrate it to themselves. They describe their consumption as "reasonable," comparing themselves to those who have more wealth rather than less. They seek to portray themselves as worthy of their wealth, constantly dialing down the way they talk about it—despite spending lavishly on things like renovations, private chefs, nannies, and private schools for their children. Some even describe themselves as "working-class" because they, you know . . . work. As one wealthy real estate agent said, "I work hard . . . my husband works hard, my kids work hard." Indeed, three out of every four millionaires consider themselves part of the 99 percent rather than the richest 1 percent of American society.[3]

But as Sherman argues, this constant attempt by the wealthy to reposition themselves vis-à-vis their wealth has real consequences. It constantly resets the bar for wealth. And in the context of rising inequality, this resetting is dangerous. It justifies the questionable social behaviors of the rich by allowing them the same worries as everyone else. Indeed, in an interview with Kerry Hannon of the *New York Times*, a former Wall Street executive worth millions complained, "I still feel, to some extent, that I don't have enough money . . . I still worry—do I have enough, if I live longer than I thought?"[4] This is paradoxical insecurity in real time.

Paradoxical insecurity has consequences. Evidence suggests that, despite their wealth, the rich are actually less charitable than the average American. An audit of IRS data by the Chronicle of Philanthropy between 2006 and 2012 found that while giving among the lowest-income Americans increased as a proportion of their overall salaries, giving among the richest Americans decreased.[5] Although the rich still give more in overall dollars, the poorest quintile of Americans gave more than twice as much to charity as a proportion of their salaries.

Indeed, studies suggest that the propensity to give actually declines with wealth. Professor Paul K. Piff leads the Morality, Emotion & Social Hierarchy Lab at the University of California, Irvine. His team studies the way that social hierarchy shapes human behavior. One study featured a rigged game of

Monopoly (kind of like our national economy), in which one participant was set up to grow far wealthier than the others. Piff and his team found that the wealthier the rigged winner got, the meaner he became to his opponent—adopting postures that signaled power, explaining the "winning strategy" to his opponent, and even eating more of the free pretzels.[6] In another series of studies, they found that drivers in more expensive cars were significantly more likely to cut off other drivers at four-way stop signs and to cut off pedestrians at crosswalks.[7]

Taken together, these findings paint a picture of the paradoxical insecure: via a stepwise inflation of their lifestyle desires, they are driven to acquire ever more, perpetuating the inequality that robs so many others of the means of a dignified life. They drift further and further away from the experience of the average American, but they cannot see—or cannot admit—how different their experiences have become. Yet with wealth comes greed, the need for more, which drives them to leverage their wealth to gain yet more of the overall spoils. All the while, they're just "working hard," like everyone else.

This has serious implications for the spread of insecurity, as the wealthy sit high atop the summit of our unequal economic system—helping set the rules by which the rest of us are forced to live. From financialization to corporate capture, each of these tactics exists because of the choices of the wealthy and privileged. And each is justified out of a sense of para-doxical insecurity. It's dog eat dog, after all. Eat or be eaten, they reason. And so our inequality accelerates because the wealthy have their feet on the gas.

* * *

Paradoxical insecurity is contagious. First, it spreads vertically by inheritance. Social scientists Stephen Haseler and Henning Meyer, writing about the 950 global billionaires in 2009, argued that "many, indeed most, of these bil-lionaires . . . would not be in the mega-rich category without the aid of a sub-stantial inheritance—for 'inheriting' remains the well-trodden route to great multimillion dollar wealth."[8] One out of every three billionaires globally inher-ited his wealth—billions passed along from generation to generation.[9] Many others may not have inherited their wealth in full, but their accumulation of wealth was aided in large part by the access to capital that their parents afforded them.

Consider one Donald Trump. As he tells it, his father gave him a "small loan" that he, through his business insights and deal-making prowess, turned into a real estate empire worth over $10 billion. The *New York Times* investigative team looked into just how "small" his father's loan had been—and they estimate that his total inheritance was about $413 million in today's dollars.[10] He was earning more than $200,000 a year—enough to put him in the top 5 percent of earners in the United States—at age three.

But it's not just wealth that transfers across generations. In her book *The Sum of Small Things: A Theory of the Aspirational Class*, Professor Elizabeth Currid-Halkett, who teaches public policy at the University of Southern California, argues that today's wealthy are far more focused on investing in the next generation's human capital than ever before. Today's rich are choosing to invest in nannies, tutors, and private schools, hot yoga and barre classes, organic broccoli and cycling vacations across the European countryside— hoarding more opportunity for their children than children without their means could ever afford. These investments exacerbate wealth inequality.

Indeed, some wealthy families aren't even satisfied with these advantages alone. In 2019 an intricate operation to defraud the admissions system at prestigious colleges by wealthy and influential parents was uncovered by investigators. The investigation into their case—dubbed Operation Varsity Blues—outlined how parents used fake nonprofit organizations, paid standardized exam takers, and doctored photos and other forms of ID to con the college admissions system.

* * *

With wealth and prestige comes its cultural trappings. In his groundbreaking 1899 work *The Theory of the Leisure Class: An Economic Study in the Evolution of Institutions*, Norwegian-American social scientist Thorstein Veblen coined the term "conspicuous consumption" to refer to the phenomenon in which the rich spend inordinately on certain items to display wealth. Real estate, luxury cars, fine art, designer clothes—all of these items have become status symbols in our society, a clear, intentional signal of wealth. Along with the requisite wealth, this culture of signaling is transmitted downward between generations.

This signaling also spreads paradoxical insecurity laterally through a perverse version of "keeping up with the Joneses." Mr. Jones just bought a Mercedes—I need a BMW. Mrs. Jones is rocking a new bag on her arm—I need one too. The social pressure of this arms race drives the need to fuel the purchases that sustain it—driving paradoxical insecurity among those with means.

But "keeping up with the Joneses" may also drive *material* insecurity. One evening, while driving down the freeway, I noticed billboards advertising Rolex watches every few miles. I had driven along this route too many times to count—but because it was after midnight, I wasn't on the phone dialing for dollars but was instead free to look up.

The cheapest of those watches sells for at least $3,000, even when they're used. *How many people who drive this road can actually afford one of those?* I thought. And yet Rolex continues to put up the advertising, meaning it must make financial sense to do it. Perhaps their profit margin on any one watch is so high that they can afford to advertise to thousands of people to attract one more marginal buyer?

Or maybe it's something else. Luxury brands like Rolex have often opted for more traditional mass-market forms of advertising—like billboards—rather than more micro-targeted forms of advertising, like social media.[11] This makes a perverse kind of sense when you consider Veblen's argument about conspicuous consumption. The whole point of these luxury brands is to signal wealth. To do that, they have to be marketed to both the wealthy, who can afford them, and everyone else who has to know that their wearers can afford them.

Consider the perverse psychological consequences of this signaling. For the 99 percent of people driving down I-94, that advertisement has little real financial impact: most can't purchase a Rolex no matter how many billboards they see; they can't afford them. And yet these advertisements have real power. They are a reminder to almost everyone on that highway that although they cannot afford one, someone driving on that same highway can. This signaling exacerbates material insecurity. It renders poorer people in more unequal societies more likely to pursue luxury items that they are less able to afford.

Economists agree that luxury cars are uniquely important in signaling wealth because they are both highly visible and portable, which means that, for the most part, you can take them with you wherever you go as a signal of your social status.[12] I learned that lesson on a cold, gray February morning. I pulled into the parking lot of a small community center on a campaign stop in Detroit's North End, one of the city's hardest-hit communities by the financial decline of the past five decades. I was driving a gray Ford Focus. When I decided to run for governor, I had to leave my role as health director, losing my salary along with it. Even on Sarah's salary, though, we were earning more than the median Michigan family. My Focus was a trade-in for the pricier Ford I had been driving. I did get the version with the juiced-up sound system, though, crucial in a car in which I'd be spending twelve-plus hours a day. Having put more than fifty thousand miles on it over fifteen months of campaigning, I'm thankful for the trade-in, both for my pocketbook and for the earth—and the tight beats.

As I walked in, the local pastor overseeing the center pulled me aside. He looked me in the eye to make sure I was going to hear his message: "Son, you gotta get yourself something more than that little gray compact you're driving around. You're a doctor; people expect a little more from you. It's embarrassing."

On my way out, I scanned the lot: Cadillac and Lincoln SUVs abounded. My little Focus did look out of place. *How do folks afford these?* I thought to myself. Inside, I had just finished talking about housing affordability and water access—both issues driving poverty in the country's poorest city. And yet the parking lot, to an untrained eye, would have told a very different story about the wealth in that room.

Peddlers of the myth of "personal responsibility" point at stories like these to argue that poverty is simply a matter of individual choices. "If poor people didn't spend so much money on frivolous things like cars, they wouldn't be poor," their argument goes. There is a naive conventional wisdom to these arguments that belies a complete failure to account for human nature—the social shame of poverty that often motivates our behaviors well beyond poverty itself. Rather than the wholly rational automata of economics textbooks, human beings are social and emotional beings. That's why keeping up appearances is as old as time—and why study after study has shown it to be a powerful motivator of our economic choices.

But inequality increases the cost of keeping up appearances. In 2017, economists started to note some interesting things about our national recovery from the Great Recession.[13] Our total debt, as American consumers, can be used as a measure of our belief in the robustness of the economy. After all, the willingness to take on debt implies a certain level of belief that we'll be able to pay it back—and that the economy will be robust enough to employ us to do that. By the first quarter of 2017, the total amount of debt Americans owed had reached $12.73 trillion, surpassing the debt owed before the onset of the Great Recession for the first time—an important milestone in our recovery.

However, there was something different about the debt that consumers were taking on. In the past, the amount of debt that consumers assumed for cars was relatively stable. By 2017 it had increased 50 percent. Auto debt was even increasing faster than home mortgage debt.[14] Those taking on auto debt tended to be poorer and had worse credit. In the post-recession economy, new regulations had frozen many of these people out of securing the kinds of bigger, riskier home loans that had helped cause the recession in the first place. So instead they were leveraging their incomes into auto loans for new cars. But homes appreciate, while cars depreciate, exacerbating wealth inequality over time.

* * *

If paradoxical insecurity is contagious, so is material insecurity. Professor Raj Chetty, who leads the Opportunity Insights project at Harvard University, set about to answer how likely is it for a child born in poverty to escape it. Chetty and his team traced the probability of a child earning more than her parents over time. For children born in 1940, more than 90 percent earned more than their parents by the same age. By 1984, the year I was born, that number had fallen to 50 percent.[15]

This is particularly troubling in America. Chetty and colleagues also compared the probability of being born in the bottom 20 percent of the income distribution and then earning in the top 20 percent of the income distribution as an adult in the United States and Canada. They found that in the United States only 7.5 percent of children born in the bottom quintile of the income distribution will achieve that—compared to 13 percent in Canada.[16]

* * *

Fearmongering is another mechanism that spreads material insecurity—one, with which, unfortunately, we have become all too accustomed in polarized political times. Fearmongers fix attention upon small relative differences in access to wealth, power, resources, or treatment between groups who are all generally poor and materially insecure. By constantly harping on these differences, they attribute poverty entirely to these small differences, rather than the broader system that has created it. They are obsessed, for example, with the small few who "cheat" a given system, whether "jumping the line" in immigration or defrauding programs like welfare or SNAP (formerly "food stamps"). And although the evidence suggests that fraud is minimal in systems like these, they hold up the exception as the norm. This is what Ronald Reagan did when he created the image of the "welfare queen," an imaginary figure living the life of luxury on welfare and food stamps, all paid for by the hardworking American taxpayer. Today, fraud in the SNAP program adds up to a mere 1.5 cents on the dollar.[17] And yet the image persists.

Images like these are so powerful because they often map onto deeply held, often racist stereotypes. They prey on and drive our insecurities, tempting us to ask why we're playing by the rules when everyone else is so obviously cheating them, which exacerbates racism and xenophobia. The attitude of "Why them and not me?" sets in. This builds animus for the other—the racial, geographic, religious, ethnic, sexual, or generational group being targeted. Next, insecurity tempts us to blame the other for what we don't have. *I don't have X*—a job, affordable housing, good schools for my kids, healthcare—*because of them*, the logic of insecurity whispers to us. Blame begets blame as material insecurity builds. And finally, blame begets hatred. The false perception that "we" must protect ourselves and people like us from "them" drives this escalating war of insecurity.

When she accosted me at the "Three Ex-Terrorists" event, that woman had hit the last stage of insecurity: the logic of insecurity had convinced her that I—an Arab- and Muslim-American and a stand-in for a whole horde of immigrants to this country—was the reason why her child hadn't been accepted to the University of Michigan and why his opportunities would be limited.

To be sure, once fear turns to blame—and then turns to hatred—it drives seemingly counterintuitive choices: insecurity leads to actions more focused on taking something away from another, rather than building for oneself and one's family.

Fearmongering is meant to distract from the systems that actually cause oppression. Don't forget, in addition to the "welfare queen" iconography, the lasting consequence of Reagan's presidency was a massive tax cut for America's wealthiest.

Donald Trump is playing heir to Ronald Reagan. He is today's fearmonger in chief. He rode to power on the narrative that "they"—the Muslims, the Jews, the Blacks, the immigrants, whoever (but oddly not the Russians)—were the reason why so many had lost so much. Only he could "make America great again." His Muslim Ban, his separation of children from their parents at the southern border, his wall, his obsession with murders at the hands of undocumented immigrants—each of these serves as a symbolic testament to his commitment to that future, founded in that past. And yet, like Reagan, his only real legislative victory has been to usher through one of the biggest tax cuts in American history, accruing disproportionately to the rich and corporations, and heaping more of the burden of funding American government onto the people whose insecurity he exploited into voting for him.

This power to divide and conquer through material insecurity is why fearmongering is a choice tool for the paradoxically insecure—people like Trump and his backers. Powerful industries have used fearmongering to destroy nearly every effort to achieve universal healthcare coverage in the United States. For example, facing the specter of a major threat to their profits through comprehensive healthcare reform legislation in the early 1990s, health insurers launched one of the most devastating political advertising campaigns in American history. It featured "Harry and Louise," a fictitious couple having a stressful conversation set "sometime in the future" about how their new government healthcare program didn't cover all of their needs. "When they choose," says Harry, "We lose," responds Louise. In a craven effort to protect their billions in profit, industry executives played on material insecurity to torpedo the reforms.

And yet the exploitation of fearmongering by the rich and powerful doesn't absolve the rest of us. Fearmongering works because we allow it to: we play our part in the cycle of fear, blame, and hatred. We allow ourselves to respond in kind to hatred and to hit back, even though we know our actions will only escalate the hatred. We learn hate, too. We become the equivalent opposite of those who hate us. Yet we think that our hate is righteous, excused by the hatred we have so long endured. But hatred is still hatred. It is still cold. It is still dead. And it is still dehumanizing.

* * *

In this section, I've laid out the American epidemic of insecurity—its symptoms, the miasma that causes it, and the contagion that spreads it. Insecurity threatens that which is most personal: our health, our households, and the dreams we have for our children. It chokes our communities and turns us inward, against each other. It has fundamentally reoriented our economy and robbed us of agency in our politics. And it perpetuates itself as those with means accelerate the inequalities that leave so many without them. It spreads between us as it tears us apart. It creates an insatiable drive to acquire that ultimately leaves us wanting.

It is impossible to understand our politics outside of this epidemic, although we often try. Because insecurity is the lens through which so many view the political world, it fundamentally shapes our collective preferences. A fundamental fear about our future, founded in the material deprivation that so many face, hijacks our goals and the way we go about achieving them.

Our insecurity prioritizes short-term thinking and convinces us to cede yet more power to institutions that promise a reprieve, only to take even more. It convinces us to cut our safety net for the promise of just a little more today. It opens us up to manipulation and exploitation. It convinces those with much that they have little—and that they ought to continue to acquire lest they end up like the others whom their acquisitiveness has marginalized.

Appreciating the dominant role that insecurity plays in our collective political attitudes and motivations should also encourage us to rethink how we engage the project of American politics. When we realize that so many of our worst instincts and worst decisions are rooted in a fundamental insecurity that is driven by the circumstances of our lives, how do we begin to rethink what we are doing and how we are doing it? Treating the insecurity epidemic—cutting the roots of insecurity—will require us to rethink our politics. In the next section, I lay out a vision for what that politics can be.

PART III

HEALING POLITICS

CHAPTER 20
Toward a politics of empathy.

Our American ideals are—and have always been—lofty. Take the preamble to the Constitution: "We the People of the United States, in Order to form a more perfect Union, establish Justice, insure domestic Tranquility, provide for the common defense, promote the general Welfare, and secure the Blessings of Liberty to ourselves and our Posterity, do ordain and establish this Constitution for the United States of America."

These words are a call to action about how we ought to be, what we ought to strive for. They are a striking synthesis of what America ought to aspire to—starting with the call to union. It's tempting to limit this to the union between states. But in its grandest interpretation, it also has to mean the union between *people*. And we shouldn't lose sight of the fact that this whole project, the whole American system, was established to further justice, peace, security, welfare, and the future.

As you may remember from your high school math class, an asymptote is a function that creates a graphical curve that approaches a line but never actually touches it. We approach our ideals like asymptotes. We have never lived up to our lofty ideals. In fact, those words were written by people who robbed Native people of their land and enslaved Black people, and that constitution was used to protect those original American sins.

We may never fully live up to our ideals—and yet, only the future is within the agency of our making. We have no choice but to commit ourselves to reaching—infinitely—for that America. That, to me, is the political work ahead. And if we are to do that work, it will take something that we have lacked in our politics for some time: empathy.

* * *

When I was in medical school, I helped care for a patient with an actively bleeding gunshot wound. The wound was just over his left knee—gruesome and bleeding terribly. As he was rushed in, screaming in pain, his hands had to be immobilized so that he wouldn't try to swat away the medical personnel who were actively working to save his life. Hands immobilized, he kept shaking his leg to ward them off—every poke and prod causing immense agony.

Imagine the fear, the pain, the anxiety of this man in this moment. Had you asked him if he wanted lifesaving treatment, his rational brain would surely have screamed, "Of course!" Yet had you asked him if he wanted to have surgery—to have someone cut open the skin and tissue around this extremely painful wound—his anxiety and fear might have told you to get the hell away from him. To be sure, his emotions were contradictory: surgery *is* lifesaving treatment. But then, that's how emotions work: they're rarely rational, rarely consistent.

The man struggled, writhing in pain. Then the emergency physician on duty that night looked him in the eye, putting her hand on his chest, and said, "Sir, I know this *really* hurts you. And we don't *want to* hurt you. I'm sorry you have to go through this. But if we can't treat you, you could die. I need you to work with me. We're going to get you something for the pain right now. But we don't have much time, so I need you to let us help you. If something hurts too much, I want you to say, 'Break, please.' And we'll give you a break, okay?" Before long, the man was carted off to surgery to remove the slug lodged in his leg.

* * *

"Empathy"—first coined more than a century ago—is one of those overused terms that's often thrown about by self-help gurus and pop-psych authors. Usually it's something about the ability to put yourself in someone else's shoes.

I want to consider the definition more critically, though. A recent review article by psychologists at Coventry University identified forty-three different definitions for "empathy."[1] After reviewing each of these definitions, they concluded that empathy is a response in thought and feeling to someone else's emotions—both automatic and motivated by one's conscious thought—that is a function of both one's personality and the circumstances one is in.

I shared the story about the doctor and her patient struggling with his gunshot wound because it is the best example of empathy I have ever seen.

Rather than engage from her own frame—i.e., *I'm a doctor: Doesn't this guy realize I know what I'm doing?*—she engaged him in his: *This is a man in pain. How would I feel if people kept touching my wound?* She took the time to understand and appreciate what the man was feeling, what he was thinking, by imagining what she might be thinking and feeling in the same circumstances.

Daniel Coleman and Paul Ekman, psychologists who have done a lot of thinking about how we apply empathy in the real world, argue that there are three types of empathy.[2] Cognitive empathy is the ability to understand, intellectually, how someone in a particular situation might be thinking. Emotional empathy is the ability to share feelings with the other person in that situation. Compassionate empathy is the ability to take those thoughts and feelings and turn them into action.

Empathy requires us to center each other—to work with someone rather than against them. It requires the humility to appreciate how another is thinking, how they are feeling, by asking ourselves how we might be thinking or feeling in their circumstances. But empathy isn't just a state of mind. In fact, just as the doctor demonstrated, compassionate empathy *requires* action. Empathizing with people who are doing something harmful doesn't mean that we leave them to do it. It just means that we seek to understand why they do it in order to intervene most effectively. Rather than condemn them to excuse our own inability to change the situation, empathy forces us to contend with their humanity, and therefore to reassess our actions for their likely effects.

* * *

Injecting empathy into our politics is about applying compassionate empathy— the ability to turn our engagement with the thoughts and feelings that come from putting ourselves in the shoes of another—to our political action. Never has this been more important than in the context of the insecurity epidemic, because so many of the political behaviors dividing us emerge from that far-reaching insecurity. Rather than fall prey to the fearmongering that is being used to tear us apart, empathy politics encourages us to recognize the struggle against the system of insecurity that unifies us. Ironically, it is only in centering the emotions of the other whom our insecurity might lead us to demonize that we can turn our attention to the system that has marginalized us all.

Empathy centers our collective humanity. It forces us to ask ourselves, *Why do they do what they do?* In putting ourselves in their position, we can appreciate their own logic in their actions, even in the case of the paradoxically insecure. Only in understanding their logic, however perverse, can we start to engage them in a way that can actually dismantle that logic and the behavior it drives.

Make no mistake: empathy politics is not silent. It is not inactive. Rather, it is the politics of righteous action. It is about embracing our collective humanity in the work of reforming the system that is robbing us of it. It is aggressive—but rather than against individuals, it is aggressive against the system. It recognizes our lived experiences as a means of unity rather than division. It does not dwell on resentment, but it appreciates how resentment might shape one's view of the world. It recognizes that responding to resentment with resentment just breeds more resentment. Responding to hate with hate just multiplies hate.

* * *

Recognizing the syndrome of insecurity, and its consequences for our politics, forms the core of the politics of empathy.

Below, I try to summarize this politics in five principles:

1. Empathy politics seeks to understand and heal insecurity rather than ignore and inflame it.
2. We must have the humility to empathize with pain. At the same time, we must have the courage to speak truth to power.
3. Reforming the systems that have driven our insecurity, inequity, and pain must be the target of our political action.
4. Kindness matters. Meanness is the tool of hatred, and hatred only begets hatred.
5. Representation matters, but we must center ideals and substance in our pursuit of identity representation.

These principles have implications for all aspects of our politics—the outcomes we push for, the strategies we plan, and the tactics we employ.

Empathy politics demands deep, structural reform of the system that has become the miasma for insecurity. It does not accept "pragmatism" as an argument for accommodating a system whose outcomes are deadly, oppressive, and inequitable.

Our leadership centers on the people *behind* us, not just those in front of us at the tables of power. Our politics engages with pain as a means of unification against the systems that *cause* that pain, rather than as a tool for recrimination. And we do not let our pain dominate our commitment to ideals, leading us down the path of resentment and grievance.

And rather than demonize our interlocutors, we empathize with them. Hurt people hurt other people. We recognize that even those who maintain and sustain systems of oppression are people—with all the complexities that come with that. And we believe that all people deserve empathy. We recognize that people can be both wrong and redeemable. Therefore, we do not condemn people but rather their positions, attitudes, and perspectives when they are unjust, immoral, or unethical. We believe that everyone can someday be a partner in the work of justice, equity, and sustainability, even if they may not be today. That is because we recognize that if we are not unifying, we are being divided, and that the work of unifying is what America is about.

Achieving this will be difficult. The people who suffer our peculiar American insecurities most acutely have been locked out of the halls of power for so long. Correcting this—achieving representation in the halls of power—is a fundamental challenge in American politics today. And applying empathy is hardest at our social fissures—and yet that's where it's most important. The fifth principle, the notion that in our pursuit of representation in our politics we must center ideals and substance alongside identity, speaks to how we must do that. In the next chapter, I lay out the case for representation and how empathy politics can guide us as we pursue it.

CHAPTER 21

Them and us.

The 116th Congress is the most diverse in American history—ushering in a 15 percent increase in women, a 10 percent increase in members of color, a 33 percent increase in Muslim-Americans, and a 33 percent increase in members who openly identify as LGBTQIA+.

Yet Congress is nowhere near representative of the U.S. population. In 2019 people of color comprised only 22 percent of Congress, although we make up 39 percent of America. Latinx-Americans and Asian-Americans are underrepresented by half. And even after a 15 percent increase in female members, less than a quarter of members of Congress are women. Worse still, the average member of Congress has twelve times the wealth of the average American household.[1]

This startling underrepresentation is both a cause and a consequence of the system of insecurity. One's perspective on this country as a leader is a function of this country's perspective on you. And unless you've seen America from a particular vantage point, you can't appreciate how those who see it that way may be injured by you—and could be helped by you. As Congresswoman Ayanna Pressley, elected to this historic 116th Congress, so eloquently stated, "The people closest to the pain should be closest to the power." Worse, even, than failing to represent our country adequately, far too many in power are driven by paradoxical insecurity to perpetuate and reinforce the other structures of insecurity pressing on everyone else for their own gain.

* * *

Representation matters. It matters because it *is* empathy in institutional form—assuring that our government, the institutional embodiment of America, knows what it's like to stand in its people's shoes and can act to represent them.

And because representation matters, identity matters, too. The necessary focus on identity to achieve representation has emerged as one of the most critical fault lines of our politics. Indeed, even in the most diverse Congress in American history, 60 percent are cis straight white men—despite constituting only 31 percent of America today.

Some see representation as an existential threat to their grip on power, eliciting rabid, violent opposition. Yet others—including many who identify with dominant groups in power—believe deeply in representation as a matter of *justice* and have stood up to demand it. Yet others are caught in the middle.

Regardless, the discourse about identity politics in America has hit fever pitch. And this is where the politics of empathy is needed most. So how do we apply empathy politics to understand representation—and how should identity shape our politics?

First, let's agree that identity is complex. That's because all of us hold multiple identities. Some of our identities are privileged with respect to physical ability, whiteness, maleness, cis gender, heterosexuality, and Christianity. And some are not. Importantly, privilege doesn't necessarily mean superiority or advantage: it usually means non-inferiority and no disadvantage. Let me explain using myself as an example. Here are a few of my identity groups, in no particular order: non-white, Arab- and Egyptian-American, Muslim, cis, straight, young, abled, male.

As a person of color whose name is ethnically distinctive, my many experiences with police, the TSA, and other agencies of the state have reminded me of these things time and again. And then there are the endless microaggressions—some more blatant, and some less so. For example, my name is Abdulrahman Mohamed El-Sayed. It doesn't matter how many degrees you to affix to it: in America, my name will always leave some people wondering if I even speak English. However, although I am not white, I'm also not Black. My racial identity doesn't expose me to the deep levels of structural, institutional, and individual racism that Black-Americans experience daily.

My name also advertises my faith. And so my allegiances will always be questioned. Throughout my campaign, I wore the requisite flag lapel pin on my jacket, opting for a pin with the crossed flags of the Stars and Stripes and the state flag of Michigan. Our state flag features a moose and an elk flanking a shield with an image of a man by a lake. A bald eagle perches atop the shield. The whole graphic is set over a dark blue backdrop.

While I was touring the Upper Peninsula, an entirely well-meaning elderly white man came up to me. Pulling my lapel closer to inspect it, he asked, "Is that the Egyptian flag?"

"No, sir," I said in my most chipper voice. "I'm afraid there are no moose or elk in Egypt."

I chose to wear my lapel pin on my right side—mostly because men's jackets have a buttonhole on the left lapel, making the placement of a lapel pin there somewhat confusing. Does it go above the buttonhole? Inside?

One morning I was the featured guest on a Detroit-based AM talk radio show, when a gentleman called in and asked if I wore my lapel pin on my right side because I had some kind of aversion to the United States of America. After all, he reasoned, wearing it on the left meant that the flag was close to your heart. By wearing it on the right, I must be signaling where my *real* allegiances lay.

One well-meaning columnist wrote describing what my name might cost me politically. In "Great Candidate, Not So Great Name," he described a candidate named "Andy Smith" who had my life story and credentials.[2] Of course, this candidate's *real* name wasn't Andy Smith but Abdul El-Sayed. His penultimate sentence read, "I find it hard to believe that Abdul El-Sayed can win a statewide election." These are but a few ways in which my ethnic and faith identities leave me susceptible to unfair treatment in our society.

Yet, I am also a cis straight man: both my gender and sexual identity make me a member of multiple privileged identity groups. Beyond this, what sociologists call my "gender performance" is clearly masculine: I look, talk, and behave in accordance with accepted male gender norms. Because of these identities, I walk through the world having inherited centuries of patriarchy that place me in a position of privilege relative to both women and sexual minorities.

The most salient aspect of my privileges here is, quite simply, and in direct contrast to my faith and ethnic identities, that I am perceived as "normal"— with all of the privileges and trappings that come with that. In professional settings, my competence is rarely questioned (at least, not because of my gender), and I am excused if I speak for or over others. After all, we've been conditioned to accept that behavior as "normal" for "masculine" men.

In many ways, I'm not even aware of all the ways I am privileged as a cis straight man. And that's just it: I don't have to be. I can enumerate all of the ways that society will engage me as a person of color, a member of a religious minority, a young person—because that otherness is incessantly felt. But when it comes to the ways that I *am* privileged, I am allowed to go on ignoring the dynamics at play, because, well, knowing them is not a matter of survival. In that respect, my privilege isn't so much about particular advantages I can enumerate; it's about disadvantages that I don't have to. But in a world where some are systematically disadvantaged, not having these disadvantages is an *advantage*. Hence the word "privilege."

* * *

The focus on abled, cis, straight, wealthy, older white men emerges from the aggregation of identities of privilege. These men belong to almost every privileged identity and have never had to walk through the world any other way. They've never had to be "different" or "other," which allows them to ignore the burdens imposed on everyone else—just as I can when it comes to my gender or the fact that I have no disabilities.

And yet these aggregated privileges have deep power. When they succeed, white men tend to be credited for their individual attributes of "hard work," "determination," or "brilliance." Never mind their inherited wealth, their opportunities, or their presumed competence. And when they fail or do horrible things, such as commit acts of violence, we say they are "troubled" or suffering from mental illness. When Black men commit murder, they are held up as a testament to reinforce their racial stereotypes. And when Middle Eastern or South Asian men commit murder, they must have been "radicalized."[3]

There is something almost childlike in this. I conjure the image of my daughter standing on a step stool, turning on the water faucet to brush her teeth—the rest of us applauding her small achievement. She basks in the glory of having done it "all by herself." We know she's standing on a stool her grandparents provided her. We know she's being steadied by her father's reassuring hand. We know that her mother applied the toothpaste to her brush. We know she's not paying the water bill. But we'll never tell her. "You did it all by yourself," we reassure her.

We permit children these exaggerations because they build a sense of self, of agency—important in this world, particularly for a Brown girl who'll be told so many times why she can't.

But if my little girl grows up and still wants me to congratulate her for doing it "all by herself," I'm going to remind her of what her great-grandmother would tell her father: "The only difference between you and them is your opportunity." I'm going to remind her of that rooftop where her grandfather studied between shifts at the fish market so that his dream might be made manifest—in her. No achievement is entirely "all by yourself."

* * *

This assumption of agency is how privilege builds its narrative. The official history of our country hails the achievements of white men—and struggles to hide the scars of their sins. We all know the mythos because it's been written into the history we learn in grade school: Columbus sailing the ocean blue in 1492; the Jamestown settlers and the First Thanksgiving; the Continental Congress; Paul Revere and the Revolutionary War; the Founding Fathers . . . All white men.

But this country was built on the backs of enslaved Africans who were forcibly removed from their homes to till the soils in lands that had been stolen from Native peoples who had tilled and hunted them long before the first white man ever landed here.

These are America's original sins: that a country that holds equality as self-evident should have been founded on the systematic oppression of Black and Brown people. After all, "this Government was made on the white basis," then-senator Stephen Douglas reminded his listeners while debating Abraham Lincoln in 1858. "It was made by the white men, for the benefit of the white men and their posterity forever."[4] These weren't extreme statements at the time: Douglas was reelected to the Senate.

No one but white men could vote until 1870, when the ratification of the Thirteenth to Fifteenth Amendments abolished slavery and finally extended citizenship to Black-Americans and granted suffrage to Black men. Women weren't granted the right to vote until 1920. And because voting was—and remains—a function of state rather than federal government, Black-Americans were then systematically denied the vote through impossible literacy tests and excessive poll taxes. The Voting Rights act of 1965 was intended to do away with that, yet even today systematic discrimination at the polls persists.

The results at the ballot box have been clear. There had never been any-one elected to the country's highest office who wasn't white and male until 2008—a full 232 years since the country's founding. And the backlash to President Obama's presidency has redefined American politics. Even though Hillary Clinton won more votes than any candidate in American history, we have yet to have a female president.

American narratives that cast the history of this country in terms of the achievements of white men, hiding their systematic efforts to exclude every-one else—these are the *true* origins of "identity politics" in America. Indeed, identity politics has been a fact of American political life since the inception of this nation. But this has been an identity politics of insecurity, one waged by white men to protect their privilege.

This identity politics of insecurity—the politics of Stephen Douglas and Jefferson Davis and George Wallace—did not end with slavery or Jim Crow. It links slavery to "America First" today. It is the identity politics of insecurity that Donald Trump continues to pump back into the American psyche. It is a politics of resentment, of anger, of hatred, of exclusion, and of symbolism. It believes in zero-sum power—that the inclusion of others comes at the neces-sary cost of their own exclusion. It subscribes to the "us-versus-them" logic that is the basis of fascism. "Their wins are our losses," they tell themselves.

* * *

But there is another identity politics—the identity politics I believe in. Begin-ning in the 1960s and 1970s, recognition of the fact that people of color, women, religious minorities, disabled people, LGBTQIA+ people, and others who were excluded from full civic and social participation in American society were often kept out by the same forces, and for the same reasons, led to the rise of a new order of social and political organizing on the left. These movements were by no means the first to advocate for equity. They built on a long history of work by trade unions and legal organizations such as the NAACP and the ACLU.

In his book *Engines of Liberty: The Power of Citizen Activists to Make Constitutional Law*, ACLU legal director David Cole lauds the role of these movements in shaping the contours of key legal battles for equal rights.[5] The feminist movement, the Black Power movement, the Pride movement—each can claim a critical role in legislative and judicial wins. These include *Roe v. Wade*, upholding a woman's right to choose; *Obergefell v. Hodges*, upholding the constitutional right to same-sex marriage; and the Twenty-Fourth Amendment, abolishing poll taxes, to name a few.

These movements on the left crystalized what would come to be coined as identity politics by the Combahee River Collective, an organization of Black women agitating for equal rights that included poet Audre Lorde and New York City first lady Chirlane McCray. In "A Black Feminist Statement,"[6] they articulated their mission and means: "We realize that the only people who care enough about us to work consistently for our liberation is us . . . This focusing on our own oppression is embodied in the concept of *identity politics*. We believe that the most profound and potentially the most radical politics come directly out of our own identity." These identity-based social movements emerged as a means of fighting for liberation and social change. They were implicitly "intersectional"—started by a group of women of color—and sought to connect across oppressed groups to advocate for broad social change. The third sentence of the "Statement" states: "We are actively committed to struggling against racial, sexual, heterosexual, and class oppression and see as our particular task the development of integrated analysis and practice based upon the fact that the major systems of oppression are interlocking."

This is the identity politics of empathy—an inclusive, intersectional politics that necessarily opposes systems that oppress and centers those who have been oppressed by them.

I think about this from the perspective of my little girl: the existence of Congresswomen Alexandria Ocasio-Cortez and Rashida Tlaib and Ilhan Omar and Ayanna Pressley is necessary in an America that has any chance of treating her—a Brown Muslim-American girl—fairly. That's because people like AOC, Ilhan, Rashida, and Ayanna, young women of color, are more likely to think about people like my daughter when they propose and vote on legislation—and more likely to understand her lived experience when they do. That's because they *were* her. This is the identity politics of empathy because it calls on our government to empathize with people like Emmalee, to put itself in her shoes. Only when there are people in positions of power who have been in those shoes before—who represent *all* of America—can it do that.

What's more, it matters to me that she grows up in a world where she can see people like her represented in the body responsible for creating the laws that govern her country—to know that she is represented. Because what does it even mean to *be American* if the institutional manifestation of America— its government—doesn't include people like you? Indeed, representation is critical to inspiring people who've been marginalized in our politics to feel included in this system—and our country. At least, it was for the elderly Yemeni-American man whom I met on Election Day. He came out to vote, to participate in the making of America, because it was the first time he could cast a ballot for someone who he felt could relate to his experience.

* * *

But if there are two identity politics—one of insecurity and one of empathy— they differ in more ways than the identities they represent. Donald Trump's identity politics of insecurity isn't just about sustaining the dominance of white people and men. It's also about a politics of resentment, hatred, and exclusion. And our identity politics of empathy isn't simply about promoting representation for people of color, women, religious minorities, disabled people, or LGBTQIA+ people. It also centers empathy, inclusion, and substance in the process. We cannot forget these crucial differences.

The primary tool of the identity politics of insecurity is collective resentment. It has a corrosive quality to it. It seeks to foster anger, hatred, and destruction. If we allow our movement of empathy, inclusion, and substance to be corroded by the emotions evinced by their exclusion and hatred, we risk borrowing their tools. And as one of the chief architects of the "Black Feminist Statement," poet Audre Lorde, reminds us, "the master's tools will never dismantle the master's house."

Collective resentment—the tool of insecurity—opens a gateway to justifying hatred for those who hate us. It is, after all, too easy to become an equivalent opposite to those who hate you—equal in hatred, opposite in direction. Every "us" has an equal and opposite "them." In falling into this insecurity-driven identity politics, we risk losing the factual and moral terms of the debate. That simple "us-versus-them" articulation of our aims gets reduced to the tribalism they crave. Every win for them becomes a loss for us; every win for us, a loss for them. Worse, when their losses become as valuable as our wins, tearing them down becomes as valuable as building ourselves up. "Us versus them" reframes our discourse in all-or-nothing terms. And because we can never have all, we might settle for nothing.

And this is exactly what the identity politics of insecurity and the demagogues who wield it are after. Fascism is, in fact, on the rise globally. Tribalism and ethno-nationalism are gaining, posing an existential threat to marginalized communities, poor and working people, and the rule of law. As we fight it, we must protect ourselves from unwittingly adopting its central logic in direct opposition.

Fascism is a direct outgrowth of insecurity: people struggling with material insecurity turn to their belonging to a certain powerful identity group to assuage it. President Lyndon B. Johnson summed it up: "If you can convince the lowest white man he's better than the best colored man, he won't notice you're picking his pocket. Hell, give him somebody to look down on, and he'll empty his pockets for you."[7] The system is self-reinforcing: material insecurity drives the need for security based in identity belonging, which drives the system that deprives people of material resources in the first place. In the end, fascists achieve power by driving dependence on the state for identity validation in the absence of anything else. Fascists seek to frame *all* identity politics around exclusion. They argue that the only way to maintain superiority and power is to exclude some from the means of power—us or them.

We have to be particularly careful never to assent to this logic of exclusion—seeking to exclude certain groups of people because they have had power for too long. Rather, achieving real representation happens when we *include* more of the people who have been marginalized out of power.

Furthermore, seeking to exclude others based on their identities leaves us excluding people who lack power—and could be allies in the struggle for justice. That's because calculating privilege isn't simple arithmetic. You can't just add up a person's demographic characteristics to calculate an "identity privilege score." People are far too complex for that. As I discussed, I am a person of color and a religious minority—and that has robbed me of certain privileges. I am also an abled, cis, straight man, which has provided me so many other privileges. But what my crude "identity privilege score" wouldn't capture particularly well is this: because of my educational and work opportunities, I am, by many standards, deeply privileged—more so than the vast majority of white men in America. I have a greater earning potential, and access to many institutions that most couldn't dream of. At the same time, my barrier to entry into some institutions—like elected office—is far higher than for the least privileged white men, simply because my name isn't Andy Smith, but Abdul El-Sayed. Identity—and the privilege it bestows—is complex.

In epidemiology, we often deal with a similar problem because medical tests aren't perfect. Sometimes there are false positives, sometimes false negatives. One patient's colon cancer may be missed, while another patient may be diagnosed with a tumor they don't have—even though both got the tests they needed.

Every test has a certain probability that it is, in fact, accurate. To measure that, epidemiologists have devised a few metrics: for every test, we measure its "sensitivity" and "specificity." Sensitivity is also known as "true positivity," while specificity is "true negativity." A highly sensitive test is one that is good at ruling in a disease, i.e., if you have the disease, you'll probably test positive. A specific test is one that is good at ruling out a disease. That means if you don't have the disease, your test will probably come back negative. Another way to think about this is that sensitive tests don't have a lot of false negatives, while specific tests don't have a lot of false positives.

We can think of simple identity as a kind of "test" for privilege. Therefore, for the sake of discussion, let's apply the concepts of sensitivity and specificity here. Being an old white man is highly sensitive for profound privilege, meaning relatively few of those with profound privilege in America, particularly throughout history, have been anything else. However, it's not specific, meaning the vast majority of white men don't have profound privilege. And that's the problem with any attempt at blunt identity calculation: it confuses identity for power, individuals for systems.

Granted, it is true that members of one identity group have held far too much power in our society to the exclusion of members of other groups for far too long. It is also true that white men are more likely to hold power in any institution of which they are a part. However, it is not true that *every* older white man holds more power than every member of any other identity groups. The mistake we've made is to have assumed that a sensitive test is also a specific one. And the consequences are dangerous. If we mistakenly assume that identity stands in for the system of power that elevates certain kinds of people, our analysis risks vilifying and demonizing the wrong people.

The vast majority of white men in America, after all, hold little power. Like all Americans, they live under the same system that is driving insecurity in all of us. Indeed, many are being crushed by material insecurity. In fact, suicide has been increasing for the past decade—and among no one more markedly than white men.[8] White men account for 70 percent of all suicides and are at twice the national risk.[9] This is the insight of the identity politics of empathy: that all of us struggle under the weight of the insecurity epidemic, and all of us must be welcome in the movements to take it on.

And although they may benefit in small—or even large—ways from the system of power, their benefits alone are not, in themselves, the system. Rather than engage people based on how the system may benefit them, we should instead engage people based on how they engage the system. Indeed, some who benefit from the system recognize its injustice and inequity most clearly and have dedicated their lives to correcting it. They are necessary allies in this work.

In contrast, a simple retreat to exclusion just fans the flames of insecurity among people forced to choose between "them" or "us." Remember that insecurity's sentinel symptoms are anxiety and fear. Anger and confrontation tend to be exactly the wrong tools to change the behavior or win the hearts of people who are afraid or anxious. Rage and recrimination only make them *more* afraid. It forces them deeper into a defensive posture.

If we are serious about representation, then we have to insist upon *inclusion*, rather than borrow the tools of the identity politics of insecurity. Inclusion is, after all, the only antidote to the exclusion that has locked too many out for too long. Rather than us *or* them, we have to insist upon us *and* them. All of us.

But insecurity makes inclusion seem like a radical proposition. That's because insecurity thinks in zero-sum terms, it warns us that our resources are scarce—that we cannot invite others because provisions are already short. Insecurity makes necessary enemies out of potential allies.

Therefore, embracing inclusion means confronting our own insecurity. It means practicing empathy with ourselves and others. And it means recognizing the insecurity that sometimes shapes behavior, in ourselves and others—understanding where it comes from so that we can defuse it.

* * *

I don't just support new leaders like AOC, Ilhan, Rashida, and Ayanna because of the color of their skin or their gender; I support what they *believe* in. That's because the identity politics of empathy recognizes that true representation means that it's not enough to look like us if you don't also take a stand against the systems that oppress us. Identity has to come with ideals. That's because the other risk we face, beyond borrowing the tools of insecurity, is tokenization: the promotion of people who look like us but who sustain the systems that oppress us.

Tokenization has been, after all, a principal tool by which movements for equity and representation have been thwarted throughout history. Take British colonial rule over India, for example. The First War of Indian Independence in 1857 sought to overthrow the brutal reign of the British East India Company, which was administering India on behalf of the British crown. Having realized the risks inherent in directly administering colonial rule, the British set up a complicated administrative system called the Raj. In distant, hard-to-govern regions of India covering about 40 percent of the Indian landmass, the Raj included a system of "Princely States" that traded direct administration by British bureaucrats for administration by local rulers—themselves maintained and controlled by the British under an arrangement called "suzerainty."

By dividing communities and then installing rulers who looked like the population they were subjugating, the British maintained their domination of India and its resources for nearly a century more. Under the guise of rulers who looked like the local population, the British could exercise near-autocratic power, deposing one British puppet for another to satisfy the locals if they didn't like the decisions being made. The colonizers gave the people they were colonizing the symbols of change rather than the substance.

These tactics persist today. When I ran for governor in Michigan, some of the fiercest opposition to my candidacy came from within the Muslim community. Some had honest criticisms. But as we demonstrated the strength of the campaign apparatus we were building, and gained real momentum, they came around, many becoming my most ardent supporters.

But a few only got more strident in their opposition as we progressed. Initially, I was flabbergasted. *What more do they want?* I asked myself. Their opposition was venomous, as some resorted to spreading smears against my family and me in the community. I realized that, to a person, they tended to be the Muslims who were closest to powerful people in state politics well before I ever decided to run. They had no independent source of support except their proximity to powerful people.

Their opposition wasn't about my positions or my chances; it was about their power. And I was disturbing it. By playing the token in halls of power, they had come to symbolize the Muslim community to powerful people, elevating themselves by claiming that they "represented" our community. And yet they wouldn't dare deign to even lift a phone to advocate for the community's needs, fearing that pressing their patrons might annoy them—and lose them their coveted positions proximate to power. Their opposition boiled down to two things: First, it was often what their patrons wanted. Second, I became an implicit threat to their personal power. In succeeding, I would upset their delicate charade.

Dynamics like these replicate themselves across marginalized communities. And it's why, as we advocate representation, we cannot mistake symbols for substance. Just because people look like us, or pray like us, or have names like ours, doesn't mean that they care about us or know our experiences. Indeed, the system that has created and sustained the epidemic of insecurity in this country relies on a network of tokens to placate the communities that suffer most.

* * *

Empathy politics responds to the many ways in which the insecurity epidemic has framed our politics. It recognizes that if we are going to build a future that is more just, equitable, and sustainable, then we are going to have to engage in a politics that centers real change. The work of empathy politics must systematically deconstruct the miasma that has created our insecurity in the first place. It has to replace it with a more just, equitable, and sustainable system.

In the following chapters I will discuss empathy *policy*. Some of the ideas I will discuss are commonplace in today's public debate: things like Medicare for All and the Green New Deal. But some haven't quite penetrated. But first, I want to discuss how insecurity has corrupted our conversations about policy and how we can use empathy to have a more constructive conversation.

CHAPTER 22

Empathy policy.

If we're serious about tackling the epidemic of insecurity, then we need solutions at the same level as our problems. We cannot tinker around the edges if we aim to address some of the greatest challenges of our time—challenges that threaten our very future. How do we make sure families aren't punished for having kids? How do we guarantee those kids the best education? How do we make sure everyone has healthcare when they need it? How do we take on the fact that too few of our seniors can afford their prescription drugs? How do we rein in financialization? How do we make sure that Americans are working good jobs again, and how do we address the economy-wide consequences of automation? How do we begin to heal racial inequities?

These are big questions that deserve bold, comprehensive, and thoughtful solutions. The challenge, however, is that our insecurity gets in the way. Insecurity, by definition, scares us away from risk. Do you remember back in Chapter 5 when I introduced the concept of complexity—the fact that, in most real-world situations, there is feedback, where the outcome of a thing can loop around to change that thing? Well, the way insecurity interrupts our public policy conversation is a classic example.

Being willing to invest in a solution hinges on believing that government can accomplish what it sets out to do. But as a society, we seem to have given up on government as a critical component of the solution. That leaves key problems unsolved, which drives our insecurity. But our insecurity keeps us from believing that government can take on those problems. Rinse and repeat. Insecurity perpetuates itself.

But if we're going to address the many causes of our insecurity, it will require us to think and act big, taking bold steps toward the kind of future we want for our children and grandchildren. We need reassurance.

* * *

If we think of our insecurity as an anxiety of sorts, it's worth asking how we treat people with clinical anxiety disorders. One of the most common and effective therapies is called cognitive behavioral therapy (CBT). According to the American Psychological Association, CBT is based on some core principles. Mainly, that psychological problems are based, in part, on faulty or unhelpful ways of thinking. If one can learn better ways of thinking, one can relieve anxiety's grip and become more effective.

CBT is about changing patterns of thinking—recognizing the faulty patterns and replacing them with new, more adaptive patterns of thought. If we know that our insecurity is hijacking our thought patterns, convincing us that we can't address the problems we face, then it's worth considering what, in fact, we should be asking ourselves. What are the faulty lines of reasoning that insecurity is leading us down? Conversely, what are the correct lines of reasoning that would allow us to cut through the anxiety of insecurity?

* * *

First, let's consider the faulty line of reasoning that is driven by insecurity. To do so, let's imagine the usual pattern of thinking that plays out when anyone proposes a bold solution to any of the big problems I named above. It usually goes something like this:

> INSECURITY: "You say you want to take on [insert big issue here]. Well, how are you going to do that?"
> BOLDNESS: "Well, [insert specific policy proposal here]."
> INSECURITY: "Well, how are you gonna pay for that?"
> BOLDNESS: "Well, [insert specific funding proposal here]."
> INSECURITY: "Well, now you're saying you're going to fix [policy proposal 1], [policy proposal 2], [policy proposal 3]. You can't possibly pay for all of them. And even if you could, I don't think the American people would go for that kinda thing. That sounds like socialism."

Too many of our policy conversations devolve into some form of the above—although usually the word "socialism" gets pulled out only as a scare tactic when you've cleared the other two hurdles with a sufficiently competent answer. This conversation is designed to tear down. That's what insecurity does. Let's identify the flaws in this reasoning. I'll start in reverse order.

"Isn't that socialism?" No. It's not.

First, "socialism" is a loaded word: it carries a whole host of historical references, personal experiences, and political innuendo. As a scientist, I was taught that words are a tool for communicating concepts across diverse people. So words that mean different things to different people are not the most useful. "Socialism" is one of those words.

If you're talking to a baby boomer, "socialism" usually refers to that system of government and economics practiced by our Cold War adversary; it was right there in the name of the Union of Soviet Socialist Republics. To them, the word is a non-starter. Not only did we fight the whole Cold War—and many very hot wars—against the spread of socialism, but it failed once already in Russia and its satellites. After kneeling under their desks in the event of a nuclear attack from "the socialists," and tens of thousands of good American boys lost in Vietnam and Korea, they'll be damned if we ever practice such a thing in America.

If you're talking to a millennial, who came of age in post–Great Recession America but may not remember the Cold War—socialism usually refers to democratic socialism, the idea that workers should have a greater share of ownership over the companies that they work for, and that society should provide a basic slate of public goods, like healthcare, transportation, education, union protections, and jobs. According to the Democratic Socialists of America, "Democratic socialists believe that both the economy and society should be run democratically—to meet public needs, not to make profits for a few. To achieve a more just society, many structures of our government and economy must be radically transformed through greater economic and social democracy so that ordinary Americans can participate in the many decisions that affect our lives."

The concept of a "more just society" through more "economic democracy" makes a whole lot of sense in an era when more and more Americans are being locked out of the economy. But frankly, I find the overuse of the word "socialism"—by both its supporters and detractors—distracting. Because the word doesn't mean the same thing to everyone, leaning on it leaves us talking past each other.

And the truth is that the word is often *intended* to distract. Harry Truman—by no means a socialist—said in 1952, "Socialism is a scareword they have hurled at every advance the people have made in the last 20 years. Socialism is what they called public power. Socialism is what they called social security. Socialism is what they called bank deposit insurance. Socialism is what they called the growth of free and independent labor organizations. Socialism is their name for almost anything that helps all the people."[1] That point is as true today as it was back then.

Beyond President Truman's list, consider other public goods, like libraries, and public parks, and publicly funded scientific research. Each of these reflects society coming together through government to solve a problem we cannot solve for ourselves. And they have been wildly successful. The idea that we should not unite to solve some of our most pressing public challenges today is frankly absurd.

* * *

Which brings us to the second flaw in thinking: "How are you going to pay for that?" People assume one of two things: either you want to raise taxes on people, or you want to reallocate funds that have already been allocated elsewhere, meaning that, in effect, you want to cut services in some other area. Sometimes that *is* the answer. I don't believe we should be fighting trillion-dollar endless wars. I'd rather we spent that money on healthcare, or schools, or a twenty-first-century green infrastructure. But usually, that's an oversimplification.

Medicare for All offers a perfect illustration of why. Nearly one-sixth of our healthcare insurance dollars in the most expensive healthcare system in the world goes to overheads that exist simply because we have a system based on having multiple insurance companies. Each has its own marketing budget, an army of billing staff, and, of course, a CEO making many millions of dollars. In addition, multiple billing systems force healthcare providers, like the doctors and hospitals that actually provide you care, to have far more personnel dedicated to sorting them all out.

Medicare for All reorients that system so that we abrogate the necessity for all of this overhead and focus our resources where they need to go: taking care of people. This of course means that the way we pay for care will change. Rather than our employers and us sending a premium check out to some insurance company every month, we might pay a payroll tax, but the overall costs will decrease. And the everyday American will be just a bit richer and far more secure for the reform. But when the "How do you pay for it?" question is asked, these added efficiencies of reform are never baked into the new price.

Second, in an era of profound inequality, one of the most egregious facts of our American system is the absurd level of corporate subsidies that result from corporate capture. It leaves wildly profitable corporations like Amazon paying literally nothing in income taxes. What makes this all the more ridiculous is that corporations have made a habit of claiming the rights of people. But shouldn't the rights of people come with the *responsibilities* of people?

If I made as much as Amazon in 2018, I would owe Uncle Sam more than $4 billion. Amazon somehow gets free speech, like I do, *and* the right to pay nothing in taxes. But then, if I made as much as Amazon, even as a real-life human being, I'd be in that rarefied class of mega-billionaires who also, somehow, get to pay less in taxes. Like others in my earning stratosphere, I'd get to exploit a spate of tax loopholes for the very rich that would allow me to move money into different assets and holdings that, in effect, leave me like Donald Trump, paying an effective tax rate that is far lower than what I actually pay as little old me. Billionaire investor Warren Buffett penned an op-ed in the *New York Times* in 2011 in which he described paying a lower effective tax rate than anyone else in his twenty-person office.[2] And that was before Donald Trump's tax cut, which favored the super-wealthy further still.[3]

Asking the richest Americans and the corporations they control to pay their fair share is just fair. It's also not unprecedented. It hasn't always been this way. In the 1950s and 1960s, widely agreed to be among the most productive period in American economic history, the top marginal income tax rate was 91 percent.[4]

And Americans by and large support raising taxes on the wealthy and corporations. In 2016 an American National Election Studies analysis found that fully two in three Americans favored raising taxes on millionaires.[5] Similarly, a 2017 Gallup poll found that 67 percent of Americans believed that corporations pay too little in taxes.[6]

Only after we've jumped these two hurdles in our flawed thinking can we start talking about actual solutions. Which we'll get to in the next chapter.

* * *

But first, if we've identified the flawed thinking that has hijacked our policy conversations, let's consider the questions that we *should* be asking instead:

1. Is this a serious problem that the government should be solving?
2. Are we, as a society, willing to invest in a solution?
3. What is the most effective, efficient, and sustainable solution to the problem?

In its simplest form, government exists to solve problems that we as individuals or the organizations we create cannot solve on our own. Classic examples of this include policing and a military—which protect private property—but if these were the only things government did, we'd be missing a lot of important responsibilities. Simply focusing on private property seems to miss the point. It's not about property; it's about people. Focusing on property, in effect, limits the attention of government to those who own property—and heaps more attention on those who own more of it. Rather, I think that government ought not to simply solve problems that we as individuals or organizations cannot solve on our own but rather solve problems that we cannot solve on our own *equitably for everyone living under that government.*

What does it mean to focus the responsibilities of government on providing a set of critical public goods that we cannot provide for ourselves or through our organizations *equitably for everyone*? It means that government takes on broader responsibilities for things like clean air, potable water, working infrastructure, urban planning, public health, and basic healthcare, to name a few. If this sounds an awful lot like providing the things I brought up in the last section when discussing the causes of insecurity, it's because it's basically the same list. In effect, the epidemic of insecurity exists today because we as a society, acting through our government, have failed to provide the basic public goods and services that are so critical to living a dignified life to too many in our society. Our government is failing its responsibilities.

It's important to distinguish between "equitably" and "equally." When we speak about equity and equality, we can be referring to both the outcomes that we desire and society's investments to attain those outcomes. I believe in equity at both ends. When it comes to outcomes, I don't believe it's possible to provide for equal outcomes. Rather, one ought to attempt to correct systematic and structural obstacles imposed on some people and not others.

Similarly, I don't believe that everyone should be given exactly the same investment. Circumstances have dealt some people particular challenges, and society should help address them. Disabled people, for example, deserve accommodations above and beyond those of us who are blessed not to have been challenged in that way. Similarly, correcting structural inequality is a government responsibility.

Back to the first question we should be asking: Is this a serious problem that the government should be solving? Well, if it's something that all of us need in order to live a dignified life—and something that government has a unique capacity to provide *equitably for everyone*—then the answer is yes.

On to the second question we should be asking: Are we, as a society, willing to invest in a solution?

This is where our insecurity tends to hijack the conversation. One simple way to cut through this is to ask whether or not there are societies that have accomplished this or something like it—even if ours has not. We Americans love to boast that we are the greatest country in the world. I firmly believe this to be true. However, being the "greatest" implies that if something is possible, the greatest ought to be able to do it. If a society can provide its people high-quality, accessible, affordable healthcare—which many societies in the world do every day—then we ought to be able to, too. If many societies are on their way to cutting their greenhouse gas emissions, we ought to be able to as well. If many have figured out how to build reliable public transit systems that connect urban, suburban, and rural communities . . . well, you can guess the answer.

* * *

Once we correct the flaws in our thinking that break us out of the insecurity death spiral, we can have a serious conversation about bold solutions to solve big problems. In the next chapter, I will lay out thirteen ideas that I believe we ought to be pursuing right now. This isn't intended to be a comprehensive list. For lack of space, there are a lot of important reforms I do not engage with—and some that I engage with less deeply than they deserve. Rather, I offer a basic collection of necessary policy proposals to tackle our insecurity epidemic, reverse our growing inequality, and provide every American with the means to a dignified life.

Each is bold, requiring us to remember that big problems require big solutions. We can't continue to dawdle at the edge of the miasma of our insecurity and think that we are going to solve it. Rather, we have to aim at the very foundations of the structures that have created our problems.

CHAPTER 23

Thirteen ideas to heal our insecurity.

1. Medicare for All

We live, on average, five years less than those in the longest-lived country in the world. We pay nearly twice as much as the average in other high-income countries for our mediocre health outcomes[1]—although our system rewards its corporate honchos handsomely. This is because of a fundamental misalignment in healthcare. Rather than caring for us as patients, it is focused on us as customers. It eliminates our choices, jacks up our prices, and misses the opportunity to protect us from getting sick in the first place.

Medicare for All is a simple, elegant approach to providing everyone with health insurance. It would provide for a single government-owned and -operated insurance program that covers necessary healthcare, vision care, dental care, mental healthcare, and long-term care.

Medicare for All would, first and foremost, achieve the goal of universal coverage: healthcare for every American. But that cannot be the only goal of real, lasting health reform. And that's where Medicare for All shines. The fact that 5 to 10 percent of Americans don't have healthcare on any given day isn't the only problem; it's just a symptom of a far bigger disease. Medicare for All is the only proposal that cures that disease.

The disease is a relatively unregulated market of private health insurers that are focused on private gain rather than the public good. These health insurers (called "payers," because they're the ones who actually pay for healthcare) create a tremendous amount of redundancy in the system. Because there are so many insurance programs, each hospital and doctor's office has to have the billing staff to be able to interface with all of them, vastly increasing costs. The overhead on health insurance in the United States is upwards of 15 percent.

By contrast, the overhead for Medicare—the popular government health plan for people over sixty-five or living with disabilities—is much lower, between 3 and 4 percent. Medicare doesn't have to market, it doesn't have to lobby, and it doesn't have executives who earn millions. Medicare for All would reduce the number of payers to one, thereby vastly reducing the overhead costs in American healthcare.

Furthermore, it would make the U.S. government the only buyer of health-care. That's powerful. We all know what a monopoly is: when there is only one seller of a good. And we know that a monopoly allows the single seller to dictate the price of that good for their profit. But there's an inverse relationship, too—when there's only one buyer. That's called a monopsony. In a monopsony, that buyer has supreme market power, too, allowing it to, in effect, dictate the price of the good in question. Under Medicare for All, the U.S. government would become the monopsony buyer of healthcare on our collective behalf, allowing it to vastly reduce the costs of care for all of us.

This is important when it comes to all kinds of care, but it is particularly important when it comes to prescription drugs, which are costing Americans way too much, as already discussed. Medicare for All would have the ability to negotiate drug prices on our behalf—that is, of course, if we are willing to stand up to the pharmaceutical lobby and repeal the legislation that is currently prohibiting it from doing so.

Gone would be the premiums, co-pays, and deductibles that make private health insurance so hard to understand—and such a headache to use when we actually need it. Although opponents of Medicare for All often argue that, in opinion polls, private insurance is quite popular among those who have it, what they miss is that most people on private health insurance don't actually have to *use* their insurance all that often. They are healthy. But ask anyone with a serious chronic illness how happy they are, and you'll get a very different answer.

That's because private insurance makes money by denying people care. After all, in any business, the goal is to take in more money than you spend. That's why insurers put up all kinds of hurdles to actually paying out, betting against the likelihood that you will keep calling their 1-800 number, keep waiting on hold, and keep haggling with some feckless corporate bureaucrat in a faceless row of cubicles.

Remember the whole debate about preexisting conditions? It concerns patients who, by virtue of a previous illness, insurance companies know will cost them more money. Before the Affordable Care Act, the insurance companies just booted those people off their rolls. Today they're forced to keep them on, but often at exorbitant costs.

This business model is also why private insurance companies often limit the doctors you can see. They'll only pay for the doctors with whom they've worked out deals. And that's why, contrary to the corporate talking points, Medicare for All would actually *increase* our choice. Under Medicare for All, the government would become our insurer and pay doctors on our behalf. There would be no shady backroom negotiations between insurers and hospital systems for preferential rates, so you would not be limited to the doctors with whom your insurer has agreements.

Those preferential rates are also responsible for massive hospital and insurance sector consolidations that have shut down so many hospitals and left us all with less choice. Those shutdowns have decimated rural healthcare in particular, forcing rural Americans to drive hours to get medical care. That has had important implications for addressing rural healthcare crises like the opioid epidemic.

Medicare for all solves all of these problems. It guarantees everyone healthcare. It reduces costs by obviating the massively bloated overhead on both the payer and provider side. And it increases choice by reducing consolidation and eliminating in- versus out-of-network coverage.

Another challenge that we have with our current healthcare system is that it incentivizes medical school graduates to go into more lucrative specialties, like plastic surgery. Although there are plastic surgeons who do incredible work treating accident victims and people with congenital deformities, that's not where the money is. That trend toward the more lucrative specialties leaves us with chronic doctor shortages in specialties like psychiatry and family practice. Many more students might choose other fields if they didn't have to worry about huge levels of student debt. Medicare for All can help solve this by funding medical education from medical school through fellowship. And because Medicare would become the monopsony for healthcare under Medicare for All, it can reprogram reimbursements to make more public-spirited specialties more lucrative, too.

And there's another, perhaps even more important benefit of Medicare for All. Beyond healthcare, public health is about what we do as a society to foster the conditions under which people can be healthy.[2] It's about doing what we can to keep ourselves healthy in the first place—to prevent the diseases that ail us.

One of the hardest things about public health is that it has to go beyond healthcare. After all, people only come to the clinic or hospital *after* they get sick. But they get sick in the places where they live their lives, and to prevent that illness, public health has to go there, too. So, while it keeps one foot firmly planted in health, it leaves the other free to roam into other areas of public policy that are so critical to keeping us healthy. The environment, housing, water infrastructure, and public schools are all places where public health should operate—if we choose to appreciate how they impact our health.

In that respect, there has been a focus in public health circles on a "health in all policies" approach. That means advocating with health in mind as we discuss why we need to rebuild our water infrastructure so that it doesn't poison small children, for example, or why we have to articulate the consequences of climate change in terms of life expectancy. I believe deeply that if we were to take this approach to our health—if we were to consider the human cost of the various policy choices that we make as a society—that we would make vastly different choices. When you think about transit infrastructure in terms of life-years it could save by reducing obesity, hypertension, diabetes, and heart disease, it definitely changes your perspective.

But right now we have caged public health because we lack the incentives to really prevent disease in the first place. Our system is uniquely bad at investing in prevention. In fact, the Centers for Disease Control and Prevention's entire prevention budget amounts to a measly four dollars per person per year.[3] Prevention requires some investment now to produce a payoff at a later time. But in our multi-payer healthcare system, people change insurance too often for the payoffs to be realized by the insurance company that made the initial investment. Medicare for All realigns the incentives for prevention: investments today mean savings tomorrow.

Our insecurity will tell us that Medicare for All is too expensive, that we cannot possibly pay for it, and that it will send our taxes sky-high. But consider what we discussed earlier. First, reorienting the system will vastly reduce its overall cost and probably, more importantly, reduce the rate at which its costs are growing.

Furthermore, in this case, there's good reason to charge big corporations a large proportion of the costs: Medicare for All would replace the healthcare costs they already have to incur as a result of paying for private health insurance for their employees. Finally, although it may raise our taxes, it would eliminate the out-of-pocket costs that render private health insurance so expensive to begin with.

And then there is the added value to society: I've met countless people who told me that if it weren't for the healthcare benefits at their dead-end jobs, they'd have left a long time ago—started that business or gone back to school for an advanced degree.

2. Green (and Blue) New Deal

Climate change is the most critical, most alarming, and most imminent challenge with which we have had to contend. According to the UN's Intergovernmental Panel on Climate Change, we have until 2030 to put in place real structural changes to the way our energy system works to avoid permanent increases in global average temperatures.[4]

Yet global governments are largely failing to act for three reasons. First, we are destroying lives and livelihoods to protect a system of energy production that is the main cause of climate change. This should be bewildering, but unfortunately it's easily explained by the fact the oil and gas industry spends millions lobbying federal, state, and local officials. Second, it's hard to perceive slow change—or to tie slow change to an actual cause, just like that poor frog we keep talking about boiling. Even though we are being hit by storms or wildfires that we call "once-in-a-century" at a yearly rate, there are too many ways to ignore them. This gives room for climate deniers and industry sympathizers to wedge doubt in people's minds. Third, the global rise of the far right has left us backsliding on global climate policy just when action is needed most. Beyond Donald Trump's disastrous choice to pull us out of the Paris climate accords, the election of Jair Bolsonaro in Brazil, home to the world's largest patch of rain forest, threatens that critical country's policies on climate action. Indeed, in the summer of 2019, wildfires ravaged swaths of the Brazilian rain forest, and evidence indicates the Bolsonaro regime was indirectly responsible.[5]

We have no choice but to face head-on our country's role in perpetuating this system. What is clear is that we are already starting to see the consequences of climate change in storms and wildfires and droughts worldwide. Poor and working people, usually in coastal urban communities around the world, will suffer worst. This, like so many of our challenges, is a generational problem, one that will hit our kids and grandkids harder than it is hitting us. That's, perhaps, why we're seeing the most urgent leadership coming from our youngest people. People like Greta Thunberg, a Swedish teenager who kicked off a global climate strike, and the young people of the Sunrise Movement are leading the way on advocacy and activism on the Green New Deal.

I support the Green New Deal. The framework would have us offer a federal job guarantee to build the national infrastructure we require to move our energy system to 100 percent renewable energy. Leveraging a big-bet investment in a green future and our own ingenuity, determination, and potential to guarantee it offers our nation the framework to solve three mutually reinforcing challenges at the same time.

While the speed with which our economy can transition is, in part, a technical question, most answers to technical questions devolve, in the end, into questions of political will. How fast can we go to the moon? That was a technical question, too, when President John F. Kennedy proposed it. At the time, nobody would have said nine years—which was the remarkably short time it ultimately took. The trick was that JFK didn't just ask us—he dared us. Given the startling rapidity with which our climate is changing, the Green New Deal is like a dare at gunpoint.

Do we have the political will to break down the political and economic obstacles to achieving 100 percent renewable energy? That is the real question. No doubt this transition will require a massive investment in technical innovation and infrastructure—not just the wind turbines and solar panels and geothermal rigs we will need to harvest renewable energy, but the batteries and disseminated grid that we will need to store and allocate it against broad variations in supply and demand. There is no doubt that this kind of mass-scale investment will create more than enough jobs to guarantee work for everyone looking for it.

I believe that the framework also needs to add a greater focus on water: a Blue New Deal. Perhaps that's because I'm from a state that is defined by its fresh water—and because my state is also known for its failure to provide that water to its people in places like Flint and Detroit. But water scarcity has implications for our global future too. Today, 2.7 billion people face water scarcity—and 2.4 billion are exposed to unsafe wastewater.[6]

Those numbers are expected to grow. At current consumption rates, by 2025, two-thirds of the world's population is likely to experience water shortages.[7] Wall Street—you know, the folks who take bets on what is going to be valuable in the future—has already started to forecast the commodity implications. Goldman Sachs called water "the petroleum of the next century."[8]

A Blue New Deal will require us to rethink the way we govern, preserve, and protect water. We need a massive investment to improve our technology and infrastructure for water purification, such as desalination, water delivery to reduce wastewater, and wastewater processing. We must also think critically about water governance, both within and between countries—about how much water we are willing to allocate to large corporations for exploitation for profit or use in wasteful industrial processes, and about how we enforce the efficient, effective, and equitable use of water.

Will the Green (and Blue) New Deal be expensive? You bet—but I invite you to consider the cost of *inaction*. In 2018 alone, the top ten biggest climate-related disasters cost $85 billion.[9] And it's getting worse. Furthermore, the Green New Deal calls for investments in infrastructure and people—both of which generally generate huge returns. Also, if the earth becomes uninhabitable for our progeny sometime in the future, I do hope they won't look back and ask why we put such a small price tag on their wellbeing.

But let's be honest: at core, most of the opposition against the Green New Deal isn't about the cost. It's not even about the policy solutions themselves. It's about the fundamental premise that climate change is real and poses an existential threat to humanity as we know it. Unfortunately, climate change denial has become a hallmark of the right. And the clock ticks away while they balk at any form of action, instead appeasing the energy corporations that fund them and whose financial incentives keep us wedded to the status quo.

3. Comprehensive Education Guarantee

There's something uniquely human about knowledge. With most goods, giving some to someone else necessarily reduces the amount that you have for yourself. But knowledge never decreases when you share it; it increases. As a former professor, I often found that teaching something, even if I had taught it many times before, improved my own grasp of it. In working to answer a student's question or mentor another through a problem, I often came to see the material in a new light. My knowledge, in fact, got *stronger* because I shared it. That is perhaps why the greatest human breakthroughs occur through collaboration. Increasing our collective knowledge *requires* that we share it.

Beyond that, innovation is the engine of our growth. We must realize that corporations, as entities, matter far less for economic growth than do the people who work in them. And assuring that those people are as well stocked with knowledge as possible should make common sense.

Finally, education is the most important and enduring driver of a person's life trajectory. A college education is worth $1.3 million in additional lifetime earnings[10]—and even more in terms of its contribution to the economy. The benefits extend well beyond earnings. One study considered differences in a number of activities, behaviors, and outcomes among college-educated Americans compared with their non-college-educated peers.[11] The college-educated were more likely to volunteer in their communities and participate in civic organizations.[12] They were more likely to report that they were happy. They were more likely to rate their health as "good" or "very good"—and more likely to exercise, be a healthy weight, and wear a seat belt. In fact, a white man with a college degree in America will outlive his counterpart without one by twelve years on average.[13] And that gap is widening.

And it's not just a college education that matters. Studies on the effects of education as early as pre-K on children's long-term life trajectories are equally convincing. One study tracked people at age thirty-five who had been enrolled in a structured pre-K through third grade program as children and found that they had nearly a 50 percent greater probability of finishing an associate's degree or higher.[14] Another followed kids enrolled in a universal pre-K program through middle school and found that they had better math scores, were more likely to be taking honors courses, and were less likely to have to repeat a grade.[15]

I believe that in order for Americans to engage the full benefits of the opportunities our country ought to afford, people deserve unlimited access to whatever education they can take on: it improves their lives and our lives. If information is value in this "information age," then we should be offering it wherever, however, and whenever we can.

And yet, never has education been harder to get. What is astounding is that our federal government spends eight times as much on the means of ending a life abroad via the military than it does on the means of making one through education. Even when you factor in state and local spending on education, we still spend nearly $100 billion more on the military than on education.[16]

To address this, we need a comprehensive education reform package. First, we need federally funded universal pre-K. That will require a massive investment in the physical and human infrastructure that we will require— the space, the buildings, and the teachers—to expand nationwide access by 150 percent of what is currently offered. Much of this physical infrastructure could be funded through a public bank, which I'll discuss below. It will also require dedicated funds to ensure that the four million children who are eligible every year get access. With a return of about $17 per dollar invested in pre-K,[17] there is no doubt that this is an investment worth making.

Because our education system is funded locally, school districts in poorer communities suffer, perpetuating a cycle of poverty. Therefore, education funding ought to be federalized and it ought to follow each student, independent of where that student grows up. A child in Detroit should get the same quality public education that I got growing up in an affluent suburb a short drive away.

More pressingly, U.S. K–12 education simply needs more investment. While our military budget grows by the year, we're watching education funds stagnate or decline. That's why I believe that we should pass a federal law pegging our country's education funding to its military funding.

Schools are a lot more than the places where our children learn; they're also the places where our children play and eat and build relationships. Therefore, we need to expand our concept of what schools should be and fund them accordingly. Schools need to be places that serve healthy, high-quality meals, and the school meals program should be expanded. Rather than threaten to remove children from their parents' custody, as one district in Pennsylvania did in 2019 when students were incurring steep school meal debts, we need to ensure that our kids are getting the nourishment they need regardless of their ability to pay. To remove the stigma from children getting assistance, we should make the program available to all, regardless of family income.

Para-educational professionals ought to be empowered and invested in. Social workers, for example, are some of the most important staff in a school, empowering students to deal with some of the challenges they may face outside the classroom and allowing teachers and students to do what they do best: teach and learn. One study of the one hundred largest high schools in America found that more social workers in a school predicted a higher probability of graduation.[18]

School infrastructure investments should account for the fact that school buildings are community spaces that bring people together. They should be built that way. And rather than rely on local funds, school infrastructure funding should also be federal.

Public education should stay public. Although there are a few exceptions, the charter school model has failed. Proponents of charter education frequently cite uniquely highly achieving charter schools to prove their point. But such schools often benefit from either explicitly or implicitly cherry-picked students. Often run by for-profit management companies, these schools spend an inordinate amount of money on marketing—money used on glossy billboards rather than to educate children. They do this to compete with public school districts for per-pupil education funding, which follows children to the schools they attend. That has a crippling impact on public school districts. Worse, charter schools often fail. This cycle of schools opening and shutting down destabilizes communities.

This is why I join the NAACP and several other prominent education and racial justice organizations in calling for a ban on for-profit charter schools. For-profit charter operators should not be allowed to privatize public funds, pocketing public money for private gain.

Finally, I believe in college for all. That means debt-free and tuition-free college education—for everyone. We would pay the cost of every student's tuition, and we would ensure that lower-income students are not forced to take on debt to pay their living expenses while they study. Importantly, this should include all forms of college, including associates degrees, junior college, community college, and skilled-trades courses.

Some argue that this would amount to a wealth transfer to the richest families, who, in our deeply unequal education system, usually get to go to college today. But they fail to account for the fact that one reason that many lower-income students don't go to college is because it is so expensive in the first place. Further, our current system has failed to address deep inequities in our pre-K–12 education that leaves lower-income students worse prepared to succeed academically and aspire to a college education.

We have to build the system we need, that we know is possible, not hold ourselves down with the one we have, however much our insecurity tells us that we can't. And in the system we need, no student should have had any obstacles to achieving her maximal educational potential. In that respect, this proposal should be viewed in the context of the other education reform ideas I proposed earlier.

Even if we halted all new college debt today, it would remain a national crisis. If you were to combine the GDPs of Australia, New Zealand, and Ireland, they'd be less than the total student debt in the United States.[19] College debt pins people down just as they're supposed to start climbing. And that's why it's not enough for us to just solve the problem for future students; we have to do something about those who are struggling today. And that's why we should simply cancel college debt.

Isn't that really expensive? Yes, but not as expensive as the overall impact on the economy of the massive debt people are carrying. Think about it this way: the dollars that would be freed from going to service student loan debt would instead be used to buy stuff in our economy or invest in it. And that throughput is what makes the economy churn.

4. Worker Rights and Corporate Responsibilities

Inequality is a scourge that is driving American insecurity. It is a consequence of the system of corporate excess and the capture of our political system by corporate lobbying. Our national mythos contends that anyone can find a great job in America, and if they're willing to work hard and play by the rules, they can make it.

And yet our economic system is failing that notion. If we are going to address our extreme inequality, empower real people, and hold corporations accountable, we need a slate of deep reforms. We have to make sure the rich pay their fair share in taxes. We need to re-empower unions, the bulwark of workers' rights. We need to ensure that all workers earn a living wage. We have to pivot to address the economic consequences of automation. If corporations want to have the rights of individuals, they should also be forced to bear the responsibilities. And finally, we need to change the way that corporations are governed so that workers are included in decision-making and political engagement is done with the whole corporation's knowledge and approval.

Much of our climbing wealth inequality is driven by the very rich using tax loopholes to avoid paying an equitable amount of taxes. If we're going to be specific, we should differentiate between income and wealth. Income is what a worker is remunerated for her labor. Whereas wealth is the capital one has accumulated. For example, Warren Buffett pays himself $100,000 as CEO of Berkshire Hathaway. However, he's worth about $84 billion in assets. His income is high, but his wealth is astronomical.

With respect to how we tax income, it's important to remember our history. The highest marginal rate in U.S. history, in the 1950s and '60s, was 91 percent. That's far higher than Congresswoman Alexandria Ocasio-Cortez's proposed maximal marginal tax rate of 70 percent for each additional dollar earned above $10 million. (Importantly, a marginal rate is what you pay in taxes above a certain earning threshold. So the marginal tax rate of 70 percent over $10 million applies to the 10-million-and-first dollar rather than the $10 million before it—which would be taxed at whatever lower rate is consistent with their marginal rates.) Seeing as our economy was both extremely productive and most equitable during the 1950s and '60s, I support the Ocasio-Cortez proposal.

Furthermore, I believe that we should be charging an additional wealth tax on accumulated income, as Senators Elizabeth Warren and Bernie Sanders have proposed. Warren suggested a 2 percent wealth tax on those with wealth greater than $50 million, and 3 percent for those worth more than $1 billion. Although enforcement would be challenging, it's the kind of proposal that has a real shot at addressing our accelerating inequality.

To empower the American worker, reinvigorating unions is a critical first step. The assault on unions, in the form of Right to Work laws, prevailing wage repeals, and old-fashioned union busting, has decimated the union movement and it's political and organizing power. We have to continue to drive efforts to overturn the disastrous Right to Work laws, which have stripped away workers' rights. In 2019, Democrats introduced the Protecting the Right to Organize Act (PRO) to protect union rights. It would allow workers to directly sue employers who bust unions and allow the National Labor Relations Board to fine employers who interfere with employee unionizing efforts. I support this proposal.

Nearly six in ten Americans earn an hourly wage—meaning many families are trying to survive on them. Nearly half a million are living on the federal minimum wage. As noted earlier, if minimum wage had kept pace with inflation since the late 1960s, it would be more than twenty dollars today, *so that's what it should be*. It should also be indexed to the consumer price index thereafter, so that it grows automatically every year with inflation—as is the case in seventeen states already.

Some argue that these policies would destroy small businesses, but that takes a narrow-minded view of how the economy works. The driver of our economy is consumption; offering minimum wage workers that kind of bump would vastly increase the amount of money they would use to consume, circulating it right back to small businesses through our economy.

The other argument that detractors make is that it would accelerate automation, as employers would have more incentive to automate higher-priced labor. However, economist David Autor of MIT, who studies automation, suggests that full automation is less likely at the lowest end of the income distribution.[20] That's because those jobs are more likely to rely on manual dexterity, which is extremely expensive in a robot. Automation is more likely to replace a paralegal than a hotel worker.

* * *

And yet automation has already decimated millions of jobs, and addressing that is going to be critical to building a more equitable economy. In some respects, the most important structural response to automation may have already been discussed above: rebuilding our troubled education system. In an automated economy, we have to equip people to take the jobs that will become available. And it may still not be enough.

First, while automation is, in some ways, an unstoppable process—the product of new technology being applied to facilitate the demands of consumers—it shouldn't be accelerated, either. We are going to need all the time we can get to deal with the economic and political ramifications of automation as it is. Therefore, tax incentives that reward businesses for automating should be repealed. The federal jobs guarantee I discussed in the context of the Green New Deal is one approach to addressing the consequences of automation, ensuring that workers displaced by automation have jobs waiting for them rebuilding our crumbling infrastructure and helping allay climate change. Alternatively, others, like Andrew Yang, have proposed a universal basic income (UBI), a sort of "social security for all" program that would replace the current welfare-based system as we know it with a guaranteed basic minimum income for every citizen.

My only challenge with both the guaranteed job and the UBI is that citizens would lose their financial stake in our government. Rather than fund the bulk of government through our taxes, corporations—and not citizens—would fund the bulk of government. The citizen's role in the economy would be reduced simply to consumer. This is potentially dangerous. Under this scenario, what is to stop the most powerful economic and government organizations from intruding upon the basic rights of the citizen? As we contend with the way that automation will shape our economy, we need to think more deeply about how it will shape our civics as well.

* * *

But in many ways that all-important firewall between civics and economics is already crumbling. Because of the concept of corporate personhood, corporations have used their heft and power to "rent seek"—using their influence on government to reduce competition within their sectors, harming real people in the process.

Let me say it again: *corporations are not people.* They never will be. But if they want the rights that are guaranteed to people, they ought to be willing, also, to bear the responsibilities. In that respect, real people pay their taxes—and real people don't get offered sweetheart land deals and other corporate subsidies to consume the tax dollars of others.

In that respect, corporations should be required to pay a progressive tax rate based on size and revenue. I also support the Corporate Tax Dodging Prevention Act of 2017 proposed by Senator Bernie Sanders and his colleagues in Congress.[21] The proposed legislation would eliminate deferral, the process that allows so many corporations to defer paying taxes on profits of offshore subsidiaries. It would also impose a onetime 35 percent tax on all offshore profits. It would eliminate loopholes that allow American corporations to benefit from foreign tax credits in an effort to reduce the U.S. taxes they pay. Further, it would prevent inversion, where a U.S. corporation merges with a foreign corporation to avoid paying U.S. taxes, or claiming foreign status based on a foreign address. It also prevents foreign corporations from avoiding paying U.S. taxes by manipulating their debt expense sheets and prevents oil companies from disguising their royalty payments to foreign governments as taxes to avoid paying the same amount in taxes in the U.S.

I believe that local and state corporate tax subsidies—the kind that Amazon tried to elicit with its HQ2 gambit—ought to be banned. They encourage a race to the bottom that ultimately hurts everyone—except, of course, the corporations.

Furthermore, today's corporate governance system has promoted the kind of financialization I discussed earlier that has devastated workers and stoked insecurity. That has to be reformed as well. To address this, I support the Accountable Capitalism Act proposed in 2018 by Senator Elizabeth Warren.[22] This legislation aims to tackle the fact that corporate boards have aimed to drive all of their earnings into shareholder returns, spurning their responsibilities to their workers, customers, and business partners. And because more than half of Americans have no stocks at all, this gross misalignment has contributed to our booming inequality. This legislation would require all corporations to obtain a federal charter obligating them to pursue the interests of all of their stakeholders, not just their shareholders, and creates a legal commitment to which they can be held accountable in court. It also provides for a process to revoke a corporation's charter for "repeated and egregious illegal conduct." The legislation mandates that 40 percent of corporate board members be elected by employees to ensure that the will of labor is considered in board decisions. To disincentivize short-term stock manipulation, it creates a five-year moratorium on stock sales by corporate executives from the time of receiving them. Although it cannot limit corporate political expenditures given the Supreme Court decision in *Citizens United*, it would require all political expenditures to be approved by 75 percent of directors and shareholders.

While it's not included in the package above, I would also support a ban on lobbying or electioneering from corporations or their subsidiaries or assets that compete for or have received federal grants—such as weapons manufacturers and pharmaceutical companies—given obvious conflicts of interests.

Finally, corporations shouldn't be permitted to get a free ride at government expense by paying less-than-subsistence wages that force their workers to go on federal benefits. Corporations whose workers go on federal benefits should be fined the value of those benefits.

5. Election Reform

The way we vote goes to the very heart of what it means to be an American. And yet the simple principle underlying our democracy—one citizen, one vote—is violated in nearly every election because of the arcane and manipulated systems by which we do it.

We need fundamental electoral reform. First, federal elections should be overseen and administered by the federal government. The system today—administered by state and local government—creates huge variations in election law and election administration. Federalizing the system would standardize it. Furthermore, congressional districts should be apportioned by a nonpartisan committee of experts who are appointed for defined terms on a rolling basis and who work alongside the U.S. Census Bureau, similar to the Federal Reserve Board. This would come as close as possible to eliminating the partisan gerrymandering that exists because of apportionment by partisan state governments in most states.

Our voting system should encourage as many people as possible to make their voices heard. I believe in mandatory voting in all federal elections, making voting day a holiday, and allowing for no-reason absentee and early in-person voting. Voters should be automatically registered to vote when they turn eighteen and reregistered automatically when they move. And in an era where you can do almost anything on your smartphone—like deposit a check in a bank account, buy your groceries, or register to vote—we should develop the cybersecurity needed to enable online voting, too. Although election hacking remains a concern, paper ballots are vulnerable to election fraud, too.

The electoral college is an anachronism designed to empower the elite over everyone else. It restricts the decision about who our president and vice president will be to a small number of relatively nonrepresentative voters. We need to abolish it.

And lastly, we need comprehensive election spending reform. Ideally, elections should be publicly funded—barring election spending by anyone, real person or fake corporate person alike. Alternatively, there should be limits placed on how much a candidate committee can spend in a race. And although we need to overturn the horrendous *Citizens United* decision to do this and to eliminate corporate campaign contributions and outside spending, in the interim we should at least force all forms of election accounts to fully disclose where they got their money and how they spent it.

6. Comprehensive Public Safety Reform

Our failed drug policies, our permissive gun laws, and the epidemic of mass incarceration combine to form a vicious cycle that emerges from our broken approach to public safety. Rather than invest in treating the mental illness that drives drug use, we've watched several drug epidemics mushroom before our eyes. And rather than curtail gun access as the drug trade got violent, we declared the War on Drugs, invested in massive, militarized police forces, and passed minimum sentences and three-strikes laws and elected overeager prosecutors and judges who threw millions behind bars, fueling mass incarceration. Meanwhile, nearly 20 percent of people in jail have diagnosable mental illness that should have been treated in the first place.

First, if we are serious about addressing the current opioid epidemic, we have to think holistically about it, addressing the supply *and* the demand for opioids as well as targeting the mechanisms by which people die of opioid overdose.

We have to dismantle the harmful stigma of drug addiction. We don't stigmatize people who have cancer, so why stigmatize people who suffer addiction, which is also a disease? And it's not just about having public, heartfelt conversations where people share their stories of addiction; it's about deconstructing the structural and institutional stigma of drugs. That means systematically dismantling the system of mass incarceration that has targeted people of color. We need to change the culture of militarized policing, ending the 1033 program, a federal program that sells military weapons to local police departments and moves war matériel onto our streets. If we limit the number of guns on our streets, law enforcement can draw down their weapons as well.

As we do this, transparency matters. Every officer should wear a body camera, and every police homicide should be fully investigated by an independent body, and when wrongful action is identified, offenders must be prosecuted to the full extent of the law.

We must end the money bail system that forces over-policed people to pay for their poverty. And we have to invest in public defenders so that everyone's right to a trial is respected—not just those who can afford a good lawyer. We've got to end three-strikes laws and habitual offender laws, and reverse minimum sentencing, truth-in-sentencing, and oppressive drug sentences to reduce prison time. We have to stop treating children like imaginary "superpredators" and raise the minimum age to be tried as an adult—and eliminate the use of solitary confinement.

We've got to treat every incarcerated person as an education policy failure, meaning we must invest in quality education and work-training programs that start on day one in prison. And because so many incarcerated people suffer from mental illness, we need to invest in universal access to psychiatric and addiction treatment for incarcerated people, to prepare them for their best possible life outside the system.

And once they get out of prison, we need to treat the parole system as a way to keep returning citizens out of jail, rather than a way to throw them back in. Empathy requires us to believe in people again rather than dooming them to the circumstances in which Ammu Othman found himself, unable to get a good job and reliant on the charity of others because our criminal justice system had marked him as a criminal for life, even though he'd done his time. That means "banning the box"—ending the practice of asking formerly incarcerated people to out themselves on applications—not just for employment but for housing, education, healthcare, and access to financial institutions.

We have to legalize marijuana nationally. Marijuana legalization is a racial justice issue. Black-Americans are nearly four times as likely to be arrested for marijuana possession, despite no higher likelihood of use.[23] And after they land in the system, systematic differences in sentencing and parole exacerbate the impact. The consequences rob families of Black and Brown men, creating generational impacts that reverberate across our American social fabric.

And it's not enough just to legalize—because that only addresses the future. We also have to correct the past. That means expunging marijuana-related offenses.

Let's not forget why people often turn to chemicals in the first place. We have to rebuild our crumbling mental health infrastructure. That means investing in the mental health clinics that we'll need to treat the scale of addiction that Americans are experiencing because of the opioid epidemic. It also means addressing the artificial barrier that has existed between "mental" health and every other kind of health. Right now, for example, Medicaid cannot reimburse for in-hospital mental healthcare at hospitals with more than sixteen beds. This "inpatient mental disease" exclusion is an unnecessary, wrongheaded barrier to care for too many Americans.

Further, we have to eliminate barriers to addiction treatment. Although methadone and buprenorphine are controlled substances, and critics argue that we're trading one addiction for another, these interventions are the best available evidence-based treatments for opioid addiction that reduce the risk of overdose. These treatments need to be fully reimbursed and made accessible and affordable.

Meanwhile, the consequences of the opioid epidemic extend beyond the direct consequences of opioids themselves. The epidemic has driven a new resurgence in HIV and hepatitis C transmission through syringe use. However, some argue that providing people needles will promote drug injection—just like providing condoms will promote sex. But the science disagrees. Clean syringes and condoms allow people who are going to do these things anyway to reduce harm to themselves or others. We have to invest in harm reduction strategies like syringe exchange programs and supervised injection sites, which would reduce both needle sharing and overdoses.

We need better prescribing guidelines. The CDC still lacks the kinds of guidelines that prevent unnecessary opioid prescriptions while accommodating the rare group of patients whose chronic pain actually requires opioids for treatment. The CDC's 2016 prescription guidelines were an important step to reducing over-prescription, although it was forced to release new guidelines in April 2019 to accommodate certain chronic pain patients.[24] Other interventions, like mandated prescriber training and limits on a patient's first prescription, should be implemented as well.

It's critical to take on the manufacturers who set this crisis ablaze. But we need a thoughtful strategy. Right now a string of massive class-action lawsuits against opioid manufacturers have delivered historic settlement payouts, including a record $1.4 billion payout from the UK-based corporation Reckitt Benckiser.[25] But the effort has been disorganized and unfocused. The main problem is that it remains unclear what the payouts will be used to do. For example, $200 million of a roughly $270 million payout to the state of Oklahoma from Purdue Pharma, manufacturer of OxyContin and one of the key players in the origins of the epidemic, was earmarked to set up a new addiction research center at Oklahoma State University rather than directly support Oklahomans who've suffered directly from the crisis. To prevent that, the Oklahoma state legislature passed a law requiring the funds to go to the state's general fund in the hope that the money will be directed to benefit those most directly affected by opioids.

These settlement funds need to support the victims of the opioid epidemic and to build the means of preventing anything like this from happening in the future. In that respect, the single most important potential long-range benefit of these funds would be rebuilding our national mental health and substance use treatment infrastructure for the twenty-first century. The funds would then be used not only to directly address the consequences of this epidemic, but also to construct infrastructure that would set us up to be ready for future mental health crises should they arise.

Finally, gun violence is a national epidemic. It's time to solve it. Although I respect the Second Amendment to the Constitution, it was never intended to mean anyone could carry any gun, anywhere, at any time. This extremist interpretation is killing people. We need a ban on military-style semiautomatic assault rifles like the AR-15 as well as on large-capacity magazines and accessories meant to increase their rates of fire. These weapons are intended for one purpose only: to shoot many people quickly. No more weapons of war on peaceful streets. But handguns are, by far, the deadliest type of gun. Handguns should require technology that personalizes them, disabling them from firing in the hands of an unauthorized user.

We also need to close the background check loophole and impose a necessary waiting period between when a gun is purchased and when it is delivered. Guns make domestic violence twelve times as deadly,[26] so people who are reasonably suspected of domestic abuse shouldn't be able to get guns. We need risk protection order laws that allow authorities to take guns away from people who might use them to hurt others. All gun owners should be licensed, and all firearms should be registered. Owners should be responsible for reporting lost or stolen guns. Openly carrying guns in certain public places should be outlawed, and carrying concealed weapons should be limited.

7. Public Banking

To most folks, a bank is a place we go to, physically or virtually, to transact day-to-day financial business. We might keep a checking and/or savings account and have a few credit cards, but too many Americans don't have that luxury. And even for those who are adequately banked, credit card debt can be predatory.

Americans deserve a public bank. That bank would allow Americans who are unbanked access to a trusted financial institution with vastly lower fees and cash balance minimums, breaking the dependence that the un- and underbanked have on alternative providers.

Beyond offering the usual checking and savings options, it could also offer low-limit credit cards and low-interest loan options that may be critical to unlocking the latent potential of people whom the corporate banking system has failed. Even for those who are adequately banked, this banking "public option," which would compete with the private banking industry, could bring down fees and rates.

But personal banking, the kind that most of us engage with, forms a tiny slice of the actual banking sector. By volume, most banking is the kind done on Wall Street, involving million- or billion-dollar deals that shuttle capital around in the corporate infrastructure.

At best, banking is about the efficient allocation of capital resources to where they're needed to create value. Government also requires this kind of financing to thrive. The problem is that it rarely has it. And it could really use that kind of capital right now. Government financing is slow, inefficient, and limited, encumbered by a laborious budgeting process. This often interferes with government's ability to finance major infrastructure projects, the kind that require serious up-front investments but yield significant long-range returns. To solve this problem for Michigan, I proposed building a public infrastructure bank when I ran for governor. It would have provided the state with the means of financing these sorely needed improvements without overstressing the state's limited budget.[27]

In that same spirit, America's public bank should also take on the role of providing innovative and accessible public financing for major government infrastructure projects. This is particularly critical for state and local governments, which often have very limited budgets, without much slack for long-range planning and construction. A major public bank that could finance infrastructure projects across state and local governments could allow these entities to, in effect, collectivize their resources.

Finally, because of America's growing debt crisis, far too few people are saving enough for retirement. This problem will become particularly acute for people working jobs that don't come with retirement benefits. It's critical that workers of all stripes have the ability to retire with dignity. In that respect, the public bank could house a federal pension program for these workers. That program could be funded by a required per-hour fee imposed on employers for workers who don't earn retirement benefits. In addition, the pension fund could provide an alternative investment avenue for gig workers who may not have stable retirement benefits, either.

8. Real Family Values

I believe deeply in family values—not the kind that judge families in crisis for failing to meet some stereotyped ideal, but the kind that actually empower families to build, grow, and thrive. America needs to make its commitment to family values clear in the form of a Twenty-First-Century Family Values Act.

First, if we believe in family, then we need to make sure that we protect the right of every person to choose when and with whom to start one. That means protecting comprehensive family planning services—including abortion services—and investing in providing these services accessibly.

To address the undue burden placed on families to provide childcare, the Twenty-First-Century Family Values Act would include guaranteed paid family leave for both parents. It would also guarantee every family childcare access for children up to three years old, allowing parents to stay in the workforce if they wished. One approach might be through a voucher program. For parents who are employed full-time and earning above a certain threshold, it could offer the benefit through an employer, with the cost split between employer and employee. For those earning below the threshold, it could provide full vouchers directly, covering the cost through a per-employee fee on corporations that do not offer the benefit.

The other challenge in family care we have to address is long-term care for the elderly or disabled. I believe that is best covered through Medicare for All, as discussed earlier. But in its absence, it should be included in any comprehensive family support program.

At first blush, this program may seem expensive. But don't forget how many people are railroaded out of the workforce because of childcare, costing our economy \$57 billion annually.[28] This is almost certainly a low estimate, counting only the costs of lost wages at the time that people, usually women, are forced to leave the workforce. But average earnings usually increase with time, and the setbacks accrued at such an early moment in someone's career compound.

9. Housing Reform

Our homes are the foundation of our lives; our homes are the places that we trust to protect ourselves and our families. And too few Americans are secure in their housing. It's time we used housing policy to right those wrongs. We need housing reform. First, we ought to establish a national Renter's Bill of Rights to guarantee renters protection from predatory landlords. One of those rights ought to be the right to collectively bargain through tenant unions. Second, rent control protects low-income people. However, in many states, state law prevents local communities from passing rent control ordinances. We need a federal law that would make rent control bans illegal. Third, we need to expand the federal housing choice voucher program—and we should pay for it by reducing the homeownership tax subsidies that are funneling money to the wealthiest Americans. In fact, of the $190 billion that the federal government spent on housing in 2015, 60 percent went to households earning more than $100,000.[29]

10. Reparations and Equal Rights

Even if we address the shocking economic inequality that has come to define the epidemic of insecurity, we will not have fully addressed the massive racial inequities in American life. No matter the measure of wellbeing, Black- and Native-Americans suffer worse, whether it's education, income, wealth, infant mortality, or life expectancy. This is a direct, and indelible consequence of American policies that systematically targeted these groups, whether slavery or Jim Crow, Indian removal or draconian reeducation and assimilation policies.

If we are serious about empathy, then we must be serious about equity. That means that we cannot mistake an even playing field today—something we are still very far from—for an even start to the game. Worse, we cannot hold up symbols of the potential for Black or Native American achievement to implicitly blame members of these groups who have not attained those achievements because of the structural, institutional, and individual racism that has and continues to set them back. Like a trench in the American civic geography, even with layers upon layers of backfill, structural racism still forms the essential groove within which our modern experiences fall.

America is long overdue in paying the damages for its original sins. We need a policy of reparations for Black- and Native-Americans. And although it won't ever make it right, it may make a difference. In his essay "The Case for Reparations," author Ta-Nehisi Coates argues, "To celebrate freedom and democracy while forgetting America's origins in a slavery economy is patriotism à la carte."[30] Yet talk of reparations from all but the very left of American political discourse tends to invoke the same relapse to technical fatalism that we know all too well from debates about Medicare for All or the Green New Deal. Coates again: "Broach the topic of reparations today and a barrage of questions inevitably follows: Who will be paid? How much will they be paid? Who will pay? But if the practicalities, not the justice, of reparations are the true sticking point, there has for some time been the beginnings of a solution."

Even race-based affirmative action, which simply provides access to colleges and universities for students who otherwise might suffer institutional racism in admissions decisions is under assault. But affirmative action forms only a small subset of the reparations that are required to secure true equity in our country. While the policy landscape for reparations remains undefined, the idea has gained traction. In the 2020 Democratic primary, several high-profile candidates came out in support of reparations, at least in theory.

More practically, we need thoughtful policy research to make these political commitments mean something. A tangible suite of reparations policies could include anything from direct investments in majority Black school districts or communities, to conditional use investment funds that can be flexibly used for housing, healthcare, food, or long-term wealth investments, to unconditional cash transfers. But we need to study what the opportunities and demerits of these and other proposals might be.

Opponents argue that this policy would inflame the identity politics that have torn us apart. Perhaps. But empathy politics requires a commitment to the ideals of justice, equity, and sustainability. Supporting reparations is not just about identity; it's first and foremost about correcting injustice.

* * *

We are long past due for equal rights for women. We are nearly a century beyond the moment that Alice Paul first introduced the concept of an Equal Rights Amendment in Seneca Falls, New York, in 1923. It was introduced into Congress that year, and it read, "Men and women shall have equal rights throughout the United States and every place subject to its jurisdiction." And by the 1940s it became a widely accepted plank of both the Republican and Democratic Parties. In 1972, Congress passed an amended form, sending it out for ratification as the Twenty-Seventh Amendment. Although it garnered twenty-two ratifications in its first year, it ultimately failed to pass, just three ratifications short of the required thirty-eight.

In 2019, it is shocking that we still don't have a constitutional amendment guaranteeing equal rights across sex, sexual orientation, and gender identity lines. And although, thanks in large part to the legal work of Supreme Court justice Ruth Bader Ginsberg, the Fourteenth Amendment has been interpreted to preclude unequal treatment based on sex, loopholes persist. Furthermore, the right to nondiscrimination ought to be enshrined specifically in the Constitution as a matter of course.

11. A Values-Driven Immigration and Foreign Policy

If we believe, truly, in the ideal that all people are created equal, we must be willing to extend our empathy beyond our own national borders. That means advocating against systems that don't just drive insecurity at home but drive insecurity abroad.

When the Trump administration chose to rip thousands of children from the arms of their parents under their "zero tolerance" policy—some still breastfeeding—they crossed a moral red line that should alarm those of us who believe in empathy. There is something profoundly human about our bond to our children, the violation of which should reverberate in our bones. But from the very top, all the way down to the officials who physically removed children from their parents' grasp, there was a collective inability or unwillingness to appreciate the shame, the horror, the evil, of what they were doing—or the humanity of the people they were doing it to.

We must oppose the white nationalism behind America First, Trump's Muslim ban, the Border Wall, the concentration camps on the southern border, the expanded drone war, and ICE raids.

First, we must reverse the profound backslide toward racist immigration policies that, for too long, have discriminated by race and national origin. In a country that literally prides itself on being a haven for peoples from all over the world, we need to remember that our diversity makes us stronger.

There are immediate steps we need to take. First, we need to reform Customs and Border Protection (CBP), including abolishing Immigration and Customs Enforcement (ICE) as an institution. The moral rot at the center of the organization became apparent after messages from a closed Facebook group of CBP officers surfaced in 2019 disparaging detainees and members of Congress in vile and obscene ways. That rot emanates from ICE, which needs to be dismantled. The remainder of CBP should be focused on policing the border rather than internal immigration enforcement through raids, which should be ended immediately.

Second, all concentration camps should be shut down. People shouldn't be caged, and families shouldn't be separated by the American government acting on our behalf.

Third, we need a pathway to citizenship for every undocumented person within our borders right now. We should start with Deferred Action for Childhood Arrivals (DACA) recipients—people who were brought to our country as children through no agency of their own, who are American in every way except their papers.

Fourth, border crossing should be decriminalized, downgraded from a criminal infraction to a civil one. That would abrogate the case for the vicious detentions that the Trump administration has used to maintain concentration camps at our border with Mexico. Fifth, immigration courts should be independent of the Justice Department.

* * *

Many of the people who come to our shores are fleeing violence, despotism, or war abroad—too much of it subsidized by the American war machine. In 2018, U.S. troops saw combat in fourteen countries, all under the same

2002 war authorization to fight Al Qaeda–linked militants. In 2019 we are still conducting drone strikes over Pakistan, Afghanistan, Iraq, and Yemen. Under the Obama administration, which oversaw the first major expansion of drone warfare, the administration reported all strikes and casualties under a 2016 executive order that the Trump administration repealed in 2019. That may be because in the first few years of the Trump presidency there have been 2,243 drone strikes—365 more than there were through the entire course of Obama's eight-year term.[31] Since the U.S. first initiated drone warfare, up to 1,725 civilians have been killed, 397 of them children.[32]

If we are serious about our ideals abroad, then we have to draw down the American war machine rather than continue to expand our footprint of destruction. We must seek nuclear nonproliferation as we also seek to decommission as much of our own nuclear arsenal as possible. And we must stop investing in useless projects like the ill-fated F-35 fighter jet program, into which we are expected to sink $1.55 trillion over the life of the program.

One can both oppose our wars and support the individuals who fight those wars; a politics of empathy understands this. Although our leaders are quick to sacrifice the lives of American servicemen and -women abroad, our veterans languish in terrible circumstances at home. But rather than invest the resources needed to empower the U.S. Department of Veterans Affairs to execute on its mandate, the Trump administration is looking for ways to chop it down and sell it for parts to healthcare industry executives promising more "efficiency" and "choice." We must protect Veterans Affairs and its health system. It needs to be fully funded, not destroyed. Second, all veterans should be entitled to a twenty-first-century GI Bill of Rights, including partial housing vouchers so that nobody who served our country is forced to go homeless, and a federal job guarantee.

We have to learn to empathize with the people whom our foreign policy affects, to consider the consequences of war in destroying the lives and livelihoods of millions of people who ought to have the same dignity that we do. But it's not just war; American foreign policy has toppled democratically elected leaders while sustaining dictators—all in the name of our own national interests. Empathy calls on us to ask what the consequences of these policies look like in the lives of people living under those regimes. I shudder to think what might have become of me the night those plainclothes cops came to question me in Egypt had I not been an American citizen.

The classic American defense of our embarrassing support for despots and dictators and occupations has always been "stability in the region." Alongside our shameful support of Egypt's military dictatorship, our support for the Saudi monarchy is another example of this. After the discovery of vast oil reserves, Saudi Arabia has been one of our key "allies"—irrespective of their brutal exploitation of their own people, their subsidization and export of a repressive and dogmatic interpretation of Islam, and their material support of terrorism. How do Saudi Arabia's human rights violations, its extrajudicial killings of dissident journalists, and its civil war in Yemen make the region more *stable*?

Similarly, although unquestioning support for Israel remains a point of bipartisan consensus, we must ask, at long last: Why? We're told that it's because Israel is the only democracy in the Middle East. Yet, like Saudi Arabia, Israel's government is under the control of a small cadre of extremists—and the country has perpetrated shocking violations of human rights and international law against the Palestinians, whose land it has occupied for the better part of a century. Are we not allowed to have a debate about a "democracy" that purposely maintains two classes of citizenship based on ethnicity? And perhaps there are so few democracies in the region because our country has so consistently backed dictators in the region.

Ultimately, America simply shouldn't be in the business of subsidizing foreign militaries, be they in Egypt, Saudi Arabia, Israel, or anywhere else. We shouldn't be putting bombs stamped "Made in the U.S.A." in another country's hands, certainly not the hands of human rights abusers.

Beyond ending military aid, we must ask, in the long term, if it makes sense to maintain strategic alliances with countries that violate human rights at all. If we are serious about upholding the dignity of all people, we cannot continue to turn a blind eye to these violations however strong our historical alliance. Too often, our condemnation of these blatant abuses has been slow in coming—if it comes at all, it is tepid, like President Obama's response to the revolutionary uprising in Egypt. And worse, we have not followed our words with actions.

We are the world's dominant superpower, one that is unabashed in our lofty ideals. The world watches us. And every time our actions miss the mark, we leave an indelible scar on the spirit of hope. Rather than being the beacon in whom the oppressed can believe, when we fail our ideals, we become another enabler of their oppressors.

12. Social Media Reform

Through fake news, troll farms, sock puppets, and algorithmic sorting, social media has become one of the principal drivers of our intellectual and political segregation. When they became a tool for Russian election manipulation, social media companies demonstrated just how dangerous they had become. They were so bent on growth, they ignored the dangers lurking in their platforms.

Furthermore, tech giants like Facebook have become virtual monopolies, so dominant that they stifle competition and innovation—or acquire it. Consider the parallel stories of Instagram and Snapchat. As the two social media start-ups began to gain in popularity—and all-important market share among younger social media users—they began to rival Facebook, a platform that had started to age. Facebook easily acquired Instagram for $1 billion in 2012. And then, in 2013, it tried to buy Snapchat, too, rumored to have offered a whopping $3 billion. But Snapchat creator and CEO Evan Spiegel declined the offer. So, in 2016, Facebook simply copied it. "Don't be too proud to copy," Mark Zuckerberg told his minions, adding Snapchat's now-famous "stories" feature—which allows users to post photos that disappear in twenty-four hours—to Facebook, Messenger, WhatsApp, and Instagram. They also began mimicking Snapchat's lenses, a popular augmented reality feature that allows users to alter pictures by adding things like sparkles and bunny ears.

Facebook has behaved in ways that should force us to think twice about the power that we've allowed them to have over us. In 2019, Facebook was slapped with a $5 billion fine for privacy violations, including handing over users' phone numbers—which users had been asked to provide for security reasons—to advertisers.

The fundamental problem is that social media users aren't the customers. We are the product. We are being sold to advertisers who use our information to sell us stuff that they think we want. And they're really good at it. On the day Facebook was slapped with that fine, it reported earnings of $16.9 billion; that's $7.05 per user. These fines are just another cost of doing business.

It's time to regulate tech in a serious way. Chris Hughes, one of the Facebook cofounders, articulated this sentiment in a *New York Times* op-ed: "Mark [Zuckerberg] may never have a boss, but he needs to have some check on his power. The American government needs to do two things: break up Facebook's monopoly and regulate the company to make it more accountable to the American people."[33] I agree with Hughes. Tech giants like Facebook and Amazon should be broken up, and mergers and acquisitions ought to be considered with far more scrutiny in the future.

Beyond this, however, I believe that social media content ought to be regulated. This is challenging, because it's hard to tell where free speech ends on these platforms. And if done wrong, establishing the precedent for social media censorship may invite repressive governments to suppress free speech, as well. Indeed, attempts to do so already by the Singaporean and Russian governments are alarming. But we already trust the Federal Communications Commission to make these decisions with other forms of media, and it ought to establish a new bureau focused specifically on social media.

There are a few clear responsibilities here. First, we all agree that privacy is a critical concern. However, there are no clear guidelines, leaving social media giants to make it up as they go—with very problematic results. There ought to be clear guidelines about privacy expectations that are aggressively enforced, the same way we protect sensitive medical records.

Second, some of the most dangerous fake content on social media isn't created or pushed directly by people at all but by armies of fake accounts. In fact, Facebook took down 2.2 billion fake accounts in the first quarter of 2019 alone.[34] Although Facebook claims that only about 5 percent of its daily users are fake, there's good reason to believe that number is higher.[35] On Twitter, up to 15 percent are fake. But, as with Facebook, it's hard to know.[36] In some respect, these companies don't know how many of their users aren't real because they haven't had to figure it out. That ought to change. Social media platforms should be required to shut down fake "bot" profiles or else face fines. This would vastly reduce the sharing of fake content without harming any (real) person's free speech.

Finally, fake news is a serious challenge and is threatening to become even worse with the advent of "deep fakes" (videos portraying real people saying things that they in fact have never said). Social media companies should be required to create tags for content that is highly likely to be fake that alert users clearly of that fact.

13. Food Reform

The advent of the obesity epidemic—now tipping the scales at nearly 40 percent of adult Americans—is one of the most important healthcare crises of our time. Obesity is a key driver of some of the most important diseases we suffer: hypertension, diabetes, heart disease, and cancer. Addressing this epidemic would be the single most impactful intervention we could make for the state of American health.

And behind obesity was the sudden advent of high-caloric density corn at artificially low prices in the late 1970s. If we want to address the obesity epidemic, we ought to rethink the way our food is processed, which will mean addressing the harmful consequences of our farm subsidies on our food environment. Although the 2019 Farm Bill passed with important measures to increase funding for "specialty crops," such as fresh fruits and vegetables, it failed to renew funding for programs that encouraged local and organic foods and largely continues the status quo.[37][38] At core, this new law does little to shake the profound impact that our farm subsidies have had on driving the artificially low price of commodity crops, like corn. Furthermore, a draft version of the Farm Bill would have imposed strict work requirements for eligibility on SNAP (formerly "food stamps") that would have forced an estimated 1.1 million households off the rolls. While the bill was signed without these requirements, the changes are being proposed as rule changes under the USDA, which oversees the program.[39] If these reforms are enacted, they will spell a food security catastrophe for more than a million families.

If we want to address our obesity epidemic, we have to rethink the nature of farm subsidies. It's critical to support American farmers, but we need a subsidies regime that prioritizes small and independent farms and local and environmentally sustainable food providers to grow crops that are healthier—like fruits and vegetables. Rather than subsidize commodity crops such as corn and soy, we ought to be subsidizing the foods that we recommend Americans be eating.

Furthermore, in an era of bad jobs and food insecurity, the SNAP program must be protected. Although these programs have been targeted by Republican administrations, of all the public benefits in America, the SNAP program and its partners, Women, Infants, and Children (WIC) and the National School Lunch Program, have been critical to assuring that low-income Americans—children in particular—have access to the foods that they need to grow and thrive.

But these programs, too, require an upgrade. To appreciate why, remember that food in America is a big business, dominated by large corporations with serious lobbying power. And those corporations—brand names like Coca-Cola and Pepsi—have wielded that power to make sure their products are subsidized by the American government. Right now about 10 percent of all SNAP dollars are spent on sugar-sweetened beverages.[40] Not only do these drinks fail to provide any nutritional value, but there's ample evidence that they are accelerating the obesity epidemic. We need to rethink the way that these benefits operate in order to ensure that we aren't yet again inadvertently subsidizing disease. One study, by nutritionists at Harvard's T. H. Chan School of Public Health, showed promise for a SNAP incentive that would make SNAP benefits worth 30 percent more for healthy foods like fruits, vegetables, and whole grains and 30 percent less for sugar-sweetened beverages.[41]

Furthermore, several local communities have stood up to the power of these corporations and passed taxes on sugar-sweetened beverages. For example, in 2016, the city of Philadelphia passed a comprehensive reform package, including a 1.5-cent-per-ounce tax on soda to fund the city's universal pre-K program, public schools, and an initiative to rebuild public parks and libraries. Although some city residents started to buy their soda in neighboring communities to escape the tax, the program reduced overall soda consumption by 38 percent[42] and raised an average of $120 million a year for the city.[43]

Soda taxes have been a prime target of lobbying by the beverage industry, which seeks to shape public opinion by arguing that they are an affront to our freedom. They follow a well-worn pathway trod by manufacturers of another harmful product: tobacco. Both the tobacco industry and the beverage industry prey disproportionately on low-income young people, and both have argued that their products are harmless if consumed in moderation. But both have contributed to death and disease in America and require regulation. Today the federal tax rate on cigarettes sits at $1.01 per pack, with additional local and state taxes that are often far higher. Although there is no federal sugar-sweetened-beverage tax, there is no doubt that such a policy is justifiable and proper.

EPILOGUE

Empathy for our future.

I was back on the road within a few weeks of Emmalee's birth, going days on end without seeing her. I missed her first word. I missed her first crawl. I missed *her*.

On August 8, the morning after I had lost the Democratic nomination for governor of Michigan, I woke up to the stunned feeling of having my chest hair pulled out and the sight of a big gummy smile and bright brown eyes. "*Baba!*" she exclaimed, and grinned again. The best thing about losing was that I was going to spend most of my day with her.

Emmalee had no idea I had lost a big election—that I would be held up in the national press as a poster child for how the Left was losing ground. To her I was just her Baba, and she loved me for it. That sustained me in many ways through the grueling days of the campaign. It would sustain me now. I pray someday I get to tell her that she was the levity—the hope—I needed through one of the most challenging experiences of my life.

Since losing my primary, I have had a lot of time to spend with Emmalee. One does not have to be a parent to appreciate how much parents love their children. Most parents would do absolutely anything for their kids, working hard to provide them with the comforts and opportunities they may or may not have had.

We cannot control all of the circumstances of our children's lives. From the day they are born, they are endowed with a particular personality—with certain skills and deficits. And they are set upon this path of life. We hope that they will experience love, but we know they will experience loss, and heartbreak, and pain, and sorrow. They will be hurt, and they will probably hurt others. They will win and they will lose.

As I've struggled to make heads from tails on parenting, I think I've come to believe that the only real thing a parent can shape is what her child considers "normal." Normal isn't defined in what we *tell* our children is normal; it's in the habits of behavior and place and culture and interactions to which our children are exposed.

Their normal is a function of repetition, of consistency. So while we may want to set normal to one thing, it is set out of the cumulative outcomes of the circumstances in which our children find themselves.

These are not normal times. We are bombarded with messaging and counter-messaging, taught to hate or fear what we do not know, although knowing may just mean knocking on the next door over. Dominated by insecurity, we are told that we suffer it alone. Forget trying to keep up with them: the Joneses are actively trying to keep us down. Insults are injuries; the only way forward is the offensive.

Donald Trump—a man who talks about demeaning women and banning people of my faith from this country—was president when my daughter was born. This is the America in which we are raising our Muslim half-Indian, half-Egyptian and 100 percent American little girl.

* * *

To be sure, the work ahead is vast and treacherous. Young people today are inheriting the full miasma of our insecurity, which has so polarized and deprived generations before them. Millennials are the first generation who won't exceed our parents in educational attainment, who won't earn as much as they did. The imminent consequences of climate change are threatening to become permanent in our lifetimes. Inequality is at an all-time high, with automation threatening to decimate traditionally high-skill jobs. The power of corporations to bully government has never been greater, since *Citizens United*.

Perhaps worst of all, we have never been more divided, our conversation more broken. Growing up as Internet natives means that the lines have blurred between what happens online and on the streets. Not only does the cacophony of rage reshape the tone and tenor of discourse but it tricks us into thinking that a few likes or retweets means change. No generation has ever been more accustomed to immediate gratification, leaving us vulnerable to institutions that bait us through our addiction to it.

We owe young people the empathy of working in this moment, showing them that "normal" can mean unusual action in the face of the abnormal. It means being willing to listen, and unify, and engage with others. It means opposing a culture of hate and outrage. It means showing them that the time spent on a Friday night or Saturday afternoon to go and help clean up a park is an act of justice. It means taking the time to understand your interlocutor, even if you may never agree with what he's saying. It means embracing empathy even when it's hard.

Finally, we owe the empathy of handing over the reins of power. As this next generation of leaders flowers, it will show us a view on leadership we have never seen: more diverse, more authentic, and more emphatic about the imminence of the challenges we face and the work we need to do to face them.

I have found that with age can come a certain brand of jadedness—of cynicism—with what is possible in the world. There is a nonchalance with which older people treat younger people, a belief that because they have watched failure—even taken part in failure many times before—success is not possible.

We hide this cynicism behind a veneer of "experience," which is what older people always lord over young people for having simply lived in the world or having worked on an issue longer. But there ought to be some humility in recognizing that having "worked on" a problem implies having never solved it. And past failure shouldn't mean we give up trying. If you see the world that way, it may be time to hand over the reins and move aside. The most devastating consequence of the deep miasma we have allowed to fester will fall hardest on this next generation of leaders. Maybe we can avoid passing on cynicism as well.

And lastly, perhaps most of all in these abnormal times, the most important "normal" we can pass along to our young ones is the belief that they are the greatest living manifestation of the hope we see in the world. They need to know that we value them, we embrace them, and we believe in their ability to move us. This, I believe, is the most important act of empathy for our future: to steel them against the insecurity that has so divided us by empowering them to believe that they can emerge beyond it.

Our young are, after all, our *hope*.

Notes

Prologue

1. Julie Mack, "Michigan Living Costs 11% Below U.S. Average and 6 Other Facts on Cost Index," MLive, February 29, 2016, https://www.mlive.com /news/index.ssf/2016/02/michigan_living_costs_11_below.html.
2. "Income Tax Calculator, Michigan, USA," Neuvoo, https://neuvoo.com /tax-calculator/?iam=&salary=49847&from=year&region=Michigan.
3. Jimmy Karnezis, "How to Estimate Monthly Payments for an Average Student Loan," Credible, last modified June 28, 2019, https://www.credible .com/blog/refinance-student-loans/how-much-will-you-actually-pay-for-a -30k-student-loan/.
4. Lacie Glover, "What You Can (and Can't) Learn from the Average Car Payment," NerdWallet, December 21, 2018, https://www.nerdwallet.com/blog /loans/auto-loans/average-monthly-car-payment/.
5. Julie Mack, "New Census Data Offers In-Depth Data on Poverty in Michigan," MLive, September 17, 2018, https://www.mlive.com/expo/news /erry-2018/09/d4b42cc89a7672/new-census-data-offers-indepth.html.
6. Tyler Clifford, "Meijer Brothers Lead *Forbes* List of Michigan Billionaires," *Crain's Detroit Business*, March 20, 2017.

Chapter 2: An Imperfect Science

1. Alfredo Morabia, "Epidemiology's 350th Anniversary: 1662–2012," *Epidemiology* 24, no. 2 (March 2013): 179-83, https://doi.org/10.1097/EDE .0b013e31827b5359.

2. Ibid.

3. John Graunt, *Natural and Political Observations Made Upon the Bills of Mortality* (1662), http://www.edstephan.org/Graunt/bills.html.

4. "Father of Modern Epidemiology," University of California Los Angeles, https://www.ph.ucla.edu/epi/snow/fatherofepidemiology.html#ONE.

Chapter 4: Privilege

1. Myron Schultz, "Rudolf Virchow," *Emerging Infectious Diseases* 14, no. 9 (September 2008): 1480–81, https://dx.doi.org/10.3201/eid1409 .086672.

2. Diane S. Lauderdale, "Birth Outcomes for Arabic-Named Women in California Before and After September 11," *Demography* 43, no. 1 (February 2006): 185–201, https://doi.org/10.1353/dem.2006.0008.

3. Abdulrahman M. El-Sayed, Craig Hadley, and Sandro Galea, "Birth Outcomes Among Arab Americans in Michigan Before and After the Terrorist Attacks of September 11, 2001," *Ethnicity & Disease* 18, no. 3 (Summer 2008): 348–56.

4. Abdulrahman M. El-Sayed and Sandro Galea, "Explaining the Low Risk of Preterm Birth Among Arab-Americans in the United States: An Analysis of 617,451 Births," *Pediatrics* 123, no. 3 (March 2009): 3438–45, https://doi .org/10.1542/peds.2008-1634.

5. Abdulrahman M. El-Sayed and Sandro Galea, "Community Context, Acculturation and Low Birth Weight Risk Among Arab-Americans: Evidence from the Arab-American Birth-Outcomes Study," *Journal of Epidemiology and Community Health* 64, no. 20 (August 2009): 155–60, https:// doi.og/10.1136/jech.2008.084491.

Chapter 5: Complex Causes

1. "World Life Expectancy," LeDuc Media, https://www.worldlifeexpectancy .com/.

2. National Geographic Staff, "If You're an Average American, You'll Live to Be 78.6 Years Old," National Geographic, December 7, 2018, https://www .nationalgeographic.com/culture/2018/12/life-expectancy-united-states/.

3. "Poverty Rate by State 2019," World Population Review, accessed September 14, 2019, http://worldpopulationreview.com/states/poverty-rate-by-state/.

4. Julie Mack, "Which Michigan Counties Have the Longest, Shortest Life Expectancy?," MLive, March 27, 2018, https://expo.mlive.com/erry-2018/03/07f0cf7208/what_michigan_counties_have_th.html.

5. "Life Expectancy at Birth by Sex and Race: Michigan Residents, Selected Years, 1950–2017," Michigan Department of Health & Human Services, last modified June 2018, https://www.mdch.state.mi.us/osr/deaths/life sxrctrend.asp.

6. "Infant Mortality," Reproductive Health, Centers for Disease Control and Prevention, last reviewed March 27, 2019, https://www.cdc.gov/reproductivehealth/maternalinfanthealth/infantmortality.htm.

7. "Number and Rate of Infant Deaths by Race for Residents of Michigan, Detroit City, Wayne County (Excluding Detroit City) and Michigan (Excluding Wayne County), 1990–2017," Michigan Department of Health & Human Services, accessed September 14, 2019, https://www.mdch.state.mi.us/pha/osr/InDxMain/Tab5.asp.

8. "Achievements in Public Health, 1900–1999: Control of Infectious Diseases," *Morbidity and Mortality Weekly Report* 48, no. 29 (July 1999): 621–29, https://www.cdc.gov/mmwr/preview/mmwrhtml/mm4829a1.htm.

Chapter 6: Ideals and Institutions

1. "Full Text: President Barack Obama's Speech to the Muslim World," *Time*, June 4, 2009, https://content.time.com/time/politics/article/0,8599,1902738-5,00.html.

2. Jeevan Vasagar, "Twenty-one Oxbridge Colleges Took No Black Students Last Year," *Guardian*, December 6, 2010, https://www.theguardian.com/education/2010/dec/06/oxford-colleges-no-black-students.

Chapter 8: Contagion and Miasma

1. John Snow, *On the Mode of Communication of Cholera* (London: John Churchill, 1855), https://books.google.com/books?hl=en&lr=&id=-No_AAAAcAAJ&oi=fnd&pg=PA1&dq=on+the+mode+of+communication+of+cholera&ots=mWQjFlNvPS&sig=EjrwIvaOHVdWeFzZQt4Gsr MdV34#v=onepage&q=on%20the%20mode%20of%20communication%20of%20cholera&f=false.

Chapter 9: Home Again

1. Paul Eagan, "Flint red flag: 2015 report urged corrosion control," *Detroit Free Press*, January 21, 2016, https://www.freep.com/story/news/local/michigan/flint-water-crisis/2016/01/21/flint-red-flag-2015-report-urged-corrosion-control/79119240/.
2. Ted Roelofs, "Michiganders Say Emergency Managers Wield Too Much Power," Bridge, March 21, 2017, https://www.bridgemi.com/michigan-government/michiganders-say-emergency-managers-wield-too-much-power.
3. Jennifer Manlove and Hannah Lantos, "Data Point: Half of 20- to 29-Year-Old Women Who Gave Birth in Their Teens Have a High School Diploma," Child Trends, January 11, 2018, https://www.childtrends.org/half-20-29-year-old-women-gave-birth-teens-high-school-diploma/.
4. Maartje Basten et al., "Preterm Birth and Adult Wealth: Mathematics Skills Count," *Psychological Science* 26, no. 10 (October 2015): 1608–19, https://doi.org/10.1177/0956797615596230.

Chapter 10: Doctoring Detroit

1. Editorial Board, "Battle over Detroit Air Quality Won—but Not the War," *Detroit Free Press*, April 5, 2016, https://www.freep.com/story/opinion/editorials/2016/04/05/marathon-air-detroit/82616308/.
2. "School Lead Screening Project," 2017 Model Practices, National Association of County & City Health Officials, https://application.naccho.org/Public/Applications/View?id=138.
3. Kevin Elliott, "Has Regional Water Board Lived Up to Expectations?," *Downtown Newsmagazine*, July 23, 2019, https://www.downtownpublications.com/single-post/2019/07/23/Has-the-regional-water-board-live-up-to-expectations.
4. "Detroit: Disconnecting Water from People Who Cannot Pay—an Affront to Human Rights, Say UN Experts," United Nations Human Rights, June 25, 2014, https://www.ohchr.org/EN/NewsEvents/Pages/DisplayNews.aspx?NewsID=14777.
5. "Detroit Demolitions," City of Detroit, last updated September 17, 2019, https://data.detroitmi.gov/Property-Parcels/Detroit-Demolitions/rv44-e9di.

6. Matt Helms, "Detroit Reaches Blight Milestone: 10,000 Demolitions," *Detroit Free Press*, last updated July 19, 2016, https://www.freep.com/story /news/local/michigan/detroit/2016/07/19/detroit-reaches-blight -milestone-10000-demolitions/87284392/.

7. Dynamo Metrics, *Estimating Demolition Impacts in Ohio*, report on the Ohio Housing Finance Agency's Neighborhood Initiative Program, 2016, 1–80, https://ohiohome.org/savethedream/documents/BlightReport-NIP .pdf.

8. Dynamo Metrics, *Estimating Home Equity Impacts from Rapid, Targeted Residential Demolition in Detroit, MI: Application of a Spatially-Dynamic Data System for Decision Support*, report, the Skillman Foundation/Rock Ventures, July 2015, http://www.demolitionimpact.org/.

9. Steve Neavling, "Detroit Is Razing Houses with Money Intended to Save Them," *Detroit Metro Times*, July 19, 2017, https://www.metrotimes .com/detroit/detroit-is-razing-houses-with-money-intended-to-save-them /Content?oid=4619015.

10. Christine Ferretti, "Feds: Demolition Costs 'Skyrocketing' in Mich., Ohio," *The Detroit News*, April 26, 2017, https://www.detroitnews.com /story/news/local/michigan/2017/04/26/demolition-costs/100939320/.

11. Steve Neavling, "Mayor Duggan's Administration Dodges Charges in Federal Demolition Probe," *Detroit Metro Times*, April 10, 2019, https:// www.metrotimes.com/news-hits/archives/2019/04/10/mayor-duggans -administration-dodges-charges-in-federal-demolition-probe.

12. Ibid.

13. Harolyn Baker et al., *Task Force Recommendations for Improving Demolition Safety and Health Standards*, report for City of Detroit Health Department, 2017, 1–30, https://www.bridgemi.com/sites/default/files/task_force _recommendations.pdf.

Chapter 11: Running for Our Lives

1. Maximillian Alvarez, "The Vital Possibility of Abdul El-Sayed," *The Baffler*, August 3, 2018, https://thebaffler.com/the-poverty-of-theory/the-vital-pos -sibility-of-el-sayed-alvarez.

Chapter 12: The Syndrome

1. "New ACC/AHA High Blood Pressure Guidelines Lower Definition of Hypertension," American College of Cardiology, November 13, 2017, https://www.acc.org/latest-in-cardiology/articles/2017/11/08/11/47/mon-5pm-bp-guideline-aha-2017.

2. Anne Case and Angus Deaton, "Mortality and Morbidity in the 21st Century," *Brookings Papers on Economic Activity* (Spring 2017): 397–476, https://doi.org/10.1353/eca.2017.0005.

3. *Behavioral Health Trends in the United States: Results from the 2014 National Survey on Drug Use and Health* (HHS Publication No. SMA 15-4927, NSDUH Series H-50), Center for Behavioral Health Statistics and Quality, U.S. Department of Health and Human Services, 2015, https://www.samhsa.gov/data/sites/default/files/NSDUH-FRR1-2014/NSDUH-FRR1-2014.pdf.

4. "Majority of Americans Say They Are Anxious About Health; Millennials Are More Anxious Than Baby Boomers," American Psychiatric Association, May 22, 2017, https://www.psychiatry.org/newsroom/news-releases/majority-of-americans-say-they-are-anxious-about-health-millennials-are-more-anxious-than-baby-boomers.

5. Mark Moran, "APA Poll Finds Americans' Anxiety Is Increasing, Especially About Health, Safety, and Finances," *Psychiatric News*, May 29, 2018, https://psychnews.psychiatryonline.org/doi/10.1176/appi.pn.2018.6a36.

6. "Living Paycheck to Paycheck Is a Way of Life for Majority of U.S. Workers, According to New CareerBuilder Survey," CareerBuilder, August 24, 2017, http://press.careerbuilder.com/2017-08-24-Living-Paycheck-to-Paycheck-is-a-Way-of-Life-for-Majority-of-U-S-Workers-According-to-New-CareerBuilder-Survey.

7. Ibid.

8. Ibid.

9. "When Is Enough . . . Enough?," UBS, 2Q 2015, 1–12, https://www.ubs.com/content/dam/WealthManagementAmericas/documents/investor-watch-2Q2015.pdf.

10. Ibid.

11. William Emmons and Bryan Noeth, "The Middle Class May Be Under More Pressure Than You Think," Federal Reserve Bank of St. Louis,

April 2, 2015, https://www.stlouisfed.org/publications/in-the-balance /2015/the-middle-class-may-be-under-more-pressure-than-you-think.

12. Kim Carollo, "Worldwide Obesity Doubled Over Past Three Decades," ABC News, February 4, 2011, https://abcnews.go.com/Health/global-obesity -rates-doubled-1980/story?id=12833461.1.

13. Mark Weinraub, "U.S. Set to Lose Top Spot as Global Corn Exporter to Brazil," Reuters, February 16, 2018, https://www.reuters.com/article/us -usa-corn-exports-analysis/u-s-set-to-lose-top-spot-as-global-corn-exporter -to-brazil-idUSKCN1G01VW.

14. "Agricultural Adjustment Act 1933, Reauthorized 1938," The Living New Deal, accessed September 14, 2019, https://livingnewdeal.org/glossary /agricultural-adjustment-act-1933-re-authorized-1938-2/.

15. "Bushels and Cents: Corn and the Farm Bill," King Corn, PBS, last modi- fied April 14, 2008, http://www.pbs.org/independentlens/kingcorn /bushels.html.

16. Peter Kilborn, "Cut in Farms Exports at Core of Problem in Prices and Supply," New York Times, December 16, 1983, https://www.nytimes.com /1983/12/16/world/cut-in-farm-exports-at-core-of-problem-in-prices-and -supply.html.

17. Allison Aubrey, "Does Subsidizing Crops We're Told to Eat Less of Fatten Us Up?," NPR, July 18, 2016, https://www.npr.org/sections/thesalt/2016 /07/18/486051480/we-subsidize-crops-we-should-eat-less-of-does-this -fatten-us-up.

18. Tim Flannery, "We're Living on Corn!" review of The Omnivore's Dilemma: A Natural History of Four Meals and Deep Economy: The Wealth of Commu- nities and the Durable Future, by Michael Pollan and Bill McKibben, New York Review of Books, June 28, 2007, https://michaelpollan.com/reviews /were-living-on-corn/.

19. Karen R. Siegel et al., "Association of Higher Consumption of Foods Derived from Subsidized Commodities with Adverse Cardiometabolic Risk Among US Adults," JAMA Internal Medicine 176, no. 8 (August 2016): 1124–32, https://doi.org/10.1001/jamainternmed.2016.2410.

20. "Bushels and Cents: Corn and the Farm Bill," King Corn, PBS, last modi- fied April 14, 2008, http://www.pbs.org/independentlens/kingcorn /bushels.html.

Chapter 13: Insecure Health

1. Christopher J. L. Murray et al., "Eight Americas: Investigating Mortality Disparities Across Races, Counties, and Race-Counties in the United States," *PLOS Medicine* 3, no. 9 (September 2006): 1513–24, https://doi.org/10.1371/journal.pmed.0030260.

2. Claudia Allemani et al., "Global Surveillance of Trends in Cancer Survival 2000–14 (CONCORD-3): Analysis of Individual Records for 37,513,025 Patients Diagnosed with One of 18 Cancers from 322 Population-Based Registries in 71 Countries," *The Lancet* 391, no. 10125 (March 2018): 1023–75, https://doi.org/10.1016/S0140-6736(17)33326-3.

3. Bradley Sawyer and Daniel McDermott, "How Do Mortality Rates in the U.S. compare to Other Countries?" Peterson-Kaiser Health System Tracker, February 14, 2019, https://www.healthsystemtracker.org/chart-collection/mortality-rates-u-s-compare-countries/#item-neoplasm-mortality-rate-2015.

4. Dan Mangan, "Medical Bills Are the Biggest Cause of US Bankruptcies: Study," CNBC, last modified July 24, 2018, https://www.cnbc.com/id/100840148.

5. Ibid.

6. Derek Beres, "42% of New Cancer Patients Lose Their Life Savings," Big Think, October 17, 2018, https://bigthink.com/politics-current-affairs/how-much-does-cancer-cost.

7. Adrienne M. Gilligan et al., "Death or Debt? National Estimates of Financial Toxicity in Persons with Newly-Diagnosed Cancer," *The American Journal of Medicine* 131, no. 10 (October 2018): 1189–99.e5, https://doi.org/10.1016/j.amjmed.2018.05.020.

8. Cristel E. van Dijk et al., "Moral Hazard and Supplier-Induced Demand: Empirical Evidence in General Practice," *Health Economics* 22, no. 3 (March 2013): 340–52, https://doi.org/10.1002/hec.2801.

9. Sharon Mason Parker, "Increase Your Medical Practice Revenue by Up-Selling and Cross-Selling," Practice Builders, January 19, 2018, http://www.practicebuilders.com/blog/increase-your-medical-practice-revenue-by-up-selling-and-cross-selling/.

10. "Average Health Care Deductible Nearly $1,500 for Individual Coverage Through an Employer Plan," International Foundation of Employee Benefit Plans, September 11, 2018, https://www.ifebp.org/aboutus/pressroom

/releases/Pages/Average-Health-Care-Deductible-Nearly-$1,500-for
-Individual-Coverage-Through-an-Employer-Plan.aspx.

11. Cory Capps and David Dranove, "Hospital Consolidation and Negotiated
PPO Prices," *Health Affairs* 23, no. 2 (March/April 2004): 175–81, https://
doi.org/10.1377/hlthaff.23.2.175.

12. Rabah Kamal, Cynthia Cox, and Daniel McDermott, "What Are the Recent
and Forecasted Trends in Prescription Drug Spending," Peterson-Kaiser
Health System Tracker, February 20, 2019, https://www.healthsystem
tracker.org/chart-collection/recent-forecasted-trends-prescription-drug
-spending/#item-among-adults-who-currently-take-any-prescription
-medicine-percent-who-report-ease-or-difficulty-affording-to-pay-the-cost
-of-their-prescription-medicine.

13. Ashley Kirzinger, Lunna Lopes, Bryan Wu, and Mollyann Brodie, "KFF
Health Tracking Poll—February 2019: Prescription Drugs," Henry J. Kaiser Family Foundation, March 1, 2019, https://www.kff.org/health-costs
/poll-finding/kff-health-tracking-poll-february-2019-prescription-drugs/.

14. Immaculada Hernandez et al., "The Contribution of New Product
Entry Versus Existing Product Inflation in the Rising Costs of Drugs,"
Health Affairs 38, no. 1 (January 2019): 76–83, https://doi.org/10.1377
/hlthaff.2018.05147.

15. John Hargraves and Amanda Frost, "Price of Insulin Prescription Doubled Between 2012 and 2016," Health Care Cost Institute, November 29,
2017, https://www.healthcostinstitute.org/blog/entry/price-of-insulin
-prescription-doubled-between-2012-and-2016?highlight=WyJpbnN1bGl
uIlo=.

16. Abby Goodnough, "Hepatitis C Deaths in U.S. Rose in 2014, but New
Drugs Hold Promise," *New York Times*, May 4, 2016, http://www.nytimes
.com/2016/05/05/us/hepatitis-c-deaths-in-us-rose-in-2014-but-new-drugs
-hold-promise.html.

17. Andrew Hill et al., "Minimum Costs for Producing Hepatitis C Direct
-Acting Antivirals for Use in Large-Scale Treatment Access Programs in
Developing Countries," *Clinical Infectious Diseases* 58, no. 7 (April 2014):
928–36, https://doi.org/10.1093/cid/ciu012.

18. Ted Alcorn, "Why Egypt Is at the Forefront of Hepatitis C Treatment," *The
Atlantic*, May 29, 2018, https://www.theatlantic.com/health/archive/2018
/05/why-egypt-is-at-the-forefront-of-hepatitis-c-treatment/561305/.

19. Ibid.

20. Maggie Fox, "Major Depression on the Rise Among Everyone, New Data Shows," NBC News, May 10, 2018, https://www.nbcnews.com/health /health-news/major-depression-rise-among-everyone-new-data-shows -n873146.

21. Susanna Schrobsdorff, "There's a Startling Increase in Major Depression Among Teens in the U.S.," *Time*, November 16, 2016, http://time.com /4572593/increase-depression-teens-teenage-mental-health/.

22. "Mental Illness," National Institute of Mental Health, https://www.nimh .nih.gov/health/statistics/mental-illness.shtml#part_154785.

23. Health Resources and Services Administration/National Center for Health Workforce Analysis; Substance Abuse and Mental Health Services Administration/Office of Policy, Planning, and Innovation, "National Projections of Supply and Demand for Behavioral Health Practitioners: 2013–2025," Rockville, MD: U.S. Department of Health and Human Services, 2016, https://bhw.hrsa.gov/sites/default/files/bhw/health-workforce-analysis /research/projections/behavioral-health2013-2025.pdf.

24. "The Silent Shortage: How Immigration Can Help Address the Large and Growing Psychiatrist Shortage in the United States," New American Economy, October 23, 2017, https://www.newamericaneconomy.org/press -release/new-study-shows-60-percent-of-u-s-counties-without-a-single -psychiatrist/.

25. "Active Physicians by Age and Specialty, 2015," Association of American Medical Colleges, https://www.aamc.org/data/workforce/reports/458494 /1-4-chart.html.

26. "How Budget Cuts Are Affecting Mental Health Care: A Look Toward Integrated Care Solutions," Cummings Graduate Institute for Behavioral Health Studies, August 5, 2016, https://cummingsinstitute.com /resources/infographics/budget-cuts-affect-mental-health-care/.

27. "Systemic Underfunding of Michigan's Public Mental Health System," Community Mental Health Association of Michigan, February 2019, https://cmham.org/systemic-underfunding-of-michigans-public-mental -health-system/.

28. Ibid.

29. Lenny Bernstein, "U.S. Life Expectancy Declines Again, a Dismal Trend not Seen Since World War I," *Washington Post*, November 29, 2018, https:// www.washingtonpost.com/national/health-science/us-life-expectancy -declines-again-a-dismal-trend-not-seen-since-world-war-i/2018

/11/28/ae58bc8c-f28c-11e8-bc79-68604ed88993_story.html?utm_term =.bd5e1f225d79.

30. Fred Schulte, "Purdue Pharma's Sales Pitch Downplayed Risks of Opioid Addiction," Kaiser Health News, August 17, 2018, https://khn.org/news /purdue-pharma-sales-pitch-downplayed-risks-of-opioid-addiction/.

31. Dennis Thompson, "Big Pharma's Marketing to Docs Helped Trigger Opioid Crisis: Study," U.S. News and World Report, January 18, 2019, https:// www.usnews.com/news/health-news/articles/2019-01-18/big-pharmas -marketing-to-docs-helped-trigger-opioid-crisis-study.

32. "Jailing People with Mental Illness," National Alliance on Mental Illness, https://www.nami.org/learn-more/public-policy/jailing-people-with -mental-illness.

33. Sara R. Collins, Munira Z. Gunja, and Michelle M. Doty, How Well Does Insurance Coverage Protect Consumers from Health Care Costs? Findings from the Commonwealth Fund Biennial Health Insurance Survey, 2016 (New York: The Commonwealth Fund, 2017): 1–22, https://www.commonwealth fund.org/publications/issue-briefs/2017/oct/how-well-does-insurance -coverage-protect-consumers-health-care.

34. Jeffrey M. Jones and Nader Nekvasil, "In U.S., Healthcare Insecurity at Record Low," Gallup, June 20, 2016, https://news.gallup.com/poll/192914 /healthcare-insecurity-record-low.aspx.

35. Cate Douglass, "Healthcare Insecurity at an All Time Low, Gallup Finds," American Journal of Managed Care, July 10, 2016, https://www.ajmc.com /newsroom/healthcare-insecurity-at-an-all-time-low-gallup-finds.

36. Mara Lee, "Majority of Americans Fear They'll Lose Health Insurance," Modern Healthcare, May 11, 2017, https://www.modernhealthcare.com /article/20170511/NEWS/170519971/majority-of-americans-fear-they-ll -lose-health-insurance.

Chapter 14: Insecure Households

1. E. Mavis Hetherington and John Kelly, For Better or For Worse: Divorce Reconsidered (New York: W. W. Norton & Co., 2002).

2. Phillip N. Cohen, "The Coming Divorce Divide," SocArXiv (September 2018): 1–6, https://doi.org/10.1177/2378023119873497.

3. Belinda Luscombe, "The Divorce Rate Is Dropping. That May Not Actually

Be Good News," *Time*, November 26, 2018, http://time.com/5434949
/divorce-rate-children-marriage-benefits/.

4. Janet Chen-Lan Kuo and R. Kelly Raley, "Diverging Patterns of Union
Transition Among Cohabitors by Race/Ethnicity and Education: Trends
and Marital Intentions in the United States," *Demography* 53, no. 4 (August
2016): 921–35, https://doi.org/10.1007/s13524-016-0483-9.

5. Richard V. Reeves and Eleanor Krause, "Cohabiting Parents Differ from
Married Ones in Three Big Ways" (Washington, DC: The Brookings Institution, 2017), https://www.brookings.edu/research/cohabiting-parents
-differ-from-married-ones-in-three-big-ways/.

6. Gretchen Livingston, "About One-Third of U.S. Children Are Living with
an Unmarried Parent," Pew Research Center, April 27, 2018, https://www
.pewresearch.org/fact-tank/2018/04/27/about-one-third-of-u-s-children
-are-living-with-an-unmarried-parent/; and Sheela Kennedy and Larry
Bumpass, "Cohabitation and Children's Living Arrangements: New Estimates from the United States," *Demographic Research* 19, no. 47 (September 2008): 1663–92, https://doi.org/10.4054/DemRes.2008.19.47.

7. "21% of Divorcées Cite Money as the Cause of Their Divorce, MagnifyMoney
Survey Shows," MagnifyMoney, February 13, 2017, https://www.magnify
money.com/blog/featured/money-causes-21-percent-divorces925885150/.

8. Claire Tsosie and Erin El Issa, "2018 American Household Credit Card
Debt Study," NerdWallet, December 10, 2018, https://www.nerdwallet
.com/blog/average-credit-card-debt-household/#foot.

9. Bill Fay, "Demographics of Debt," Debt.org, https://www.debt.org/faqs
/americans-in-debt/demographics/.

10. "Educational Attainment in the United States," United States Census
Bureau, February 21, 2019, https://www.census.gov/data/tables/2018
/demo/education-attainment/cps-detailed-tables.html.

11. Federal Deposit Insurance Corporation, *2017 FDIC National Survey of
Unbanked and Underbanked Households*, by Gerald Apaam et al., FDIC
-038-2018, FDIC, Washington, DC, 2018, https://www.fdic.gov/house
holdsurvey/2017/2017execsumm.pdf.

12. Alyssa Yun, "Financial Exclusion: Why It Is More Expensive to Be Poor,"
Wharton School of the University of Pennsylvania, June 2, 2017, https://
publicpolicy.wharton.upenn.edu/live/news/1895-financial-exclusion-why
-it-is-more-expensive-to-be.

13. Claire Zillman, "Childcare Costs More Than College Tuition in 28 U.S.

States," *Fortune*, October 22, 2018, http://fortune.com/2018/10/22/child care-costs-per-year-us/.

14. Leila Schochet, "The Child Care Crisis Is Keeping Women Out of the Workforce," Center for American Progress, Washington, DC, 2019, https://www.americanprogress.org/issues/early-childhood/reports/2019 /03/28/467488/child-care-crisis-keeping-women-workforce/.

15. John Halpin, Karl Agne, and Margie Omero, "Affordable Child Care and Early Learning for All Families," Center for American Progress, Washington, DC 2018), 1–15, https://cdn.americanprogress.org/content/uploads /2018/09/12074422/ChildCarePolling-report.pdf.

16. Schochet, "The Child Care Crisis."

17. Sandra Bishop-Josef, Chris Beakey, Sara Watson, and Tom Garrett, "Want to Grow the Economy? Fix the Child Care Crisis," Council for a Strong America, Washington, DC, 2019, 1-7, https://strongnation.s3.amazonaws .com/documents/602/83bb2275-ce07-4d74-bcee-ff6178daf6bd .pdf?1547054862&inline;%20filename=%22Want%20to%20Grow%20 the%20Economy?%20Fix%20the%20Child%20Care%20Crisis .pdf%22.

18. Zameena Majia, "Just 24 Female CEOs Lead the Companies on the Fortune 500—Fewer than Last Year," CNBC Make It, May 21, 2018, https:// www.cnbc.com/2018/05/21/2018s-fortune-500-companies-have-just-24 -female-ceos.html.

19. Heather Koball and Yang Jiang, "Basic Facts About Low-Income Children: Children Under 18 Years, 2016," National Center for Children in Poverty, January 2018, http://www.nccp.org/publications/pub_1194.html.

20. "Number of Children in Foster Care Continues to Increase," U.S. Department of Health & Human Services Administration for Children & Families, November 30, 2017, https://www.acf.hhs.gov/media/press/2017 /number-of-children-in-foster-care-continues-to-increase.

21. Gretchen Livingston, "Fewer than Half of U.S. Kids Today Live in a 'Traditional' Family," Pew Research Center, December 22, 2014, https://www .pewresearch.org/fact-tank/2014/12/22/less-than-half-of-u-s-kids-today -live-in-a-traditional-family/.

22. "ACEs Science 101," ACEs Too High News, https://acestoohigh.com/aces -101/.

23. "Got Your ACE Score?," ACEs Too High News, https://acestoohigh.com /got-your-ace-score/.

24. "ACEs Science 101," ACEs Too High News, https://acestoohigh.com/aces-101/.

25. Margaret A. Sheridan et al., "Variation in Neural Development as a Result of Exposure to Institutionalization Early in Childhood," *Proceedings of the National Academy of Sciences of the United States of America* 109, no. 32 (August 2012): 12927–32, https://doi.org/10.1073/pnas.1200041109.

26. Ryan J. Herringa et al., "Childhood Maltreatment Is Associated with Altered Fear Circuitry and Increased Internalizing Symptoms by Late Adolescence," *Proceedings of the National Academy of Sciences of the United States of America* 110, no. 47 (November 2013): 19119–24, https://doi.org/10.1073/pnas.1310766110.

27. Natalie Weder et al., "Child Abuse, Depression, and Methylation in Genes Involved with Stress, Neural Plasticity, and Brain Circuitry," *Journal of the American Academy of Child & Adolescent Psychiatry* 53, no. 4 (April 2014): 417–24.e5, https://doi.org/10.1016/j.jaac.2013.12.025.

28. Bao-Zhu Yang et al., "Child Abuse and Epigenetic Mechanisms of Disease Risk," *American Journal of Preventative Medicine* 44, no. 2 (February 2013): 101–107, https://doi.org/10.1016/j.amepre.2012.10.012.

29. "Older People Projected to Outnumber Children for First Time in U.S. History," United States Census Bureau press release, March 13, 2018, https://www.census.gov/newsroom/press-releases/2018/cb18-41-population-projections.html.

30. "Presidential Statement Signing the Social Security Act—August 14, 1935," Social Security History, Social Security Administration, https://www.ssa.gov/history/fdrsignstate.html.

31. Casey Schwarz, "AARP Survey Highlights Prescription Drug Use Among Older Adults," *Medicare Rights Center Blog*, April 28, 2016, https://blog.medicarerights.org/aarp-survey-highlights-prescription-drug-use-among-older-adults/.

32. "A Profile of Older Americans: 2017," U.S. Department of Health and Human Services Administration on Aging, Washington, DC, 2018, https://acl.gov/sites/default/files/Aging%20and%20Disability%20in%20America/2017OlderAmericansProfile.pdf.

33. "What Is Elder Abuse?" National Council on Aging, https://www.ncoa.org/public-policy-action/elder-justice/elder-abuse-facts/.

34. Richard J. Bonnie and Robert B. Wallace, eds., *Elder Mistreatment: Abuse, Neglect, and Exploitation in an Aging America* (Washington, DC: National

Academies Press, 2003), 266, https://www.ncbi.nlm.nih.gov/books /NBK98802/.

35. "Caregiver Statistics," Caregiver Action Network, https://caregiveraction .org/resources/caregiver-statistics.

36. Ibid.

37. Ibid.

38. "2019 Parents, Kids & Money Survey Results," Money Confident Kids presented by T. Rowe Price, http://www.moneyconfidentkids.com/content /money-confident-kids/en/us/media/research/2019-parents-kids-money -survey-results.html.

39. Matthew Desmond and Rachel Tolbert Kimbro, "Eviction's Fallout: Housing, Hardship, and Health," *Social Forces* 94, no. 1 (September 2015): 295–324, https://doi.org/10.1093/sf/sov044.

40. "Assembly Speaker Sheldon Silver, Housing Committee Chairman Vito Lopez, the Assembly Majority and the Community Service Society Release Groundbreaking Report Highlighting NYC Housing Crisis and the Need for Stronger Rent Laws," New York State Assembly press release, March 13, 2011, https://nyassembly.gov/Press/20110313/.

41. Renee Lewis, "Report: NYC Homelessness Soared Under Mayor Bloomberg," Al Jazeera America, March 12, 2014, http://america.aljazeera.com /articles/2014/3/12/record-breaking-nychomelessnessblamedonforprofit sheltersreport.html.

42. Desmond and Kimbro, "Eviction's Fallout."

43. "Definitions of Food Security," United States Department of Agriculture, last modified September 4, 2019, https://www.ers.usda.gov/topics/food -nutrition-assistance/food-security-in-the-us/definitions-of-food-security .aspx.

44. Justin Wolfers, David Leonhardt, and Kevin Quealy, "1.5 Million Missing Black Men," *New York Times*, April 20, 2015, https://www.nytimes.com /interactive/2015/04/20/upshot/missing-black-men.html.

45. "Criminal Justice Fact Sheet," The National Association for the Advancement of Colored People, https://www.naacp.org/criminal-justice-fact -sheet/.

46. Ibid.

47. "Race and the Criminal Justice System," Equal Justice Initiative, https:// eji.org/history-racial-injustice-race-and-criminal-justice.

48. John DiLulio, "The Coming of the Super-Predators," *Washington Examiner*,

November 27, 1995, https://www.weeklystandard.com/john-j-dilulio-jr/the-coming-of-the-super-predators.

49. *Deadly Force: Police Use of Lethal Force in the United States*, report by Amnesty International USA, 2015, 1–102, https://www.amnestyusa.org/files/aiusa_deadlyforcereportjune2015.pdf.

50. National Research Council, *The Growth of Incarceration in the United States: Exploring Causes and Consequences* (Washington, DC: The National Academies Press, 2014), https://doi.org/10.17226/18613.

51. "Criminal Justice Fact Sheet," The National Association for the Advancement of Colored People, https://www.naacp.org/criminal-justice-fact-sheet/.

52. Chris Mai and Ram Subramanian, *The Price of Prisons: Examining State Spending Trends, 2010–2015* (New York: Vera Institute of Justice, 2017): 1–27, https://www.vera.org/publications/price-of-prisons-2015-state-spending-trends/price-of-prisons-2015-state-spending-trends/price-of-prisons-2015-state-spending-trends-prison-spending.

53. John Maxwell, "Marginal Cost of Corrections: Michigan's Experience," Senate Fiscal Agency, Lansing, MI, 2015, http://www.senate.michigan.gov/sfa/Publications/Issues/CorrectionsMarginalCost/CorrectionsMarginalCost.pdf.

54. "Family Profiles," Office of Financial Aid, University of Michigan, https://finaid.umich.edu/family-profiles/.

55. "Criminal Justice Fact Sheet," The National Association for the Advancement of Colored People, https://www.naacp.org/criminal-justice-fact-sheet/.

56. "New Cigna Study Reveals Loneliness at Epidemic Levels in America," Cigna press release, May 1, 2018, https://www.multivu.com/players/English/8294451-cigna-us-loneliness-survey/.

Chapter 15: Insecure Communities

1. Solomon Greene, Margery Austin Turner, and Ruth Gourevitch, "Racial Residential Segregation and Neighborhood Disparities," US Partnership on Mobility from Poverty, August 29, 2017, https://www.mobilitypartnership.org/publications/racial-residential-segregation-and-neighborhood-disparities.

2. Ibid.

3. U.S. Department of Housing and Urban Development Office of Policy Development and Research, *Housing Discrimination Against Racial and Ethnic Minorities 2012*, Washington, DC, U.S Department of Housing and Urban Development, 2013, https://www.huduser.gov/portal/Publications /pdf/HUD-514_HDS2012.pdf.

4. Ibid.

5. Robert I. Lerman and Signe-Mary McKernan, "Promoting Neighborhood Improvement While Protecting Low-Income Families," Urban Institute, May 3, 2007, https://www.urban.org/research/publication/promoting -neighborhood-improvement-while-protecting-low-income-families.

6. Richard Fry and Paul Taylor, "The Rise of Residential Segregation by Income," Pew Research Center, August 1, 2012, http://www.pewsocial trends.org/2012/08/01/the-rise-of-residential-segregation-by-income/.

7. Beverly Daniel Tatum, "Segregation Worse in Schools 60 Years After Brown v. Board of Education," *Seattle Times*, September 14, 2017, https:// www.seattletimes.com/opinion/segregation-worse-in-schools-60-years -after-brown-v-board-of-education/.

8. Ibid.

9. Michael R. Kramer and Carol R. Hogue, "Is Segregation Bad for Your Health?," *Epidemiologic Reviews* 31, no. 1 (November 2009): 178–94, https://doi.org/10.1093/epirev/mxp001.

10. Alan Greenblatt, "Political Segregation Is Growing and We're Living with the Consequences," *Governing*, November 18, 2016, http://www .governing.com/topics/politics/gov-bill-bishop-interview.html.

11. Drew DeSilver, "How the Most Ideologically Polarized Americans Live Different Lives," Pew Research Center, June 13, 2014, http://www .pewresearch.org/fact-tank/2014/06/13/big-houses-art-museums-and -in-laws-how-the-most-ideologically-polarized-americans-live-different -lives/.

12. Alan Greenblatt, "Political Segregation Is Growing and 'We're Living with the Consequences,'" *Governing Magazine*, last updated November 18, 2016, https://www.governing.com/topics/politics/gov-bill-bishop -interview.html.

13. Filipe R. Campante and Daniel A. Hojman, "Media and Polarization: Evidence from the Introduction of Broadcast TV in the United States," *Journal of Public Economics* 100, (April 2013): 79–92, https://doi.org/10.1016 /j.jpubeco.2013.02.006.

14. Nick Newman, *Reuters Institute Digital News Report 2017* (Oxford: Reuters Institute for the Study of Journalism, 2017): 1–132, http://www.digital newsreport.org/survey/2017/.

15. Travis L. Dixon, *A Dangerous Distortion of Our Families: Representation of Families, by Race, in News and Opinion Media, report for Family Story/ Color of Change,* December 2017, https://colorofchange.org/dangerous distortion/.

16. United States Government Accountability Office, *Countering Violent Extremism: Actions Needed to Define Strategy and Assess Progress of Federal Efforts,* GAO-17-300, Washington, DC: GAO, 2017, https://www.gao.gov /assets/690/683984.pdf.

17. Juju Chang, Jake Lefferman, Claire Pedersen, and Geoff Martz, "When Fake News Stories Make Real News Headlines," ABC News, November 29, 2016, https://abcnews.go.com/Technology/fake-news-stories-make -real-news-headlines/story?id=43845383.

18. Ibid.

19. "Blue Feed, Red Feed," *Wall Street Journal,* last updated August 19, 2019, accessed February 27, 2019, http://graphics.wsj.com/blue-feed-red-feed /#/immigration.

20. Andrew Liptak, "A Military Expert Explains Why Social Media Is the New Battlefield," The Verge, October 12, 2018, https://www.theverge.com/2018 /10/12/17967544/likewar-social-media-pw-singer-interview.

21. Ryan Nunn, Jimmy O'Donnell, and Jay Shambaugh, "A Dozen Facts About Immigration," The Brookings Institution, Washington, DC, 2018, 1–18, http://www.hamiltonproject.org/papers/a_dozen_facts_about _immigration.

22. James G. Gimpel, "Immigration Policy Opinion and the 2016 Presidential Vote: Issue Relevance in the Trump-Clinton Election," Center for Immigration Studies, December 4, 2017, https://cis.org/Report/Immigration -Policy-Opinion-and-2016-Presidential-Vote.

23. German Lopez, "20 Years After Columbine, America Sees Roughly One Mass Shooting a Day," *Vox,* last updated April 20, 2019, https://www.vox .com/2019/4/19/18412650/columbine-mass-shootings-gun-violence-map -charts-data.

24. "Gun Violence in America," Everytown for Gun Safety Support Fund, last updated April 4, 2019, https://everytownresearch.org/gun-violence -america/.

25. "Gun Violence Statistics," Giffords Law Center to Prevent Gun Violence, https://lawcenter.giffords.org/gun-deaths-and-race-statistics/.

26. Sarah Mervosh, "Nearly 40,000 People Died from Guns in U.S. Last Year, Highest in 50 Years," *New York Times*, December 18, 2018, https://www.nytimes.com/2018/12/18/us/gun-deaths.html.

27. "Firearm Suicide in the United States," Everytown for Gun Safety Support Fund, August 30, 2019, https://everytownresearch.org/firearm-suicide/.

28. Ibid.

29. "Lethality of Suicide Methods: Case Fatality Rates by Suicide Method, 8 U.S. States, 1989–1997," Harvard T. H. Chan School of Public Health, https://www.hsph.harvard.edu/means-matter/means-matter/case-fatality/.

30. Nurith Aizenman, "Deaths from Gun Violence: How the U.S. Compares with the Rest of the World," NPR, November 9, 2018, https://www.npr.org/sections/goatsandsoda/2018/11/09/666209430/deaths-from-gun-violence-how-the-u-s-compares-with-the-rest-of-the-world.

31. Jonathan Masters, "How do U.S. gun laws compare to other countries?," *PBS NewsHour*, last updated November 17, 2017, https://www.pbs.org/newshour/nation/how-do-u-s-gun-laws-compare-to-other-countries.

Chapter 16: Insecure Places

1. American Society of Civil Engineers, *2017 Infrastructure Report Card: A Comprehensive Assessment of America's Infrastructure* (Reston, VA: American Society of Civil Engineers, 2017), 1–16, www.infrastructurereportcard.org.

2. Richard Florida, "How 'Social Infrastructure' Can Knit America Together," CityLab, September 11, 2018, https://www.citylab.com/life/2018/09/how-social-infrastructure-can-knit-america-together/569854/.

3. Eric Klinenberg, "Worry Less About Crumbling Roads, More About Crumbling Libraries," *The Atlantic*, September 20, 2018, https://www.theatlantic.com/ideas/archive/2018/09/worry-less-about-crumbling-roads-more-about-crumbling-libraries/570721/.

4. Heather Bellow, "York Lake Bathrooms Another Victim of State Park Cuts," *Berkshire Eagle*, July 15, 2018, https://www.berkshireeagle.com/stories/york-lake-bathrooms-another-victim-of-state-park-cuts,544832.

5. "President's Budget Proposal Damaging to National Parks as They Continue to Recover from Government Shutdown," National Parks Conser-

vation Association press release, March 11, 2019, https://www.npca.org /articles/2130-president-s-budget-proposal-damaging-to-national-parks-as -they-continue-to.

6. American Society of Civil Engineers, 2017 *Infrastructure Report Card*.

7. Ibid.

8. Andrew Kouri, "Introducing Crowdsourced Pavement Quality Maps," *Medium*, October 30, 2018, https://medium.com/lvl5/introducing-crowd sourced-pavement-quality-maps-8ddafd15a903.

9. Julie Mack, "Bad Roads Cost Michigan Drivers Average of $648 a Year in Additional Vehicle Expenses, Study Says," MLive, last updated March 12, 2019, https://www.mlive.com/news/2019/03/bad-roads-cost-michigan -drivers-average-of-648-a-year-in-additional-vehicle-expenses-study-says .html.

10. American Society of Civil Engineers, 2017 *Infrastructure Report Card*.

11. New York City Independent Budget Office, *"We Are Being Held Momentarily": How Much Time and Money Are New York City Subway Riders Losing to Delays?*, New York City Independent Budget Office, 2017, p. 1, https:// ibo.nyc.ny.us/iboreports/we-are-being-held-momentarily-how-much-time -and-money-are-new-york-city-subway-riders-losing-to-delays-october-2017 .html.

12. Michael Jackman, "Back Track," *Detroit Metro Times*, March 29, 2006, https://www.metrotimes.com/detroit/back-track/Content?oid=2184294.

13. Jonathan English, "Why Did America Give Up on Mass Transit? (Don't Blame Cars)," *CityLab*, August 31, 2018, https://www.citylab.com /transportation/2018/08/how-america-killed-transit/568825/.

14. Ibid.

15. John P. Heimlich, "Status of Air Travel in the USA," presentation, Ipsos, April 13, 2016, http://airlines.org/wp-content/uploads/2016/04/2016 Survey.pdf.

16. American Society of Civil Engineers, 2017 *Infrastructure Report Card*.

17. Nathan Bomey, "U.S. Vehicle Deaths Topped 40,000 in 2017, National Safety Council Estimates," *USA Today*, last updated February 15, 2018, https://www.usatoday.com/story/money/cars/2018/02/15/national-safety -council-traffic-deaths/340012002/.

18. Douglas W. Harwood et al., *Safety Benefits of Highway Infrastructure Investments* (Washington, DC: AAA Foundation for Traffic Safety, 2017), https:// aaafoundation.org/safety-benefits-of-highway-infrastructure-investments/.

19. American Society of Civil Engineers, *2017 Infrastructure Report Card.*

20. Ibid.

21. Ibid.

22. Ibid.

23. Shara Tibken, "Why 5G Is Out of Reach for More People than You Think," CNET, October 25, 2018, https://www.cnet.com/news/why-5gs-out-of -reach-for-more-people-than-you-think/.

24. Federal Communications Commission, *2016 Broadband Progress Report*, FCC 16-6, Washington, DC, 2016, https://www.fcc.gov/reports-research /reports/broadband-progress-reports/2016-broadband-progress-report.

25. American Society of Civil Engineers, *2017 Infrastructure Report Card.*

26. Organisation for Economic Cooperation and Development, *Education at a Glance 2017* (Paris: OECD Publishing, 2017), 179, https://www.oecd -ilibrary.org/education/education-at-a-glance-2017_eag-2017-en.

27. Drew DeSilver, "U.S. Students' Academic Achievement Still Lags That of Their Peers in Many Other Countries," Pew Research Center, February 15, 2017, http://www.pewresearch.org/fact-tank/2017/02/15/u-s-students -internationally-math-science/.

28. Ibid.

29. Suparna Dutt D'Cunha, "Modi Announces '100% Village Electrification,' but 31 Million Indian Homes Are Still in the Dark," *Forbes*, May 7, 2018, https://www.forbes.com/sites/suparnadutt/2018/05/07/modi-announces -100-village-electrification-but-31-million-homes-are-still-in-the-dark /#37b7c31d63ba.

30. Michael Hartnack, "Rising Power Outage Cost and Frequency Is Driv- ing Grid Modernization Investment," Navigant Research, June 28, 2018, https://www.navigantresearch.com/news-and-views/rising-power-outage -cost-and-frequency-is-driving-grid-modernization-investment.

31. Ponemon Institute, *Cost of Data Center Outages* (Traverse City, MI: Ponemon Institute, 2016): 1–20, https://www.vertivco.com/globalas- sets/documents/reports/2016-cost-of-data-center-outages-11-11_51190 _1.pdf.

32. George Luber and Jay Lemery, eds., Global Climate Change and Human Health (San Francisco: Jossey-Bass, 2015), 311–23, https://books.google .com/books?id=U0E1CAAAQBAJ&source=gbs_navlinks_s.

33. Thomas W. Sanchez, *An Inherent Bias? Geographic and Racial-Ethnic Pat- terns of Metropolitan Planning Organization Boards* (Washington, DC: The

Brookings Institution, 2006): 1–19, https://www.brookings.edu/research /an-inherent-bias-geographic-and-racial-ethnic-patterns-of-metropolitan -planning-organization-boards/.

Chapter 17: Insecure Economy

1. Kurt Metzger, "Demographic and Workforce Trends in Southeast Michigan," presentation, Macomb/St. Clair Workforce Development Board, August 25, 2011, https://datadrivendetroit.org/files/D3P/Macomb_St _Clair_Workforce_Bd_8_25_11.pdf.

2. Arne L. Kalleberg, Barbara F. Reskin, and Ken Hudson, "Bad Jobs in America: Standard and Nonstandard Employment Relations and Job Quality in the United States," *American Sociological Review* 65, no. 2 (April 2000): 256–78, https://doi.org/10.2307/2657440.

3. John Schmitt and Janelle Jones, *Bad Jobs on the Rise* (Washington, DC: Center for Economic and Policy Research, 2012), 1–18, http://cepr.net /documents/publications/bad-jobs-2012-09.pdf.

4. "How the Great Recession Changed American Workers," Wharton School of the University of Pennsylvania, September 10, 2018, http://knowledge .wharton.upenn.edu/article/great-recession-american-dream/.

5. David N. F. Bell and David G. Blanchflower, "Underemployment in the US and Europe," Working Paper no. 24927, The National Bureau of Economic Research, Cambridge, MA, August 2018, https://www.nber.org/papers /w24927.

6. David Autor, *The Polarization of Job Opportunities in the U.S. Labor Market: Implications for Employment and Earning* (Washington, DC: Center for American Progress and the Brookings Institution, 2010): 1–40, https:// economics.mit.edu/files/5554.

7. Henry S. Farber et al., "Unions and Inequality Over the Twentieth Century: New Evidence from Survey Data," Working Paper no. 620, Princeton University, Princeton, NJ, May 2018, 1–93, https://dataspace.princeton .edu/jspui/bitstream/88435/dsp01gx41mm54w/3/620.pdf.

8. Matthew Michaels, "Minimum Wage Will Rise in 18 States in 2018—but No One Can Agree on the Impact It Will Have," *Business Insider*, December 21, 2017, https://www.businessinsider.com/minimum-wage-increase -states-in-2018-2017-12.

9. Michael J. Hicks and Srikant Devaraj, *The Myth and the Reality of Manufac-*

turing in America (Muncie, IN: Ball State University, 2015), http://projects
.cberdata.org/reports/MfgReality.pdf.

10. Ingrid Lunden, "Amazon's Share of the US E-commerce Market Is Now
49%, or 5% of All Retail Spend," TechCrunch, July 13, 2018, https://tech-
crunch.com/2018/07/13/amazons-share-of-the-us-e-commerce-market-is
-now-49-or-5-of-all-retail-spend/.

11. Greta R. Krippner, "The Financialization of the American Economy," *Socio
-Economic Review* 3, no. 2 (May 2005): 173, https://doi.org/10.1093/SER
/mwi008.

12. Ian Thibodeau, "Ford Reports $7.6B Profit in 2017, up 65%," *Detroit News*,
January 24, 2018, https://www.detroitnews.com/story/business/autos
/ford/2018/01/24/ford-annual-earnings/109777880/.

13. Brent Snavely, "Report: Ford to Cut 10% of Global Workforce," *Detroit Free
Press*, last updated May 16, 2017, https://www.freep.com/story/money/cars
/ford/2017/05/16/report-ford-cut-10-global-workforce/324191001/.

14. David Shepardson, "Ford to Cut 1,400 White-Collar Jobs, Shares Tumble,"
Reuters, May 17, 2017, https://www.reuters.com/article/us-ford-motor-jobs
-idUSKCN18D1GN.

15. Chris Isidore, "GM's Restructuring Was Tough. Ford's Could Be Event
Harder," CNN Business, December 4, 2018, https://www.cnn.com/2018
/12/04/business/ford-job-cut-forecast/index.html.

16. "Subsidy Tracker Parent Company Summary," Good Jobs First, https://
subsidytracker.goodjobsfirst.org/parent/ford-motor.

17. Anders Melin, Jenn Zhao, and Jason Perry, "Disney Faces Fresh Criticism
After Heir Calls Iger's Pay 'Insane,'" Bloomberg, last updated September
12, 2019, https://www.bloomberg.com/graphics/ceo-pay-ratio/.

18. Diana Hembree, "CEO Pay Skyrockets to 361 Times That of the Average Worker," *Forbes*, May 22, 2018, https://www.forbes.com/sites/diana
hembree/2018/05/22/ceo-pay-skyrockets-to-361-times-that-of-the-average
-worker/#583bdfcb776d.

19. "CEO-to-Worker Pay Ratio Ballooned 1,000 Percent Since 1950: Report,"
Huffington Post, last updated May 1, 2013, https://www.huffingtonpost
.com/2013/04/30/ceo-to-worker-pay-ratio_n_3184623.html.

20. Matthew Desmond, "Americans Want to Believe Jobs Are the Solution to
Poverty. They're Not," *New York Times*, September 11, 2018, https://www
.nytimes.com/2018/09/11/magazine/americans-jobs-poverty-homeless
.html.

Chapter 18: Insecure Politics

1. Jennifer Vanasco, "Explainer: The Supreme Court, Voting Rights and New York," WNYC News, June 25, 2013, https://www.wnyc.org/story/301391 -explainer-supreme-court-voting-rights-and-new-york/.

2. Henry Kanengiser, "In New York, Where You Live Can Determine How Hard It Is to Vote," *City Limits*, April 25, 2019, https://citylimits.org/2019 /04/25/nyc-polling-place-shortage-inequality/.

3. Alan Judd, "Georgia's Strict Laws Lead to Large Purge of Voters," *Atlanta Journal-Constitution*, October 27, 2018, https://www.ajc.com/news/state— regional-govt—politics/voter-purge-begs-question-what-the-matter-with -georgia/YAFvuk3Bu95kJIMaDiDFqJ/.

4. Phoebe Henninger, Marc Meredith, and Michael Morse, "Who Votes Without Identification? Using Affidavits from Michigan to Learn About the Potential Impact of Strict Photo Voter Identification Laws," SSRN, July 2018, https://papers.ssrn.com/sol3/papers.cfm?abstract_id=3205769.

5. G.E.M., "Do Voter ID Laws Reduce Turnout Among Black Americans?," *The Economist*, February 19, 2019, https://www.economist.com/democracy -in-america/2019/02/19/do-voter-id-laws-reduce-turnout-among-black -americans.

6. Alex Vandermass-Peeler et al., *American Democracy in Crisis: The Challenges of Voter Knowledge, Participation, and Polarization* (Washington, DC: Public Religion Research Institute, 2018), 1–35, https://www.prri.org /research/American-democracy-in-crisis-voters-midterms-trump-election -2018/.

7. Vann R. Newkirk II, "Voter Suppression Is Warping Democracy," *The Atlantic*, July 17, 2018, https://www.theatlantic.com/politics/archive/2018 /07/poll-prri-voter-suppression/565355/; and Zachary Roth, "Study: North Carolina Polling Site Changes Hurt Blacks," NBC News, November 23, 2015, https://www.nbcnews.com/news/nbcblk/study-north-carolina -polling-site-changes-hurt-blacks-n468251.

8. "Party Affiliation Among Adults in Michigan," Pew Research Center, https://www.pewforum.org/religious-landscape-study/state/michigan /party-affiliation/.

9. Ibid.

10. Jonathan Oosting, "Benson: Pro-Whitmer Ads Violated Campaign Finance Law," *Detroit News*, last updated February 10, 2019, https://www

.detroitnews.com/story/news/local/michigan/2019/02/08/benson-pro
-whitmer-group-broke-law/2812710002/.

11. Santa Clara County v. Southern Pacific R. Co., 118 US 394, U.S. Supreme
Court, 1886, https://supreme.justia.com/cases/federal/us/118/394/.

12. First National Bank of Boston v. Bellotti, 435 U.S. 765, U.S. Supreme
Court, 1978, https://supreme.justia.com/cases/federal/us/435/765/.

13. Bob Biersack, "8 Years Later: How Citizens United Changed Campaign
Finance," OpenSecrets, February 7, 2018, https://www.opensecrets.org
/news/2018/02/how-citizens-united-changed-campaign-finance/.

14. "Top Industries," Lobbying, OpenSecrets, https://www.opensecrets.org
/lobby/top.php?indexType=i.

15. Lee Fang and Nick Surgery, "Lobbying Documents Reveal Health Care
Industry Battle Plan Against 'Medicare for All,'" *The Intercept*, November
20, 2018, https://t.co/gc31lnqjRb.

16. "Private Prisons in the United States," The Sentencing Project, last updated
August 2, 2018, https://www.sentencingproject.org/publications/private
-prisons-united-states/.

17. Corrections Corporation of America, 2014 Annual Report Form 10-K for
the Period Ending December 31, 2014 (filed February 25, 2015), 1–88,
http://www.annualreports.com/HostedData/AnnualReportArchive/c
/NYSE_CXW_2014.pdf.

18. Ibid.

19. "CoreCivic Inc Summary," Lobbying, OpenSecrets, https://www
.opensecrets.org/lobby/clientsum.php?id=D000021940.

20. Corrections Corporation of America, 2014 Annual Report.

21. Ibid.

22. Arne Holst, "Subscriber Share Held by Smartphone Operating Systems
in the United States from 2012 to 2019," Statista, last edited September
13, 2019, https://www.statista.com/statistics/266572/market-share-held
-by-smartphone-platforms-in-the-united-states/.

23. Anna-Maria Kovacs, "Competition in the U.S. Wireless Services Market,"
Working Paper, Georgetown Business and Public Policy, Washington, DC,
August 2018, https://cbpp.georgetown.edu/sites/default/files/Policy%20
Paper%20-%20Kovacs%20-%20Wireless%20Competition%202018-08
.pdf.

24. Washington's Blog, "America Has Been at War 93% of the Time—222 out
of 239 Years—Since 1776," Global Research, January 20, 2019, https://

www.globalresearch.ca/america-has-been-at-war-93-of-the-time-222-out
-of-239-years-since-1776/5565946.

25. Jeff D. Colgan, *Oil, Conflict, and U.S. National Interests* (Cambridge, MA: Harvard Kennedy School Belfer Center for Science and International Affairs, 2013), https://www.belfercenter.org/publication/oil-conflict-and -us-national-interests.

26. Nima Elbagir et al., "Bomb That Killed 40 Children in Yemen Was Supplied by the US," CNN, last updated August 17, 2018, https://www.cnn .com/2018/08/17/middleeast/us-saudi-yemen-bus-strike-intl/index.html.

27. "U.S. Defense Spending Compared to Other Countries," Peter G. Peterson Foundation, May 3, 2019, https://www.pgpf.org/chart-archive/0053 _defense-comparison.

28. Kimberly Amaded, "Vietnam War Facts, Costs, and Timeline," The Balance, last updated June 25, 2019, https://www.thebalance.com/vietnam -war-facts-definition-costs-and-timeline-4154921.

29. Ibid.

30. Dorian Merina, "When Active-Duty Service Members Struggle to Feed Their Families," NPR, April 19, 2017, https://www.npr.org/sections/the salt/2017/04/19/524563155/when-active-duty-service-members-struggle -to-feed-their-families.

31. Lisa K. Lindquist, Holly C. Love, and Eric B. Elbogen, "Traumatic Brain Injury in Iraq and Afghanistan Veterans: New Results from a National Random Sample Study," *The Journal of Neuropsychiatry and Clinical Neurosciences* 29, no. 3 (Summer 2017): 254–59, https://doi.org/10.1176/appi .neuropsych.16050100.

32. "How Common Is PTSD in Veterans?," PTSD: National Center for PTSD, U.S. Department of Veterans Affairs, https://www.ptsd.va.gov/understand /common/common_veterans.asp.

33. Rachel Widome et al., "Food Insecurity Among Veterans of the US Wars in Iraq and Afghanistan," *Public Health Nutrition* 18, no. 5 (April 2015): 844–49, https://doi.org/10.1017/S136898001400072X.

34. "FAQ About Homeless Veterans," Background & Statistics, National Coalition for Homeless Veterans, http://nchv.org/index.php/news/media/back ground_and_statistics/.

35. Lewei Lin et al., "Changing Trends in Opioid Overdose Deaths and Prescription Opioid Receipt Among Veterans," *American Journal of*

Preventive Medicine 57, no. 1 (July 2019): 106–10, https://doi.org/10.1016/j.amepre.2019.01.016.

Chapter 19: The Spread of Insecurity

1. "When Is Enough . . . Enough?," UBS, 2Q 2015, 1–11, https://www.ubs.com/content/dam/WealthManagementAmericas/documents/investor-watch-2Q2015.pdf.
2. Rachel Sherman, *Uneasy Street: The Anxieties of Affluence* (Princeton, NJ: Princeton University Press, 2017), https://press.princeton.edu/titles/11096.html.
3. "When Is Enough . . . Enough?"
4. Kerry Hannon, "I'm Rich, and That Makes Me Anxious," *New York Times*, November 7, 2017, https://www.nytimes.com/2017/11/07/your-money/wealth-anxiety-money.html?mabReward=CTS2&recid=ow2HM8KVTqUMhwpJFvDe9i2NpvC&recp=0.
5. Tyler Davis, Drew Lindsay, and Brian O'Leary, "How America Gives Data: Leaders and Laggards, Giving Opportunities, and More," *The Chronicle of Philanthropy*, October 2, 2017, https://www.philanthropy.com/interactives/how-america-gives.
6. Paul Piff, "Does Money Make You Mean?," TEDxMarin, San Rafael, CA, October 2013, video, https://www.ted.com/talks/paul_piff_does_money_make_you_mean?language=en.
7. Paul K. Piff et al., "Higher Social Class Predicts Increased Unethical Behavior," *Proceedings of the National Academy of Sciences of the United States of America* 109, no. 11 (March 2012): 4086–91, https://doi.org/10.1073/pnas.1118373109.
8. Alexis Brassey and Stephen Barber, eds., *Greed* (New York: Palgrave Macmillan, 2019), 26, https://books.google.com/books?id=2kjeCwAAQBAJ&lpg=PA26&ots=xbLYbiJgOs&dq=how%20much%20inheritance%20mega%20wealthy&pg=PA26#v=onepage&q=how%20much%20inheritance%20mega%20wealthy&f=false.
9. Oma Seddiq, "How the World's Billionaires Got So Rich," *Forbes*, March 10, 2018, https://www.forbes.com/sites/omaseddiq/2018/03/10/how-the-worlds-billionaires-got-so-rich/#6828db87124c.
10. David Barstow, Susanne Craig, and Russ Buettner, "Trump Engaged in

Suspect Tax Schemes as He Reaped Riches from His Father," *New York Times*, October 2, 2018, https://www.nytimes.com/interactive/2018/10/02 /us/politics/donald-trump-tax-schemes-fred-trump.html.

11. "The State of Luxury Advertising: 5 Trends to Watch," MDG Advertising, August 6, 2018, https://www.mdgadvertising.com/marketing-insights /the-state-of-luxury-advertising-5-trends-to-watch/.

12. Jesse Bricker, Rodney Ramcharan, and Jacob Krimmel, "Signaling Status: The Impact of Relative Income on Household Consumption and Financial Decisions," Federal Reserve Board, Working Paper No. 2014 -76, Washington, DC, 2018, https://www.federalreserve.gov/econresdata /feds/2014/files/201476pap.pdf; and Ori Heffetz, "A Test of Conspicuous Consumption: Visibility and Income Elasticities," *The Review of Economics and Statistics* 93, no. 4 (November 2011): 1101–17, https://doi.org/10.1162 /REST_a_00116.

13. Henry Grabar, "The Rich Are Getting More Mortgages. The Poor Are Getting More Car Loans," *Slate*, May 19, 2017, https://slate.com/business /2017/05/the-rich-are-getting-more-mortgages-the-poor-are-getting-more -car-loans.html.

14. Ibid.

15. Raj Chetty et al., "The Fading American Dream: Trends in Absolute Income Mobility Since 1940," *Science* 356, no. 6336 (April 2017): 398–406, https://doi.org/10.1126/science.aal4617.

16. Raj Chetty et al., "Where Is the Land of Opportunity? The Geography of Intergenerational Mobility in the United States," Working Paper no. 19843, the National Bureau of Economic Research, Cambridge, MA, January 2014, https://www.nber.org/papers/w19843.

17. United States Department of Agriculture Office of Inspector General, *Detecting Potential SNAP Trafficking Using Data Analysis*, 27901-0002-13, Alexandria, VA: USDA, 2017, https://www.usda.gov/oig/webdocs/27901 -0002-13.pdf.

Chapter 20: Toward a Politics of Empathy

1. Benjamin M. P. Cuff et al., "Empathy: A Review of the Concept." *Emotion Review* 8, no. 2 (April 2016): 144–53, https://doi.org/10.1177 /1754073914558466.

2. Daniel Goleman, "Three Kinds of Empathy: Cognitive, Emotional,

Compassionate," June 12, 2007, http://www.danielgoleman.info/three
-kinds-of-empathy-cognitive-emotional-compassionate/.

Chapter 21: Them and Us

1. Dan Kopf, "The Typical US Congress Member Is 12 Times Richer than
   the Typical American Household," Quartz, February 12, 2018, https://
   qz.com/1190595/the-typical-us-congress-member-is-12-times-richer-than
   -the-typical-american-household/.
2. Jack Lessenberry, "Great Candidate, Not So Great Name," Michigan Radio,
   May 17, 2017, https://www.michiganradio.org/post/great-candidate-not-so
   -great-name.
3. Rafia Zakaria, "How Media Coverage of Terrorism Endorses a Legal Double Standard," *Columbia Journalism Review*, September 15, 2016, https://
   www.cjr.org/special_report/media_terrorism_muslim_law_trump.php/.
4. "The Lincoln-Douglas Debates, Fifth Joint Debate: Mr. Douglas's Speech,"
   Claremont McKenna College, http://www1.cmc.edu/pages/faculty/JPitney
   /lincdoug.html.
5. David Cole, *Engines of Liberty: The Power of Citizen Activists to Make Constitutional Law* (New York: Basic Books, 2016).
6. *The Combahee River Collective Statement: Black Feminist Organizing in
   the Seventies and Eighties* (Kitchen Table/Women of Color Press: 1986),
   https://we.riseup.net/assets/43875/combahee%20river.pdf.
7. Bill D. Moyers, "What a Real President Was Like," *Washington Post*, November 13, 1988, https://www.washingtonpost.com/archive/opinions/1988/11/13
   /what-a-real-president-was-like/d483c1be-d0da-43b7-bde6-04e10106ff6c/.
8. Randy Essex, "Dark Side of American Dream Is Killing White Men,"
   Detroit Free Press, last updated April 15, 2019, https://www.freep.com/
   story/opinion/contributors/2019/04/12/suicide-rates-prevention-white
   -men/3436883002/.
9. Ibid.

Chapter 22: Empathy Policy

1. David Mikkelson, "Did Harry Truman Denounce the Use of 'Socialism'
   as a 'Scare word'?" Snopes.com, last updated March 15, 2019, https://www
   .snopes.com/fact-check/truman-socialism-scare-word/.
2. Warren E. Buffet, "Stop Coddling the Super-Rich, *New York Times*, August

14, 2011, https://www.nytimes.com/2011/08/15/opinion/stop-coddling-the -super-rich.html?_r=0.

3. Ben Steverman, Dave Merrill, and Jeremy C. F. Lin, "A Year After the Middle Class Tax Cut, the Rich Are Winning," Bloomberg, December 18, 2018, https://www.bloomberg.com/graphics/2018-tax-plan-consequences/.

4. "Top Federal Income Tax Rates Since 1913," Citizens for Tax Justice, November 2011, https://www.ctj.org/pdf/regcg.pdf.

5. Isabel V. Sawhill and Christopher Pulliam, "Americans Want the Wealthy and Corporations to Pay More Taxes, but Are Elected Officials Listening?," The Brookings Institution, March 14, 2019, https://www.brookings.edu /blog/up-front/2019/03/14/americans-want-the-wealthy-and-corporations -to-pay-more-taxes-but-are-elected-officials-listening/.

6. Frank Newport, "Majority Say Wealthy Americans, Corporations Taxed Too Little," Gallup, April 18, 2017, https://news.gallup.com/poll/208685 /majority-say-wealthy-americans-corporations-taxed-little.aspx.

Chapter 23: Thirteen Ideas to Heal Our Insecurity

1. Bradley Sawyer and Cynthia Cox, "How Does Health Spending in the U.S. Compare to Other Countries?," Peterson-Kaiser Health System Tracker, December 7, 2018, https://www.healthsystemtracker.org/chart-collection /health-spending-u-s-compare-countries/.

2. Centers for Disease Control and Prevention Office for State, Tribal, Local and Territorial Support, "United States Public Health 101," Centers for Disease Control and Prevention, Atlanta, GA, 2013, PowerPoint, http:// www.cdc.gov/publichealthgateway/docs/usph101.pptx.x.

3. Albert Lang, Molly Warren, and Linda Kulman, *A Funding Crisis for Public Health and Safety: State-by-State Public Health Funding and Key Health Facts* (Washington, DC: Trust for America's Health, 2018), 8, https://www .tfah.org/wp-content/uploads/archive/assets/files/TFAH-2018-InvestIn AmericaRpt-FINAL.pdf.

4. Myles Allen et al., *Special Report: Global Warming of 1.5°C: An IPCC special report on the impacts of global warming of 1.5°C above pre-industrial levels and related global greenhouse gas emission pathways, in the context of strengthening the global response to the threat of climate change, sustainable development, and efforts to eradicate poverty*, The Intergovernmental Panel on Climate Change, 2018, https://www.ipcc.ch/sr15/.

5. Alexander C. Kaufman, Travis Waldron, and Chris D'Angelo, "Look No Further than Brazil's Amazon Fire for the Dangers of Deregulation," *Mother Jones*, August 24, 2019, https://www.motherjones.com /environment/2019/08/look-no-further-than-brazils-amazon-fire-for-the -dangers-of-deregulation/.

6. "Water Scarcity," Threats, World Wildlife Fund, https://www.worldwildlife .org/threats/water-scarcity.

7. Ibid.

8. James Fergusson, "The World Will Soon Be at War Over Water," *Newsweek*, April 24, 2015, https://www.newsweek.com/2015/05/01/world-will-soon -be-war-over-water-324328.html.

9. Dana Drugmand, "Climate Costs in 2018: Top 10 Disasters Cost $85 Billion," Climate Liability News, January 2, 2019, https://www.climate liabilitynews.org/2019/01/03/climate-costs-2018/.

10. Jennifer Cheeseman Day and Eric C. Newburger, *The Big Payoff: Educational Attainment and Synthetic Estimates of Work-Life Earnings*, P23-210, Suitland, MD: U.S. Census Bureau, 2002, https://www.census.gov/library /publications/2002/demo/p23-210.html.

11. Philip Trostel, "It's Not Just the Money: The Benefits of College Education to Individuals and to Society," Lumina Foundation, Indianapolis, IN, 2015, 1–72, http://www.luminafoundation.org/files/resources/its-not-just-the -money.pdf.

12. Ibid.

13. Isaac Sasson, "Trends in Life Expectancy and Lifespan Variation by Educational Attainment: United States: 1990–2010," *Demography* 53, no. 2 (April 2016): 269–93, https://doi.org/10.1007/s13524-015-0453-7.

14. Arthur J. Reynolds, Suh-Ruu Ou, and Judy A. Temple, "A Multicomponent, Preschool to Third Grade Preventative Intervention and Educational Attainment at 35 Years of Age," *JAMA Pediatrics* 172, no. 3 (March 2018): 247–56, https://doi.org/10.1001/jamapediatrics.2017.4673.

15. Claudio Sanchez, "Does Preschool Pay Off? Tulsa Says Yes," NPR, December 12, 2017, https://www.npr.org/sections/ed/2017/12/12/568378251/does -preschool-pay-off-tulsa-says-yes.

16. Kyle Jaeger, "Here's How Military and Education Spending Compare in America," *ATTN:*, August 30, 2016, https://archive.attn.com/stories/11036 /how-military-and-education-spending-compare-america.

17. Steffanie Clothier and Julie Poppe, "New Research: Early Education as

Economic Investment," National Conference of State Legislators, accessed September 14, 2019, http://www.ncsl.org/research/human-services/new -research-early-education-as-economic-investme.aspx.

18. Kevin Tan et al., "The Impact of School Social Workers on High School Freshman Graduation Among the One Hundred Largest School Districts in the United States," *School Social Work Journal* 93, no. 2 (Spring 2015): 1–14, https://www.researchgate.net/publication /309112431_The_Impact_of_School_Social_Workers_on_High_School _Freshman_Graduation_among_the_One_Hundred_Largest_School _Districts_in_the_United_States.

19. Shelly Banjo, "American student loan debt has surpassed the GDP of Australia, New Zealand, and Ireland combined," *Quartz*, February 18, 2015, https://qz.com/346342/american-student-loan-debt-has-surpassed-the -gdp-of-australia-new-zealand-and-ireland-combined/.

20. David H. Autor, "Why Are There Still So Many Jobs? The History and Future of Workplace Automation," *Journal of Economic Perspectives* 29, no. 3 (Summer 2015): 3–30, https://economics.mit.edu/files/11563.

21. U.S. Congress, Senate, The Corporate Tax Dodging Prevention Act of 2017, S 586, 115th Cong., 1st sess., introduced in Senate March 9, 2017, https:// www.sanders.senate.gov/download/corporate-tax-dodging-prevention-act -2017-summary?inline=file.

22. U.S. Congress, Senate, Accountable Capitalism Act of 2018, S 3348, 115th Cong., 2nd sess., introduced in Senate August 15, 2018, https://www .warren.senate.gov/imo/media/doc/Accountable%20Capitalism%20Act %20One-Pager.pdf.

23. ACLU Foundation, *The Way on Marijuana in Black and White: Billions of Dollars Wasted on Racially Biased Arrests*, report, New York, NY, 2013, 1–185, https://www.aclu.org/report/report-war-marijuana-black-and -white?redirect=criminal-law-reform/war-marijuana-black-and-white.

24. Deborah Dowell, Tamara M. Haegerich, and Roger Chou, "CDC Guideline for Prescribing Opioids for Chronic Pain—United States, 2016," *Morbidity and Mortality Weekly Report* 65, no. 1 (2016): 1–48, https://www.cdc.gov/mmwr/volumes/65/rr/rr6501e1.htm?CDC_AA _refVal=https%3A%2F%2Fwww.cdc.gov%2Fmmwr%2Fvolumes%2F65 %2Frr%2Frr6501e1er.htm.

25. Alia Paavola, "UK Firm Agrees to Record $1.4B Payout in US Opioid Fraud Lawsuit," *Becker's Hospital Review*, July 11, 2019, https://www

.beckershospitalreview.com/pharmacy/uk-firm-agrees-to-record-1-4b-payout-in-us-opioid-fraud-lawsuit.html.

26. Linda E. Saltzman et al., "Weapon Involvement and Injury Outcomes in Family and Intimate Assaults," *JAMA* 267, no. 22 (1992): 3043–47, https://doi.org/«Xtags error: No such color: tag c»10.1001/jama.1992.03480220061028.

27. Abdulrahman M. El-Sayed, *Abdul for Michigan Infrastructure Plan*, policy paper, Abdul for Michigan, 2018, 1–18, https://static1.squarespace.com/static/5c93c8e3d7819e5afbf3cd2d/t/5ca7683ae5e5f049cd180865/1554475067127/Infrastructure+Bank.pdf.

28. Sandra Bishop-Josef, Chris Beakey, Sara Watson, and Tom Garrett, *Want to Grow the Economy? Fix the Child Care Crisis*, report by ReadyNation/Council for a Strong America, Washington, DC, 2019, 1–7, https://strong nation.s3.amazonaws.com/documents/602/83bb2275-ce07-4d74-bcee -ff6178daf6bd.pdf?1547054862&inline;%20filename=%22Want%20 to%20Grow%20the%20Economy?%20Fix%20the%20Child%20 Care%20Crisis.pdf%22.

29. Will Fischer, "As More Low-Income Renters Struggle, Federal Subsidies Favor Well-Off Homeowners," Center on Budget and Policy Priorities, June 23, 2016, https://www.cbpp.org/blog/as-more-low-income-renters -struggle-federal-subsidies-favor-well-off-homeowners.

30. Ta-Nehisi Coates, "The Case for Reparations," *The Atlantic*, June 2014, https://www.theatlantic.com/magazine/archive/2014/06/the-case-for -reparations/361631/.

31. "Trump Revokes Obama Rule on Reporting Drone Strike Deaths," BBC News, March 7, 2019, https://www.bbc.com/news/world-us-canada -47480207.

32. "Drone Warfare," The Bureau of Investigative Journalism, accessed March 7, 2019, https://www.thebureauinvestigates.com/projects/drone-war.

33. Chris Hughes, "It's Time to Break Up Facebook," *New York Times*, May 9, 2019, https://www.nytimes.com/2019/05/09/opinion/sunday/chris -hughes-facebook-zuckerberg.html.

34. Emily Stewart, "Facebook Has Taken Down Billions of Fake Accounts, but the Problem Is Still Getting Worse," *Vox*, May 23, 2019, https://www.vox .com/recode/2019/5/23/18637596/facebook-fake-accounts-transparency -mark-zuckerberg-report.

35. Jack Morse, "50 Percent of Facebook Users Could Be Fake, Report Claims,"

Mashable, January 25, 2019, https://mashable.com/article/report-claims
-half-facebook-maus-fake/.

36. Michael Newberg, "As Many as 48 Million Twitter Accounts Aren't People,
Says Study," CNBC, last updated March 10, 2017, https://www.cnbc.com
/2017/03/10/nearly-48-million-twitter-accounts-could-be-bots-says-study
.html?utm_source=www.cloohawk.com.

37. Gracy Olmstead, "The Farm Bill Ignores the Real Troubles of U.S. Agriculture," *New York Times*, December 14, 2018, https://www.nytimes.com
/2018/12/14/opinion/farm-bill-agriculture.html.

38. Ibid.

39. Beth Kaiserman, "Trump Signs 2018 Farm Bill as USDA Aims to Increase
SNAP Work Requirements," *Forbes*, December 20, 2018, https://www
.forbes.com/sites/bethkaiserman/2018/12/20/trump-signs-2018-farm-bill
-as-usda-aims-to-increase-snap-work-requirements/#255cf8e61b79.

40. Allison Aubrey, "Food Stamps for Soda: Time to End Billion-Dollar Subsidy for Sugary Drinks?," NPR, October 29, 2018, https://www.npr.org
/sections/thesalt/2018/10/29/659634119/food-stamps-for-soda-time-to
-end-billion-dollar-subsidy-for-sugary-drinks.

41. Dariush Mozaffarian et al., "Cost-Effectiveness of Financial Incentives
and Disincentives for improving food purchases and health through the
US Supplemental Nutrition Assistance Program (SNAP): A microsimu-
lation study," *PLOS Medicine* 15, no. 10 (2018): 1-2, https://doi.org/10.1371
/journal.pmed.1002661.

42. Christina A. Roberto et al., "Association of a Beverage Tax on Sugar-Sweetened and Artificially Sweetened Beverages with Changes in Beverage
Prices and Sales at Chain Retailers in a Large Urban Setting," *JAMA* 321,
no. 18 (2019): 1799–810, https://doi.org/10.1001/jama.2019.4249.

43. Max Martin, "Here's Everything Philly's Soda Tax Money Is (and Isn't)
Paying for," Billy Penn, December 12, 2018, https://billypenn.com/2018
/12/12/heres-everything-phillys-soda-tax-money-is-and-isnt-paying-for/.

Acknowledgments

Having become more accustomed to conveying words by tongue than by fingertip, I found the process of creating this book difficult. You can't "resay" the words you speak, but you can certainly rewrite. And it turns out that so much of the quality of a book is in the rewriting. Ironically, that makes communicating on the page that much more challenging. And, as with most things, the reward is buried under the challenge. But I am deeply grateful for the good folks who were with me throughout the process, cajoling, nudging . . . sometimes demanding better words.

I'm grateful to my editor, Jamison Stoltz, and the incredible team at Abrams Press for recognizing what this book ought to be—and for shepherding me through the writing (and rewriting). My agent, Anna Sproul-Latimer, saw the potential even earlier, helping me assemble my thoughts into a skeleton and guiding me through the fast-paced and eventful world of book publishing(!). Dara Kaye—thank you for schlepping around New York City with me as we told the story of this book!

Tara Terpstra: As with most things in my life over the past four years, this book would not have happened without your attention to detail, your care, and your support. Thank you for finding me the time and space of mind to sit my butt down and research and write. Whether clearing my calendar for another draft or managing citations right down to the period, or just offering a warm smile and some reassurance when the grind got hard, I count on you more than you know. Thank you for your effort, your honesty, your reliability, and your friendship.

Austin Fisher, you really are the ultimate utility player. Thank you for helping me manage this and other projects concurrently, all while keeping the world abreast of what we were up to: I'm grateful for your insights and your Macomb County work ethic. Thank you for being my friend.

To my readers, Lama Alzuhd, Frank Chi, Connor Farrell, Dr. Sandro Galea, Amytess Girgis, Adam Joseph, Martha McKenna, Dr. Jisung Park, Dr. Sabeel Rahman, Tara Terpstra, and Jennifer Westwalewicz: Thank you for your insights. This book is so much the better for having had your minds on it. To Amytess and Frank in particular, thank you for challenging me to step out of my words to find them.

To my colleagues at the Detroit Health Department and throughout the City of Detroit: Thank you for your courage and your leadership—and for all you've done to make the city healthier. Your grit, patience, and enthusiasm inspired me from the day I set foot into that back office at the Parking Department. It inspires me today. I hope that my words have honored the commitment we made together for Detroit's health.

To the Abdul for Michigan team: Thank you for being an extension of my family for eighteen months. You buoyed me at my lowest moments—and grounded me at my highest. Your commitment to Sarah, Emmalee, and me throughout the campaign was nothing short of an act of love. Your belief in the world we worked to build together imbues every page of this book; I only hope I did it justice.

To all the folks who made our movement—the thousands who donated, knocked on doors, sent text messages, made phone calls: You are why I believe in our future. Your enthusiasm, your commitment, and your idealism are what hope is made of. And to the 340,560 people who lent me your stake in our democracy on August 7, 2018, I'm so profoundly grateful. Though I was not elected, I hope I may yet do something to have earned the vote you gave me.

To those whose stories I shared, I hope I've done them justice. And to all of you who've shaped me—as my friend, my teacher, my student, my patient, or my constituent: Thank you for sharing yourself with me, as I have ventured to share myself with you. I hope what I have shared of us both in these pages does service to the world we are building together.

Grandma and Grandpa: Thanks for always being in my corner. No matter what. I'm so grateful for you in my life.

To my siblings—Adam, Eman, Osama, Arwa, and Samia—and my siblings in-law—Aasim, Hatifa, Mariam, Zahid, Aisha, Salim, Yousuf, Ayesha, Kamau, and Heba: Thank you for your love, your support, and your unique ability to keep me grounded.

To my second set of parents, Dr. Jukaku and Faiziya Tayeb: You cared for us in every way throughout the journey of the campaign and thereafter. You've given me my best friend and cared for my daughter when I could not. I cannot begin to thank you as much as you deserve, so, rather, know that I pray for you every day. God grant you love, sustenance, and security, as you have given us in a place greater than this one.

To my parents, Baba, Mama, and Mom—as on the campaign, I learned quickly that telling my story in these pages would be impossible without telling yours. Your unique paths intersected at one point, in one person—in me. I am grateful for all the love, time, effort, and sacrifice you've invested to build me, in ways I witnessed, and ways I did not; in ways I can comprehend, and in ways I cannot. Indeed, at best, my story is a chimera of the ones you've each written with your lives—together, if apart. God accept, uplift, and empower you as you have me.

Sarah, my companion on this journey: No one's given more and asked less. I've written 110,000 words—and none of them, in quality or quantity, do justice to what you mean to me. I cannot imagine what this path would be without your honest love and mercy—your security. God fill you with the security you've given me.

Emmalee, I couldn't have imagined that a toothless smile could change me. Yours did. And it has—and will—so long as we stay together on this earth. Please keep smiling, and I'll do everything I can to give you reasons to. God protect and raise you righteous and loving and kind, and worthy of the work we'll leave to you.

Praise be to God in all things.

Index

Affordable Care Act, 59–60, 70, 258
agent-based modeling, 54–55
agriculture, 139–40, 287–88
air pollution, 99–100
air travel, 34, 180–81
Alzuhd, Lama, 117
Amazon, 192, 209, 252, 286
American culture, 209–11, 220–23
American dream, 6, 216
American identity, 26–27
animal control, 92–96
antibiotics, 50, 80
anxiety, 135–36, 158
Arab Spring, 56
asthma, 40–41, 99–100
automation, 191–94, 268–69
automobile industry, 188–89, 193–94

banking, 154–55, 276–77
Barkan, Ady, 118–20
birth outcomes, 45–47
Bishop, Bill, 168
Black Americans, 11, 33, 162–63, 279–80
blackouts, 185
blood pressure, 133
Blue New Deal, 261–62
bridges, 178–79, 181
British rule, 245–46

Brooking, Emerson T., 170–71
Bush, George W., 211–12
Butz, Earl, 139

campaign funds, 111, 130–32, 197, 203–8
campaigning, 1–6
    decision to run, 110–11
    Election Day and, 123–26
    support team, 114–18, 120–23
    voting and, 196–99
cancer, 5, 18, 141–42
car insurance, 129–30
Carter, Jimmy, 139
Case, Anne, 134–35
catastrophic insurance, 143–44
causation, 20–23, 48–55
charter schools, 265
Chetty, Raj, 223
childcare, 155–57, 183–85, 278
childhood trauma, 158
children, 1–4, 43, 172, 223, 281–82, 290–91
    animal control and, 93, 96
    Flint water crisis and, 87–88, 100–102
    public health and, 91–92, 93, 96,
        97–102
    vaccines and, 81–82
    vision and, 92, 97–99
cholera, 20, 48, 78–80, 81, 147

climate change, 177, 186–87
    Green New Deal for, 118, 122, 260–62
Clinton, Bill, 57, 58–59
Clinton, Hillary, 120–21, 239
Coates, Ta-Nehisi, 280
cognitive behavioral therapy, 249
Cole, David, 240
Coleman, Daniel, 231
Columbia University, 67–68
Constitution, U.S., 205–6, 229
corporate lobbying, 204–8, 266–67, 271
corporate responsibility, 266–71
correlation, 20–23
cost of living, 6, 158–61
Currid-Halkett, Elizabeth, 220

death and mortality data, 19–20, 48, 134–35
death threats, 2–3, 4
Deaton, Angus, 134–35
debt, 153–54, 222–23
defensive politics, 116–17
dehumanization, 33
Desmond, Matthew, 160
Detroit, 1–4, 12–13, 114–15, 129–30
    housing demolition program in, 105–7
    as insecure community, 166–67
    public health in, 4–5, 82, 83, 87–96,
        101–7
diabetes, 50–51, 145
discrimination, health, 73–75, 103
disease. See also specific diseases
    defining, 132
    environment and, 78–82
    epidemiology and, 18–20, 49–53,
        78–82, 132–33, 137
diversity, 27–28
    education and, 43–44
    of Muslim-American identity, 34–35
divorce, 13–14, 65, 150–53
Douglass, Frederick, 33
Du Bois, W. E. B., 11
Duggan, Mike, 86–87, 100, 103–5

economy, 69, 136
    automation and, 191–94, 268–69
    insecurity in, 158–61, 188–95, 216
    jobs and, 188–94, 266–68
    market dominance and, 208–9
    stocks and, 193
education, 5, 16, 26–27, 164–65
    charter schools, 265
    diversity and, 43–44
    infrastructure and, 184–85
    medical school, 43–47, 67–69, 71–77,
        229–30, 258
    privilege and, 26, 61, 220
    public health and, 92, 97–102
    reform and guarantee, 263–66
    Rhodes scholarship and, 61–63
    segregation in, 167
    student loans for, 153–54, 266
Egypt, 11–17, 56, 60, 185, 209–10, 284
Egyptian-American identity, 11–17
Ekman, Paul, 231
election interference, 170
election reform, 271–72
emergency care, 73
emergency management, 87–88, 103–4, 202
empathy, 229–33, 245–47, 292
    policies of, 248–55
energy infrastructure, 185–87, 260–61
environment
    disease and, 78–82
    insecurity relating to, 137–40
    public health and, 99–100
epidemiology, 5
    defining, 18
    disease and, 18–20, 49–53, 78–82,
        132–33, 137
    insecurity and, 19–20
    overview and brief history of, 18–24
    politics and, 126
    public health and, 18, 44–47, 49–51,
        84–85, 107–8
    social, 45–46, 48–55

eviction, 160–61
exclusion, 242–45

Facebook, 169–70, 285–86
faith, 35–38
fake news, 169–71, 285
family
    background, 11–17
    childcare and, 155–57
    divorce and, 13–14, 65, 150–53
    poverty and, 151–53
family values, 150–51, 278
Farmer, Paul, 43
Farrell, Connor, 117
fear
    insecurity and, 134, 224–26
    politics and, 4, 109, 213–14, 224–26
    socialism and, 250–51
Flint water crisis, 4, 87–88, 100–102, 181
flooding, 175–77, 182
food, 50–52, 66–67
    insecurity and, 52, 137–40, 161, 214, 224
    reform, 287–89
foreign policy, 60, 281–85
fossil fuels, 186–87
fraud, 224
free speech rights, 26–27, 286
fulfillment, 64–65

Galea, Sandro, 44–47, 67, 83–86
gender, 5, 155–57, 236, 239–40, 281
gentrification, 167
gerrymandering, 201–2, 271
Gimpel, James, 172
giving, 40, 218–19
Glass, Max, 117
Graunt, John, 18–20, 48
Great Recession, 189, 190–92
Green New Deal, 118, 122, 260–62
grief, 65–66
Gunn-Wright, Rhiana, 117–18

gun rights, 5, 173–74
gun violence, 172–74, 272, 276

Hadley, Craig, 45
happiness, 64–65
Haseler, Stephen, 219–20
hate
    Muslim-American identity and, 37–38
    "other" and, 33, 211–12, 224–25
    politics and, 2–5, 119–20, 211–12, 225–26, 241–42
    racism and, 27–34
health care, 5, 84
    Affordable Care Act and, 59–60, 70
    discrimination in, 73–75, 103
    hospitals and, 142–44, 258
    information asymmetry and, 142–43
    insecurity and, 141–49
    mental, 146–48, 272–73
    patterns in, 141
    politics and, 42, 69–71, 207
    poverty and, 72–76, 80–82
    privilege and, 40–41, 42–47
    profiteering in, 141–46, 256
    structural inequality and, 69, 72–76
    universal, 115, 207, 251–52, 256–60
health insurance, 141–45, 207, 256–60
health reform, 59–60, 69–70, 256–60
health risk, 8, 18
hepatitis A, 175–77
hepatitis C, 145–46
herd immunity, 81
Herman Kiefer, 89–90
HIV/AIDS, 74–75
hope, 59–61, 292
hospitals, 142–44, 258
household insecurity
    banking and, 154–55
    childcare and, 155–57
    cost of living and, 158–61
    debt as, 153–54
    food and, 161

household insecurity *(cont.)*
    incarceration rates and, 162–64
    loneliness and, 164
    marriage and, 150–53
    material insecurity and, 220–23
    privilege and, 157–58
housing, 6
    cost of, 156, 160–61
    demolition program, 105–7
    eviction, 160–61
    lead and, 101–2, 105–7
    reform, 279
    segregation and, 167

identity
    American, 26–27
    complexity of, 235–36
    double-consciousness of, 11–13
    as Egyptian-American, 11–17
    gender and, 236, 239–40
    insecurity and, 234–38, 241–45
    movements in identity politics, 239–41
    Muslim-American, 2–4, 30–38, 245–46
    name and, 11–12
    politics and, 234–47
    privilege and, 236–39, 242–44
    race and, 234–36, 238–41
immigration, 169–70, 171–72, 281–85
incarceration rates, 162–64, 207, 272–74
"incels," 164
income
    banking and, 154–55
    gap, 155–57, 194
    insecurity and, 131–32, 135–36
    life expectancy and, 48–49
    marriage and, 152–53
    median household, 6
    minimum wage, 136, 191
    universal basic income, 269
infant mortality, 49–50, 91, 94
    public health and, 97–98, 102–3
information asymmetry, 142–43

infrastructure
    childcare and, 183–85
    education and, 184–85
    energy, 185–87, 260–61
    flooding and, 175–76
    funding, 178, 184, 187
    insecurity in, 175–87
    internet, 183
    race and, 187
    social, 178
    transportation, 178–81
    water, 181–82
inheritance, 219–20
insecure communities
    gentrification and, 167
    gun violence and, 172–74
    immigration and, 171–72
    racism and, 166–67
    segregation and, 167–70, 171, 174
    social media and, 168–71
insecurity
    anxiety and, 135–36
    cognition and, 249
    complexity of, 137–40
    defining, 134
    in economy, 158–61, 188–95, 216
    environment relating to, 137–40
    epidemiology and, 19–20
    fear and, 134, 224–26
    food and, 52, 137–40, 161, 214, 224
    health care and, 141–49
    household, 150–65, 220–23
    identity and, 234–38, 241–45
    income and, 131–32, 135–36
    in infrastructure, 175–87
    paradoxical, 218–26
    politics and, 5–7, 166–67, 196–215,
        224–26
    poverty and, 19, 26–27, 130, 222–23
    spread of, 216–26
    structural inequality and, 216–26
    in wealth, 131–32

institutional racism, 34
insulin, 145
Internet, 115, 183
Islam, 35–38
Japan, 48
Jim Crow, 167, 279–80
jobs
    automation and, 191–94, 268–69
    economy and, 188–94, 267–68
    gender and, 155–57
    maternal leave and, 155–56, 278
    workers' rights and corporate responsi-
        bility, 266–71
Johnson, Jackie, 14
Joseph, Adam, 117

Klinenberg, Eric, 178
Koch, Robert, 80
Krippner, Greta, 193

Lauderdale, Diane, 45
lead
    Flint water crisis and, 4, 87–88,
        100–102, 181
    housing and, 101–2, 105–7
Lead Safe Detroit, 101–2
libraries, 178
life expectancy, 48–50, 134–35, 141, 158–59,
    256
lobbying and campaign contributions,
    204–8, 266–67, 271
London, 19–20
loneliness, 164
Lorde, Audre, 240, 241
Luscombe, Belinda, 152

Malahlela, Mary, 43
marijuana legalization, 274
marriage, 64
    divorce and, 13–14, 65, 150–53
    household insecurity and, 150–53
    income and, 152–53

mass contagions, 18–19
mass shootings, 172–73
matched-pair analysis, 24
material insecurity, 220–26
maternal leave, 155–56, 278
McCray, Chirlane, 240
media, 168–71, 203–4, 213–14, 285–87
median household income, 6
medical school, 43–47, 67–69, 71–77,
    229–30, 258
Medicare, 144–46
Medicare for All, 251–52, 256–60
mega-corporations, 208–9
mental health care, 146–48, 272–73
Meyer, Henning, 219–20
miasma, 78–82, 137, 226, 291
Michigan Department of Environmental
    Quality, 99–100
Miller, Melissa, 94–95
minimum wage, 136, 191, 268
Mubarak, Hosni, 56, 60
Mukwege, Denis, 43
Muraszko, Karin, 43
Muslim-American identity, 2–4, 30–38,
    245–46
Muslim Ban, 113

name and identity, 11–12
Native American reparations, 279–80
"native informants," 32
natural disasters, 45, 175–77, 182
natural experiments, 22–24
Nixon, Richard, 139

Obama, Barack, 56, 59–61, 239
obesity, 50–51, 52, 67, 138–40, 287–88
Ocasio-Cortez, Alexandria, 112–13, 240–41,
    267
Ohye, Rick, 43
oil, 99–100, 212
opioid epidemic, 148, 273–75

"other"
    exclusion and, 242–45
    hatred and, 33, 211–12, 224–25
    politics, identity, and, 234–47
Othman, Ammu, 40, 274
overconsumption, 50–52, 138–40, 220–23
Oxford University, 61–62, 66–67

paradoxical insecurity, 218–26
parks, 178
Pasteur, Louis, 80
pathology, 42
pharmaceutical companies, 144–46, 207,
    257, 275
plague, 18–19, 48
police, 28–30
politics
    campaign funds and, 111, 130–32, 197,
        203–8
    defensive, 116–17
    election interference and, 170
    election reform and, 271–72
    of empathy, 229–33, 245–55, 292
    epidemiology and, 126
    fear and, 4, 109, 213–14, 224–26
    gerrymandering and, 201–2, 271
    Great Recession and, 191–92
    hate and, 2–5, 119–20, 211–12, 225–26,
        241–42
    health care and, 42, 69–71, 207
    hope and, 59–60
    ideals and policy reform, 256–89
    identity and, 234–47
    insecurity and, 5–7, 166–67, 196–215,
        224–26
    lifestyle preferences and, 168
    lobbying and campaign contributions,
        204–8, 266–67, 271
    Obama and, 59–61
    policy and, 248–55
    public health and, 108–11
    segregation and, 168–69

tokenization in, 245–47
    voter suppression and, 199–201
    war and, 211–15
poverty
    definition of, 6
    in Egypt, 15–16
    family and, 151–53
    food and, 51–52
    health care and, 72–76, 80–82
    infectious disease and, 78–79
    insecurity and, 19, 26–27, 130, 222–23
    privilege and, 25–26, 41
    public health and, 91–92
    race and, 41
    seniors in, 158–60
    suffering and, 25–26, 51–52, 80–81
    water access and, 103–4
preexisting conditions, 257–58
pregnancy, 20–22, 54, 92
premature birth, 20–22, 54
prescription drugs, 144–46, 257, 275
prisons, 162–64, 207, 272–74
privacy, 285–87
privilege
    education and, 26, 61, 220
    giving and, 40
    health care and, 40–41, 42–47
    household insecurity and, 157–58
    identity and, 236–39, 242–44
    poverty and, 25–26, 41
    race and, 39–40
    wealth and, 219–20
productivity-pay gap, 194
protest, 93–94, 129–30
public banking, 276–77
public health
    air pollution and, 99–100
    animal control and, 92–96
    budget and, 95, 97
    children and, 91–92, 93, 96, 97–102
    in Detroit, 4–5, 82, 83, 87–96, 101–7
    education and, 92, 97–102

environment and, 99–100
epidemiology and, 18, 44–47, 49–51,
    84–85, 107–8
flooding and, 175–77, 182
infant mortality and, 97–98, 102–3
law and, 95
life expectancy and, 134–35, 256
politics and, 108–11
poverty and, 91–92
Trump and, 109–10
public safety reform, 272–76

race
    birth outcomes and, 45–47
    identity and, 234–36, 238–41
    incarceration rates and, 162–64
    infrastructure and, 187
    life expectancy and, 48–49
    poverty and, 41
    privilege and, 39–40
racism
    hate and, 27–34
    immigration and, 281–82
    insecure communities and, 166–67
    institutional, 34
    Muslim-American identity and, 30–34,
        37–38
    by police, 28–30
    structural inequality and, 216–17
racist stereotyping, 169
randomization, 22–23
randomized controlled trials (RCTs), 22–24
Reagan, Ronald, 224–25
religion, 35–38
religious extremists, 36, 212–13
reparations, 279–81
retirement, 158–60
rights, 240
    to education, 16
    free speech, 26–27, 286
    gun, 5, 173–74
    reparations and equal rights, 279–81

to water, 103–4
    for women, 281
roads, 178–80, 181
Roosevelt, Franklin D., 159

sadness, 64–66, 134–35
safety, 27, 53, 272–76
Sandberg, Claire, 117
Sanders, Bernie, 117, 120–23, 267–68,
    269
sanitation systems, 50, 78–80, 175–76, 182
Sayoc, Cesar, 3
Scarborough, Peter, 67
science, 41–42, 44
segregation, 167–70, 171, 174, 279–80
seniors, 158–60, 278
Sherman, Rachel, 217–18
Singer, P. W., 170–71
slavery, 33, 238
smoking, 20–22, 54, 288–89
Snow, John, 20, 48, 78–80, 137
Snyder, Rick, 87–88, 147, 192
social epidemiology, 45–46
    agent-based modeling and, 54–55
    causation in, 48–55
social infrastructure, 178
socialism, 249–51
social media, 169–71, 285–87
Social Security Act (1935), 159
social status, 6, 221–23
soda tax, 288–89
sofosbuvir, 145–46
sorites paradox, 138
stereotyping, 169, 224–25
stocks, 193–94
structural inequality, 41
    health care and, 69, 72–76
    insecurity and, 216–26
    racism and, 216–17
student loans, 153–54, 266
substance abuse, 73–74, 134–35, 146–48,
    272–74

taxes, 192, 251–52, 267–70, 288–89
Terpstra, Tara, 117
terrorism, 3, 30–31, 37
Tharoor, Shashi, 117
Tlaib, Rashida, 125, 240–41
tobacco industry, 288–89
tokenization, 245–47
transportation infrastructure, 178–81
Truman, Harry, 251
Trump, Donald, 3, 4, 37, 113, 188–89, 220,
    225, 239, 241, 252, 283
    election of, 108–9
    on immigration, 171–72, 281
    public health and, 109–10
Turner, Nina, 122

unemployment, 188–91
unions, 129, 188–89, 191–92, 268
universal basic income, 269
universal health care, 115, 207, 251–52,
    256–60
universal Wi-Fi, 115
upselling, 143

vaccines, 27, 50, 80–82, 176–77
Veblen, Thorstein, 220
Veterans Affairs, 283
Virchow, Rudolf, 42
vision, 92, 97–99
voter suppression, 199–201
voting, 196–99, 202–3, 215, 238–39,
    271–72

war, 210–15, 282–85
Warren, Elizabeth, 267–68, 270–71
water, 27, 137–38
    Blue New Deal and, 261–62
    Flint water crisis, 4, 87–88, 100–102,
        181
    infrastructure, 181–82
    poverty and access to, 103–4
    sanitation systems and, 50, 78–80,
        175–76, 182
wealth, 6, 131–32, 217–20, 267–68
Welch, Leseliey, 97
white men, 244
Will, George F., 151
women
    health risk in, 8
    maternal leave for, 155–56, 278
    pregnancy and, 20–22, 54, 92
    rights for, 281
worker rights, 266–71
Yemen, 78, 81, 137